Deinstitutionalization and Community Adjustment of Mentally Retarded People

Edited by

Robert H. Bruininks
C. Edward Meyers
Barbara B. Sigford
K. Charlie Lakin

Monograph of the
American Association on Mental Deficiency, Number 4

C. Edward Meyers, Series Editor

American Association on Mental Deficiency
5101 Wisconsin Avenue, N.W.
Washington, D.C. 20016
Albert Berkowitz, Executive Director

Library of Congress Catalogue Number 80-70191

Typeset and manufactured in the United States of America by the Department of Printing and Graphic Arts, University of Minnesota

Preface

Deinstitutionalization and community placement have been under way for some years now, and so have evaluations of the procedures and problems in this movement. That movement has also stimulated careful research attending to the characteristics of clients in the community and of their careproviders and the interactions between them, not to mention the subtler issues of lifestyle and adjustment. We therefore planned *Monograph No. 4* of the American Association on Mental Deficiency to report on the issues of community placement and adjustment. Such a volume would provide more than a snapshot of our revolutionary time. Because we solicited some papers based on the work of states that had taken early initiative in community placement, these early experiences can be shared with the later starters to their profit.

This volume combines two sets of papers developed around the general issues of deinstitutionalization and adjustment of retarded people living in community settings. Several papers were initially secured by the Series Editor for a special monograph on this general topic. The other set, prepared at approximately the same time, was originally presented at a special invitational conference devoted to research on community adjustment sponsored by the Department of Psychoeducational Studies, University of Minnesota.

These manuscripts were subsequently revised for this volume. Together, the papers present a broad, in-depth examination of deinstitutionalization as a public policy, its trends and special problems in implementation, conceptual and methodological aspects of its study, and our present knowledge base regarding the consequences of community placement on the lives and living conditions of retarded citizens.

The Series Editor acknowledges assistance and support of several people, especially Charles C. Cleland, Richard K. Eyman, and Louis Rowitz.

C. E. Meyers, Editor
AAMD *Monograph* Series

Acknowledgements

It is a long road from the first conceptualization of a volume to its publication. Fortunately, we have had much generous and talented help along the way.

Partial financial support for the preparation of manuscripts was provided by a grant (54P-71173/5-01) from the Administration on Developmental Disabilities, Office of Human Developmental Services, Department of Health and Human Services. The points of view and opinions expressed in this volume, of course, do not necessarily represent the official position of that agency.

In planning this volume we were fortunate in being able to receive valuable advice, assistance and support from Christy Boswell, Jack Cockshott, Allen Cohen, Eunice Davis, Margaret Edwards, Joni Fritz, Doris Haar, Laird Heal, Gordon Krantz, Fred Krause, Toni Lippert, Gene Patterson, Robert Perske, David Rosen, Richard Scheerenberger, Joan Van Norstrand, Luke Watson, Michael Weber, and Edward Zigler.

We owe special thanks to Kathy Nicolay who prepared these papers for typesetting. Through years of experience she has developed the ability to type, proofread and edit at the same time. We do not know how she does it, but we are very pleased that she does it for us. Dewey Force and Nancy Larson of the University of Minnesota were also instrumental in shaping the final volume through their careful and very skillful copy editing of the manuscripts.

Deep appreciation is also expressed to Albert Berkowitz and Susan Yoder of the American Association on Mental Deficiency for their support for this project, and to the many skilled professionals of the University of Minnesota's Printing and Graphic Arts Departments who made our priorities and timelines theirs.

Contents

Research on Providing and Evaluating Community Placements

Summary

Introduction

This volume is concerned with an often misunderstood and poorly conceptualized issue: the community adjustment of people defined by society as mentally retarded. Its purpose is not to deal with all the myriad concerns surrounding this issue, for an adequate exploration of community adjustment would require painstaking examination of the social and psychological theory and research encompassing the entire continuum of an individual's life cycle. Instead, the papers in this volume focus on the living patterns of people who at one time lived in public institutions for the mentally retarded, or who would likely have lived in such facilities prior to the deinstitutionalization movement of recent years. The volume examines issues in research on this topic and reports on the findings of selected studies regarding this social phenomenon.

Although addressing a seemingly narrow issue, this volume deals with concerns of broad public policy, as well as social and historical significance. The study of community adjustment deals with fundamental responses of society toward the care and treatment of mentally retarded people through its social institutions. For the most part, the focus of research on community adjustment is upon the experiences of people in various residential living arrangements. Recently, research on community adjustment has assumed added significance as approaches to meeting the residential needs of retarded people have undergone substantial change under the concept and policy of deinstitutionalization.

Deinstitutionalization has primarily affected persons with problems of mental illness and mental retardation, although the impact of this policy has affected people with other handicapping conditions as well. As outlined by the National Association of Superintendents of Public Residential Facilities for the Mentally Retarded (1974):

> Deinstitutionalization encompasses three interrelated processes: (1) prevention of admission by finding and developing alternative community methods of care and training; (2) return to the community of all residents who have been prepared through programs of habilitation and training to function adequately in appropriate local settings; and (3) establishment and maintenance of a responsive residential environment which protects human and civil rights. (pp. 4-5)

The factual aspects of deinstitutionalization can be observed in various statistics regarding residential services. From most of these, deinstitutionalization appears as a sharp contrast and a definite break from past treatment practices, and in fact it has been. Nevertheless, this recent revolution cannot be totally isolated from the gradual changes in residential services occurring in the post-World War II years, and is much more easily understood within an historical context.

From the founding of the first institution for mentally retarded persons in a wing of a state school for the blind in Massachusetts in 1848, public residential facilities for mentally retarded persons steadily grew in resident population through 1967 (see Figure 1). Fiscal year 1967-1968 saw the first drop in annual average daily population of American public institutions in history when the population dropped from 194,650 to 194,000 (Lakin, 1979). As Scheerenberger will describe more fully later in this volume, a steady annual decrement in average population has followed every year since.

While 1967 has been referred to as the "watershed year," some important changes were taking place in philosophy of care and treatment of mentally retarded persons long before 1967. Some of these are worthy of passing mention.

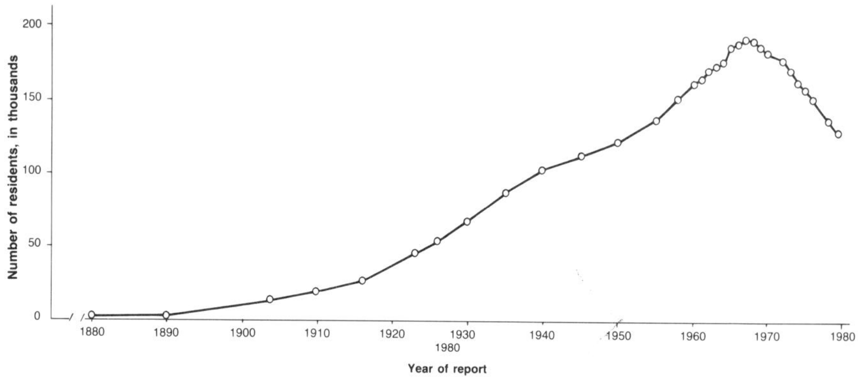

Figure 1. Total populations of mentally retarded people in public institutions for mentally retarded persons for the period 1880 to 1979. (Sources: Lakin, 1979; Krantz, Bruininks & Clumpner, 1979)

Figure 2 shows the ratio of patients to staff in public institutions for mentally retarded persons from 1915 to 1979. As the reader can see, with the exception of the depression years when money was short and the last years of the Second World War when personnel were in short supply, that ratio remained between 6.0 to 6.9 residents per one staff member. Since the end of the Second World War there has been a precipitous drop in the ratio of residents to staff members in public facilities. That ratio has only recently begun to stabilize around 1.4 residents per staff member.

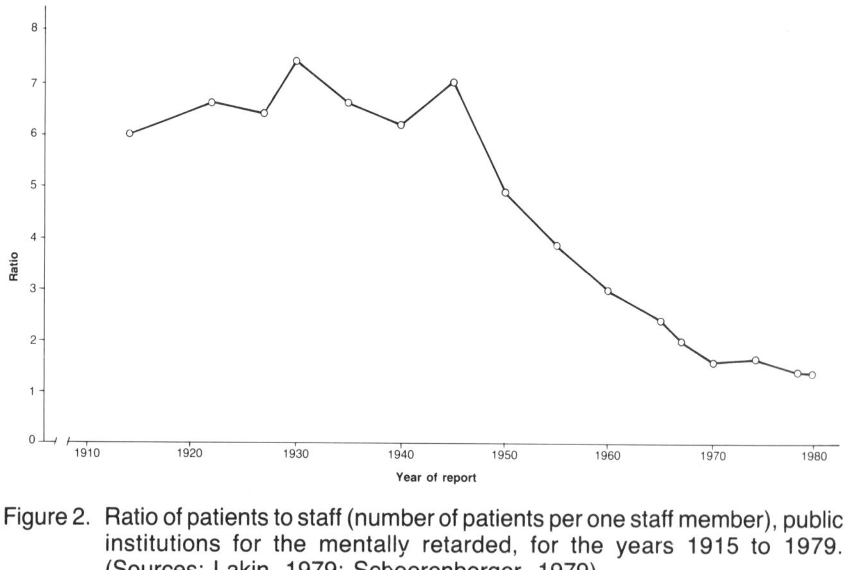

Figure 2. Ratio of patients to staff (number of patients per one staff member), public institutions for the mentally retarded, for the years 1915 to 1979. (Sources: Lakin, 1979; Scheerenberger, 1979)

There are other signs of an enormous change in commitment of our society toward the care of institutionalized mentally retarded persons immediately following World War II. Compare, for example, the annual per capita costs per resident of these facilities between the pre- and post-war years as illustrated in Figure 3. In 1915 the annual cost per resident in constant 1967 dollars was 600 dollars. By 1945 that per capita expenditure had risen only to 716 dollars. As shown in Figure 3 those expenditures have increased enormously since the end of World War II, growing more in the three years following the return to peace than they had in the previous thirty years.

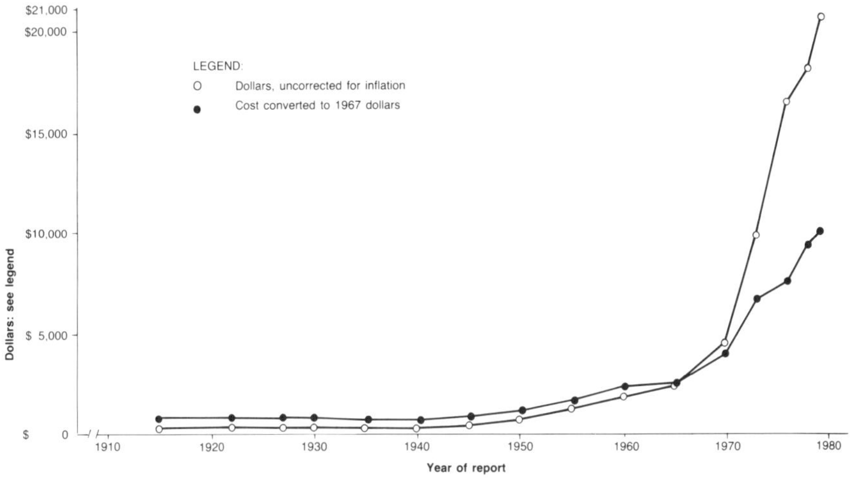

Figure 3. Annual cost per resident of care in public institutions for the mentally retarded for the years 1915 to 1979. (Sources: Lakin, 1979; Krantz, Bruininks & Clumpner, 1979)

In the early 1950s a new concept, "decentralization," was infused into the system of residential treatment of the mentally handicapped. Decentralization generally refers to the breakup of large institutions with state-wide catchment areas into a greater number of administrative units and often smaller facilities with a more regional focus. Philosophically these changes were founded on many of the same premises which are argued in support of extra-institutional residences for mentally handicapped persons: they were smaller allowing greater effort to be spent on care rather than maintenance of a monolithic unchanging organization with thousands of residents and staff. It was also assumed through decentralization that there would be a division of labor and deprofessionalization of decision making and program planning, that patients would remain closer to their home community and family, and that the facilities would be more "open," more directly in service to their catchment area.

This change, which grew out of the community mental health movement of the 1950s, had spread to mental retardation residential services by 1960. The large old institutions were not eliminated in great numbers, but the new ones were being built on the smaller, regional model. From 1960 to 1970 state-operated residential facilities for mentally retarded persons nearly doubled in number, growing from 108 to 190. During this same period the average number of residents per institution dropped from 1516 to 982, despite the fact that there were approximately 23,000 more residents in public residential facilities for the mentally retarded in 1970 than in 1960. As Figure 4 shows this trend has continued since 1970.

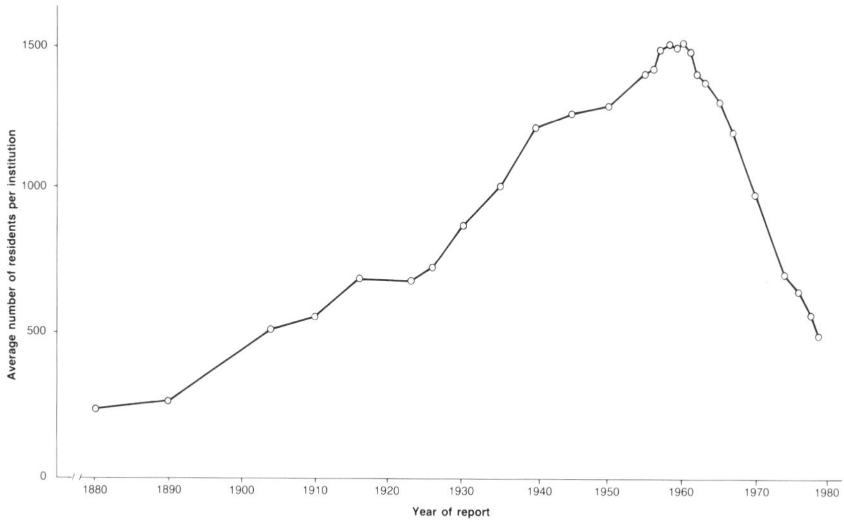

Figure 4. Average number of residents per public institution for the mentally retarded, 1880 to 1979. (Sources: Lakin, 1979; Krantz, Bruininks & Clumpner, 1979)

In short, then, the residential services system had been anything but static during the post-war years. Coinvolved with the changes described above was a progressively more impaired resident population as mildly retarded persons continued to make up nearly two-thirds of the discharges and one-third of the first admissions in the post-war years. There was also a sizable drop in the per capita death rate and an enormous demographic bulge in the resident population caused by the 1946-1960 birth cohorts. This later factor was highly influential in the growth of resident population through the mid-60s when the demographic bulge of the "baby boom" cohorts fell within the "school years," the age range where retarded individuals are most "at risk" of first admission to an institution. This bulge also had much to do with the drop in resident population in the late 1960s as this same group passed into adulthood, a period when release was much more probable. However, this early drop in institutional populations was both supported and encouraged by a fledgling system of community-based residential facilities which will be discussed subsequently. But while the first years of the progressive decrement in institutional populations may have been largely an artifact of an unprecedented demographic situation, what has followed in the 1970s can only be attributed to a philosophic and social revolution as radical and as sweeping as was the initial movement to build institutions for mentally retarded people in the late 19th and early 20th centuries.

Since the late 1960s, under the influence of deinstitutionalization, tens of thousands of mentally retarded people have been moved from state institutions to smaller residential facilities, to their natural families, to independent living, and to other types of community-based placement. Thousands more requiring residential services for the first time have been placed directly into non-institutional settings. During the 1960s and 1970s researchers and policy makers increasingly expressed concern over the evaluation of deinstitutionalization as a public policy, with a particular focus upon the adjustment and quality of life experienced by people who were released from public institutions for the mentally retarded. The research in this area, often characterized as community adjustment studies, sought to describe the living patterns, problems of living and general adjustment of retarded citizens, and often the reactions of others in society to them. Although the term *community adjustment* is as yet ill-defined, most of these studies focus upon assessing dimensions of adaptive behavior defined generally as the "effectiveness or degree with which the individual meets the standards of personal independence and social responsibility expected of his or her age and cultural group" (Grossman, 1973).

Research on community adjustment and living patterns of mentally retarded people is not new, for many studies have examined questions in this area during the past 100 years. (Excellent reviews of earlier studies have been written by Cobb [1972], Goldstein [1964], Heal, Sigelman & Switzky [1978], Heber & Dever [1970] and McCarver & Craig [1974].) What is especially significant about researching issues of community adjustment today is the added importance of current work in evaluating and adjusting public policies affecting retarded people. Perhaps more than previously, studies of the community adjustment of retarded people released from institutional settings can be characterized as policy research. According to Coleman (1972), two qualities distinguish policy research from disciplinary inquiry: the origin of the research problem outside an intellectual discipline in the world of action, and the use of research findings in the world of action outside that intellectual discipline. The characterization of studies on community adjustment and residential services as policy research has been noted also by Zigler and Balla (1977):

> In conclusion, if there is a consistent theme to this 20 years of work on the effects of institutionalization, it is a continuing and increasing emphasis on the social-policy implications of our research. We are convinced that any comprehensive program of research must take into account not only the behavioral functioning of residents but the quality of life they experience, the extent to which they maintain contact with the community, and whether they are successfully discharged to community placement. (p. 10)

The papers in this volume were developed out of a recognition of the importance of current research on community adjustment of retarded people for the evaluation and development of public policy, for understanding the quality of their life experiences, and for increasing knowledge about the important responses of agencies and people to them.

Organization of this Volume

This volume has been organized into four major sections: (1) An Overview of Deinstitutionalization and Community Placement; (2) Issues in Research on Deinstitutionalization and Community Adjustment; (3) Recent Research on Community-Based Placements; and (4) Research on the Provision and Evaluation of Community-Based Placements.

Section 1: An overview. Since 1967 the population of American public residential facilities for developmentally disabled people has been steadily decreasing. In the opening chapter of this volume, *Scheerenberger* describes the recent trends in the deinstitutionalization movement from the perspective of publicly operated residential facilities. Also discussed are specific problems now facing the residential service system in maintaining the momentum of this movement.

The following chapter by *Bruininks, Kudla, Hauber, Hill and Wieck* continues the discussion of the recent trends in the provision of residential services, focusing on the community-based service system. Described are characteristics of clients and facilities as well as the problems now facing that system.

In the next chapter *Lakin, Bruininks and Sigford* examine the early history of the deinstitutionalization of mentally retarded people. These writers note that many of the problems presently incurred in the deinstitutionalization process have been evident to researchers and administrators for a half-century, and they suggest that those interested in this contemporary social phenomenon can learn much from those who held similar interests many years ago.

In the final chapter of this section *Bachrach* also focuses on what researchers of the deinstitutionalization of developmentally disabled persons can learn from the past. She, however, focuses on the more recent past, reflecting on how the systematic application of what was learned in studying the deinstitutionalization of chronically mentally ill persons, a phenomenon now two decades old, can offer many insights to those studying this same process with mentally retarded people.

Section 2: Issues in research. The second section of this volume discusses some major methodological issues facing researchers of the community adjustment of developmentally disabled persons. Almost all recent research on post-institutional adjustment has been conducted using the traditional methods of psychology. In the first paper of this section *Taylor and Bogdan* compare this method of "quantitative" research with "qualitative" methods most often associated with anthropology and sociology. These writers make a strong case for greater application of qualitative methodologies in studying the social process called deinstitutionalization.

Returning to the problems facing "quantitative" researchers, in the second paper of this section *Seltzer, Sherwood, Seltzer and Sherwood* note that much of the past research on post-institutional adjustment has been difficult to interpret because the concept of community adjustment has been operationalized in many different ways. These writers consider the problems in the most commonly used operational definitions of adjustment and suggest an alternative model in which adjustment is measured as positive change in multiple behavioral characteristics, relative to the individual's abilities and within the context of a particular social setting.

In the following paper, *Gollay*, the primary investigator of a major study of deinstitutionalized mentally retarded people, reports briefly on the findings of her study of the extra-institutional life experiences of severely and profoundly retarded people, and then, drawing from first-hand knowledge, considers carefully the problems and issues facing researchers of post-institutional adjustment.

Whether a study of the community adjustment of developmentally disabled persons is conducted with "qualitative" or "quantitative" methods, it is very frequently the case that the most logical sources of information about extra-institutional life are mentally retarded people themselves. In a paper which reports on a large research project which used deinstitutionalized people as primary sources of information, *Wyngaarden* describes how she and her associates structured questions, trained interviewers and conducted interviews with mentally retarded respondents so as to obtain results which were as complete and reliable as possible. In a second paper on this topic *Sigelman, Schoenrock, Winer, Spankel, Hromas, Martin, Budd and Bensberg* report on a systematic study of the responsiveness of mentally retarded interviewees, as well as the validity and reliability of their responses. It is a paper which should be read by anyone considering interviews with mentally retarded people as part of a research program.

Section 3: Recent research. The third section of the volume begins with a paper in which *Bercovici* demonstrates the utility of the qualitative methods described by Taylor and Bogdan. In this paper the author looks beyond the semantics and desired outcomes of the deinstitutionalization movement to examine to what extent social reintegration actually takes place. The author raises important questions as to whether the social institutions created to break the pattern of isolation associated with large institutions are able to do so, or whether they may, in fact, serve to perpetuate the subcultural status of deinstitutionalized people.

The second chapter of this section also addresses some of the ambiguities of life as a mentally retarded person in our society. In this paper, *Edgerton* reconsiders the vacillating polarities of our societal conceptualizations of mentally retarded people: from "victim to victimizer." The results of his study suggest that usually they are neither, and sometimes they are both; and further that simple answers to complex social problems are terribly elusive.

Proponents of deinstitutionalization often put forth the argument that community-based living arrangements provide retarded people considerably greater opportunity to experience interaction and friendship with other persons. In a letter to a fictitious director of any state's developmental disabilities services, *Berkson and Romer,* two social psychologists, describe the bases of friendship and peer interaction in community-based residences and show that the nature of social activity can vary considerably among apparently similar facilities. Based on their findings, they make many recommendations that are respectful of the feelings and existing friendship patterns of those who are subject to future community placements.

The deinstitutionalization of severely and profoundly retarded persons poses enormous difficulties for the future of the deinstitutionalization movement. These difficulties as they exist in one state are discussed by *Landesman-Dwyer and Sultzbacher* in the fourth chapter of this section. Their research indicates that relatively little has been done to move severely and profoundly retarded people into community-based living and those who have been transferred have been the most capable of the severely/profoundly retarded population. A number of cautions are suggested before too much is invested into unproven residential options for this group of institutionalized persons.

To fully appreciate "community adjustment" as a process, time must obviously be considered. *Bell, Schoenrock and Bensberg* add this variable to their study of the adjustment of former residents of institutions for the mentally retarded. It proves to be an important variable, but one which does not appear to affect all aspects of community adjustment. Neither are all changes over time always in directions typically assumed to indicate greater social integration.

One seldom discussed alternative in the extra-institutional placement of developmentally disabled adults is the return to their natural family. *Willer, Intagliata and Wicks* report on the findings of their research on this type of placement and suggest that this option may be a more viable alternative than many people have thought. There are problems, however, and the authors discuss these at some length.

A persistent problem in the research on the effects of different settings on the personal growth and adjustment of their residents is that researchers have tended almost exclusively to make comparisons on the basis of "type" of facility (e.g., group home, boarding home, nursing home). Such an approach may be meaningful if there are fewer distinct differences in the nature of care offered in those facilities making up a particular type than there are among facilities selected on a random basis or on the basis of some other factor (e.g., size, location, staff or resident composition). Few researchers, however, have focused their work within one particular type of residential placement. In the final chapter of this section, *Intagliata, Willer and Wicks* address the issue of group differences among family care homes in New York State. They report on a method of categorizing the quality of care providers which in turn relates positively to a number of measures of personal growth, adaptive behavior, use of time, use of social services and personal independence on the part of the residents of these homes.

Section 4: Provision and evaluation of community placements. The fourth and final section of this volume focuses on research directly related to the providing and evaluating community programs. The range of topics covered in this section is a reflection of the multitude of complex considerations required in developing and evaluating community-based residential services.

For a half-century one community placement alternative for developmentally disabled persons has been foster family care. In recent years the number of foster care homes providing residential services to developmentally disabled persons has been growing steadily, particularly in New York and California. In the first chapter of this section *Intagliata, Crosby and Neider* discuss what has been learned about foster family care over the past 50 years and describe recent changes in this care alternative which are making it an even stronger option for the future.

As ecological psychologists have pointed out for years, adjustment within a social system involves reciprocal adjustments on the part of all members of that system. *Sutter and Mayeda* have applied this notion to the study of the community adjustment of mentally retarded people, demonstrating that compatibility of client characteristics with careprovider or employer preferences was highly related to placement success. Their chapter in this volume describes the procedures and two scales employed in their work.

It has long and often been recognized that care providers form the core of the residential services system. For a half-century researchers have been interested in isolating those variables which could predict quality environments and superior carepersons. Recently *Lei, Nihira, Sheehy and Meyers* have been reinvestigating this problem, focusing on small family care homes. In this chapter they present some of the findings of their work and discuss issues facing family care research.

With the recent growth in the use of the family care model for providing residential services for developmentally disabled people has come the realization that handicapped residents place considerably greater demands on foster families than do non-handicapped wards. To help foster parents cope with these demands, as well as to increase their effectiveness, several training programs have been developed in the past decade. *Intagliata and Willer* review some of these programs, make observations about their content and offer suggestions for their use.

One important goal of the residential services system should be to move clients as far as possible toward the highest level of independence they are able to achieve. One of the best known programs founded on this premise is the Mid-Nebraska Independent Living Training Program. In discussing this model program, *Schalock and Harper* describe how a well-conceptualized program, focused on specific independent living skills, can aid even severely retarded clients in attaining a good measure of personal independence and community adjustment.

In the sixth chapter of this section *Bjaanes, Butler and Kelly* examine the need for and provision of services to mentally retarded people of varying levels of handicap and in different forms of residential placement. This analysis suggests that when persons leave a residential setting they may often leave behind many of the services for which they retain a need. The authors caution that perhaps in the haste to place people in more normalized environments, planners have overlooked those programs which might help clients develop more normalized patterns of behavior. This, suggest the authors, ultimately may be a disservice to these same clients.

Much has been written in recent years about the differences in the quality of care offered across major types of residential facilities and for the most part explanations of these variations in the nature of care provision have focused on environmental, organizational and/or personnel differences. *Borthwick, Meyers and Eyman,* however, focus on a fourth crucial variable affecting residential facilities, the behavioral repertoires of the residents themselves. Their research shows that there are such large and systematic differences in residents' characteristics among facilities that these differences must be born in mind when considering the kind of care offered among alternative residential settings.

The term "residential services system" has been much used in recent years without much consideration of how "systematically" it operates. After tracing retrospectively the past contacts with professionals and agencies of individual residents of one facility and analyzing the paths these contacts took, *Rowitz* in the eighth chapter of this section shares both empirical data and general observations about both the complexity and efficiency of the "service system" from the perspective of consumers.

For the most part, the efforts to move large numbers of mentally retarded people out of public institutions into community-based residential facilities, to their natural homes, and other living arrangements have been remarkably successful. However, the early phase of deinstitutionalization has been much easier than will be subsequent phases, since most institution residents released in past years have been among the least handicapped. In the final chapter of this section, *Mayeda and Sutter* draw on the situation in Hawaii, a state with an early and successful program of deinstitutionalization, to reflect on future prospects for this movement. They point to the marked contrasts among previously released groups and today's residents of the Hawaiian state institution who are nominated as the best candidates for release and consider how this new reality will affect residential services.

Finally, in a summary chapter, *Lakin, Bruininks and Sigford* draw on the papers in this volume and the general literature regarding the social adjustment of deinstitutionalized developmentally disabled persons to outline a number of the more prominent issues and the research which bears on them.

As editors we have learned much from those who have contributed to this volume. While research efforts may not provide complete answers to social problems such as the one on which this volume focuses, we hope readers will find in these writings reason to believe that through careful and systematic scrutiny, the provision of residential and related community services to developmentally disabled persons can be substantially improved.

K. Charlie Lakin
Robert H. Bruininks
Barbara B. Sigford

University of Minnesota

References

Butterfield, E. Some basic changes in residential facilities. In R. Kugel & A. Shearer (Eds.), *Changing patterns in residential services for the mentally retarded*. Washington, DC: President's Committee on Mental Retardation, 1976.

Cobb, H. V. *The forecast of fulfillment*. New York: Teachers College Press, 1972.

Coleman, J. S. *Policy research in the social services*. Morristown, NJ: General Learning Press, 1972.

Goldstein, J. Social and occupational adjustment. In H. A. Stevens & R. Heber (Eds.), *Mental retardation*. Chicago: University of Chicago Press, 1964.

Heal, L. W., Sigelman, C. K., & Switzky, H. N. Community residential alternatives for the mentally retarded. In N. R. Ellis (Ed.), *International review of research in mental retardation* (Vol. 9). New York: Academic Press, 1978.

Heber, R. F. & Dever, R. B. Research on education and rehabilitation of the mentally retarded. In R. C. Haywood (Ed.) *Social-cultural aspects of mental retardation*. New York: Appleton-Century-Crofts, 1970.

Krantz, G. C., Bruininks, R. B., & Clumpner, J. L. *Mentally retarded people in state-operated residential facilities: Year ending June 30, 1979*. Minneapolis: University of Minnesota, Department of Psychoeducational Studies, 1979.

Lakin, K. C. *Demographic studies of residential facilities for the mentally retarded: An historical review of methodologies and findings*. Minneapolis: University of Minnesota, Department of Psychoeducational Studies, 1979.

McCarver, R. B., & Craig, E. M. Placement of the retarded in the community: Prognosis and outcome. In N. R. Ellis (Ed.), *International review of research in mental retardation* (Vol. 7). New York: Academic Press, 1974.

National Association of Superintendents of Public Residential Facilities for the Mentally Retarded. *Contemporary issues in residential programming*. Washington, DC: President's Committee on Mental Retardation, 1974.

Scheerenberger, R. C. *Public residential facilities for the mentally retarded, 1979*. Madison, WI: Central Wisconsin Center for the Developmentally Disabled, 1979.

Zigler, E., & Balla, D. A. Impact of institutional experience on the behavior and development of retarded persons. *American Journal of Mental Deficiency*, 1977, *82*, 1-11.

I. An Overview of Deinstitutionalization and Community Adjustment

Deinstitutionalization: Trends and Difficulties

Richard C. Scheerenberger

Central Wisconsin Center for the Developmentally Disabled
Madison, Wisconsin

Deinstitutionalization today is one of the most visible issues in the fields of both mental retardation and law. Rights of persons who are mentally retarded, least restrictive alternatives, comprehensive community services and their funding, as well as the future of residential (institutional) programming are all topics of considerable debate and controversy. The purpose of this presentation is to review briefly the current status and trends as they relate to public residential facilities (PRFs), i.e., state-sponsored and administered facilities that offer comprehensive programming to mentally retarded individuals on a 24-hour, 7-day-a-week basis. Most of the data cited are based on the results of a recent study of PRFs covering fiscal year (FY) 1978-1979 (July 1, 1978-June 30, 1979) sponsored by the National Association of Superintendents of Public Residential Facilities for the Mentally Retarded.[1]

Deinstitutionalization in Perspective

While the term "deinstitutionalization" is relatively new, its basic premises and practices are not. Though there was a brief historical moment when institutions were theoretically viewed as being the sole answer to the problem of mental retardation, the idea was quickly abandoned as both unwise and impractical. At no time have more than approximately 3% of the total mentally retarded population ever resided in an institution (Scheerenberger, 1976a, p. 17). The notion that institutions are not appropriate for most mentally retarded persons is as old as institutions themselves as evidenced by the writings and/or practices of Howe (1874) and Seguin (1846). Programs intended to offer alternatives to the congregate living associated with large PRFs were both advocated and implemented by Bernstein (1916) and Fernald (1919), two outstanding leaders in the field, as early as 1916. In many respects professionals are currently attempting to realize many of the ideas and programs outlined at least sixty years ago. (Cf. Lakin, Bruininks & Sigford in this volume for a thorough discussion of this literature.)

Further, institutions have always had a flow of population. In 1926, for example, the discharge rate was 6% in comparison to the approximate 10% rate reported for FY '78-'79, and there was considerably less reliance on public support and the simple transferring of persons to other forms of residential settings (U.S. Department of Commerce, 1931). The major difference between these two periods involves levels of adaptive behavior; more persons discharged in 1926 were mildly mentally retarded than in FY '78-'79.

---

[1]This study, which was also authorized by the President's Committee on Mental Retardation, was financially supported in part as one phase of the Developmental Disabilities Project on Residential Services and Community Adjustment, administered by the Department of Psycho-educational Studies, University of Minnesota, which, in turn, was supported by a grant (54P-71173/5) from the Bureau of Developmental Disabilities, Rehabilitation Services Administration, Office of Human Development Services, Department of Health, Education, and Welfare.

The current emphasis on deinstitutionalization is approximately eight years old, using the landmark case of *Wyatt v. Stickney* (1972) as the date of origin. Yet, concentrated efforts to place mildly mentally retarded people in the community were evident in the 1940s and 1950s as were similar efforts for the moderately mentally retarded in the 1950s and 1960s. Today, the primary concern is upon serving the more severely and profoundly multiply handicapped—physically and/or emotionally—in the community.

Current Status and Trends

During the summer months of 1979, questionnaires were forwarded to the superintendents of the 278 operational PRFs in the United States, all of whom responded. The questionnaire involved six areas of inquiry: basic demographic data; population movement; resident programs; parent visitations; services to non-residents; and administration, including budgeting and staffing. The 21-item questionnaire has been used by the National Association of Superintendents of Public Residential Facilities for four annual surveys. The data requested represent standard information maintained by each residential facility not only for internal operation but also to satisfy both state and federal regulations. The current discussion will be limited to those items and responses directly related to deinstitutionalization.[2]

The average daily population reported by the 278 PRFs (100%) for FY '78-'79 was 139,410. The range was 9 to 2,504 with a median of 389, down 41 from the median of 430 reported for FY '76-'77.[3] The resident census on June 30, 1979, was 139,329, a substantial decrease from the resident census on June 30, 1977, of 151,498. In spite of such decreases, however, 39 PRFs (14%) still served over 1,000 residents per day during FY '78-'79.

Figure 1 shows the average daily population of PRFs for six reporting fiscal years, beginning with FY '72-'73. The decrease in population between FY '76-'77 and '78-'79 was approximately 7.74%, which, distributed equally across the two years, would be 3.87% per year. This rate of decrease in average daily population was quite similar to that reported for fiscal years '72 through '76—4.37%, 4.33%, 4.32%, and 3.44% respectively. It was also significantly higher than the 1.36% reported for FY '76-77. The reduction in population from 173,775 in FY '72-'73 to 139,410 in FY '78-'79 represents a 19.78% overall decrease.

Several factors must be taken into account when considering the decrease in population in terms of deinstitutionalization. First, there would be a natural decline in new admissions simply because of the reduced birth rate in the United States. To illustrate, from 1970 to 1978 the number of youngsters under 13 years of age has decreased 11.8% (U.S. Department of Commerce, 1978). This factor plus a relatively constant annual mortality rate in PRFs of approximately 1.5% would result in a reduced census.

---

[2]Persons interested in the full report are referred to Scheerenberger (1979).

[3]Unless otherwise noted, references to FY '72-'73 and FY '73-'74 are from Scheerenberger (1975); references to FY '75-'76 are from Scheerenberger (1976b); and references to FY '76-'77 are from Scheerenberger (1978).

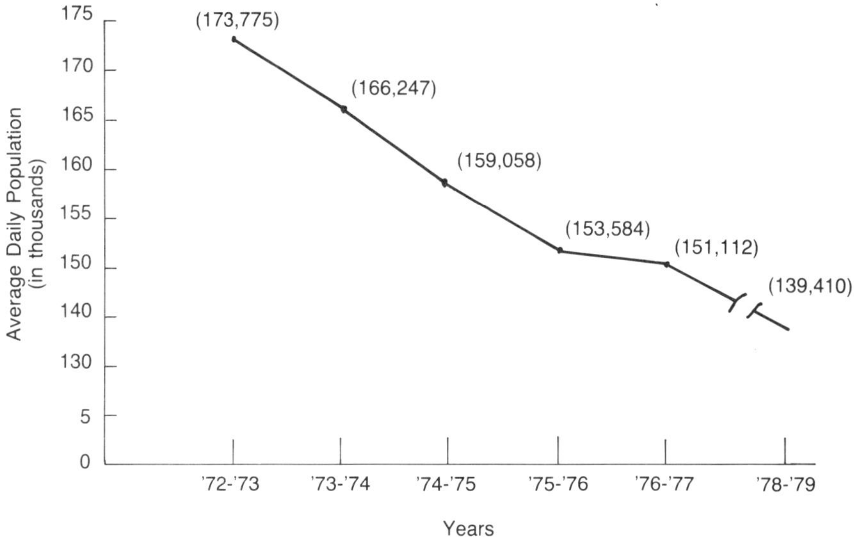

Figure 1. Average daily population in public residential facilities (FY '72-'73 through FY '78-'79).

Second, one must take into consideration the alternative placements of former residents. As will be observed from Table 1, 31% of 8,733 residents placed during FY '78-'79 as reported by 172 PRFs (62%) were, in essence, transferred to

Table 1

Alternative Placements as Reported by 172 Public Residential Facilities with a Total Resident Population of 97,180

Placement	Number of residents	Percent
Less restrictive:		
Independent living	40	.5
Own (parent or guardian) home	2,142	24.6
Other relatives	100	1.1
Foster home	643	7.4
Group home	1,620	18.6
Boarding home	271	3.1
Supervised apartment	64	.7
Work placement	132	1.5
Community ICF	989	11.3
Equally restrictive:		
Rest home	145	1.7
Nursing home	602	6.9
Penal	134	1.5
County home	25	.3
Other MR or DD residential facility	1,470	16.9
Mental hospital	320	3.7
General Hospital	26	.2
Total	8,723	100.0

another form of residential facility. The degree to which such programs are "less restrictive" than the original residential setting is unknown; however, there have been a number of disappointing reports concerning the adequacy of programming in many such facilities.

Deinstitutionalization does not simply involve the placement of mentally retarded persons into the community, it also involves the establishment of those programs intended to reduce the need for initial admission and readmission. For FY '78-'79, 222 PRFs (80%) indicated that there were 5,237 new admissions, or 4% of the total resident population of 127,975. Of marked concern was the fact that 22% of the new admissions were moderately and mildly retarded individuals of school age, and approximately 17% were mildly and moderately retarded adults. Only 61% of new admissions were severely and profoundly retarded, and 35.8% of those were of school age.

With regard to the effectiveness of community programming, it will be observed from Table 2 that approximately 40% of the new admissions came from their own homes, thus indicating either the absence of adequate natural home support programs or the availability of alternative home-like settings in the community. It also will be observed that there were a large number of interinstitutional transfers.

Table 2

New Admissions: Previous Placement

Original Setting	FY '76-'77 Number of residents	FY '76-'77 Percent	FY '78-'79 Number of residents	FY '78-'79 Percent
Work placement	21	.25	16	.32
Own home	3,399	39.50	2,060	41.04
Relatives' home	67	.78	115	2.29
Foster home	249	2.88	152	3.02
Group home	171	1.98	156	3.11
Boarding home	27	.31	36	.72
Community ICF	107	1.24	230	4.58
Rest home	24	.28	21	.42
Nursing home	136	1.58	97	1.92
Corrections	121	1.42	222	4.42
County home	14	.16	6	.12
Other MR facility	4,026	46.79	1,305	26.00
General Hospital	34	.40	148	2.95
State hospital for mentally ill	195	2.27	181	3.61
Other (unspecified)	11	.16	275	5.48
Total	8,591	100.00	5,020	100.00

In addition, one must take into consideration the pattern of readmissions. For FY '78-'79, 221 PRFs (79%) reported a total of 2,457 readmissions, 1.9% of the total resident population of 127,385. Though the readmission rate was less than that reported for previous years (e.g., 3.7% for FY '76-'77), a significant number of newly admitted residents (48%) were mildly and moderately retarded persons 3-62 years of age. Of these, approximately 17% were of school age as were approximately 25% of the severely and profoundly mentally retarded persons readmitted. These data indicate that while there is a decrease in both new admissions and readmissions, additional community services are sorely needed.

Though not directly related to the question of deinstitutionalization, it is of interest to note that the cost of residential programming continues to increase exponentially. The average per diem cost for FY '78-'79 was $60.10 per day with a range of $23.51 to $197.76. The $60.10 per diem rate represented a 36% increase over the per diem rate for FY '76-'77 and a 451% increase over the per diem rate reported in 1970 (Scheerenberger, 1979). This increase reflects both improved staffing levels and inflationary trends.

In terms of projected placements for FY '79-'80, 172 PRFs (62%) estimated that while 14,992 residents (15.4% of the total resident population) were ready for an alternative placement, only 7,853 (52%) were expected to be placed. This anticipated placement rate of 8% was slightly lower than the actual placement rates reported over the past few years. In order to gain some perspective on the nature of the placement problem, it is necessary to examine briefly the characteristics of the current resident population.

Table 3 shows an estimated distribution of the 139,329 residents in residence on June 30, 1979, extrapolated from the data provided by 175 PRFs (63%) with a total resident population of 87,451. As will be observed, the largest single population group was composed of adult severely and profoundly mentally retarded persons. Of the total resident population, 61% had at least one major multiple handicapping condition of physical origin and approximately 25% had severe emotional disorders. Thirty-three percent of the population had more than one handicapping condition or disorder. As regards adaptive behavior, 60.1% of the residents could walk without assistance; 56.3% could dress without assistance; 74.2% could eat without assistance; 81.2% could understand spoken words; 59.1% could communicate verbally, and 86.4% were toilet trained. Taking all factors into consideration, one can estimate that a sizable proportion of the current residential population probably could be served adequately in the community if appropriate services were available. In the judgment of the superintendents, however, PRFs are faced with a number of critical problems associated with the placement of mentally retarded people in the community.

Table 3

Estimated Distribution of 139,329 Residents by Chronological Age and Level of Retardation

Level of retardation	Chronological Age: 0-2	3-21	22-62	63+	Total
	Number of residents	Number of residents	Number of residents	Number of residents	Number of residents
Mild+*	15	2,550	7,670	1,063	11,298
Moderate	16	4,835	14,239	1,087	20,177
Severe/ Profound	206	32,951	70,935	3,762	107,854
Total	237	40,336	92,844	5,912	139,329

*Includes a small number who are borderline.

Problems in Placement

In conjunction with the study of national trends, superintendents were requested to respond to a companion questionnaire addressing problems and difficulties associated with community placements. The 54 items were collated according to: (1) problems and barriers to placing mentally retarded persons into the community; (2) residents most difficult to place in community-based programs; and (3) problems causing community placement failures that result in the return of an individual to an institution, taking into consideration both client and community variables. Again, this information is readily available in PRFs in order to satisfy Title XIX requirements.

For each item, the respondent was requested to record according to level of retardation (mild, moderate, and severe/profound) whether the item represented (1) a major, constant problem, (2) an occasional problem, or (3) rarely a problem. A well-designed, well-staffed, and a well-funded system of integrated, comprehensive community services should result in few problems. In other words, ideally, each of the items would receive a rating of 3. Occasional problems (rating of 2) would be less desirable but certainly acceptable in today's society. Thus, an average rating of 2 to 3 would be considered reflective of an adequate service. An average rating of less than 2, however, signaled a troublesome area, one not compatible with individual needs and/or rights and one that requires extensive remediation. An average rating of 1 to 1.5 identified an area in which a service basically was not available.

Of the 278 PRFs, 176 (63%) responded. These facilities served 103,664 residents (average daily population) during FY '78-'79, which represented 74% of the total number of residents served in all PRFs on the basis of average daily population for the same reporting period. Facilities representing each of the 48 contiguous states responded; Alaska and Hawaii did not.

Barriers to Community Placement

Table 4 shows the results concerning barriers to community placement that took into consideration seven factors: availability of alternative living facilities; quality of available community living facilities; availability of community support services; quality of community support services; funding; number of community program personnel; and adequacy of training.

As will be seen, availability of alternative community living facilities for mentally retarded persons, regardless of level of retardation, was considered to represent a major problem to deinstitutionalization. While the quality of alternative living facilities was rated rather adequate for the more mildly affected, it was considered less than adequate for the severely and profoundly retarded.

As regards the availability of community support services, educational programs for mildly and moderately retarded students were rated adequate as were medical services for the same population. Such services for the severely and profoundly mentally retarded were, however, judged to be less than adequate. Adult programming and behavior management, regardless of level of retardation, were basic services uniformly judged inadequate throughout the country. It should be noted that Public Law 94-142, which provides for the education of all severely and profoundly mentally retarded children, was relatively new at the time of this study. The quality of such services, when available, was rated slightly higher than the quantity.

Funding of community programs was considered substantially inadequate with few exceptions. Educational and medical services were considered to be ade-

Table 4

Mean Ratings of Problems Associated with Community Placement

Item	Level of Retardation: Mild mean	Moderate mean	Severe/ profound mean
Availability of Alternative Community Living Facility	1.82	1.58	1.16
Quality of Alternative Community Living Facility	2.00	1.87	1.52
Availability of Community Support Services			
Education	2.33	2.15	1.65
Adult Programming	1.27	1.21	1.03
Medical Services	2.13	2.01	1.72
Behavior Management	1.49	1.43	1.35
Quality of Community Support Services			
Education	2.28	2.07	1.74
Adult Programming	2.19	1.87	1.70
Medical Services	2.18	2.15	1.95
Behavior Management	1.73	1.54	1.45
Funding			
Alternative Living	1.71	1.70	1.59
Education	2.26	2.12	2.04
Adult Programming	1.92	2.10	1.73
Medical Services	2.24	2.26	2.15
Behavior Management	1.65	1.61	1.59
Number of Community Support Services			
Education	2.04	2.07	1.87
Adult Programming	1.91	1.81	1.60
Medical Services	2.29	2.05	2.02
Behavior Management	1.57	1.45	1.33
Adequacy of Training			
Education	2.27	201	1.74
Adult Programming	2.37	2.09	1.56
Medical Services	2.26	2.15	1.94
Behavior Management	1.57	1.60	1.41

*Data are mean scores based on a three-point rating scale of 1 for "a major, constant problem," 2 for "an occasional problem," and 3 for "rarely a problem."

quately funded as was adult programming for moderately retarded persons. Funding of alternative living community facilities, behavior management programs, and adult programming for mildly and more severely retarded persons was again considered insufficient.

The number of available community support personnel was considered adequate for educational and medical services but substantially inadequate for adult programming and behavior management. The latter held true regardless of level of retardation.

Similarly, professional personnel associated with education, adult programming, and medical services were judged to be adequately prepared when providing for mildly and moderately retarded persons but substantially inadequate when meeting the needs of the more severely affected. Behavior management personnel were considered to lack sufficient training to deal effectively with mentally retarded individuals regardless of their level of intelligence.

Characteristics of Difficult-to-Place Residents

Table 5 summarizes the results as they pertain to resident characteristics that could adversely influence community placement. As will be noted, only chronological age appeared to be of relatively little importance. Residents with behavior problems, ambulation difficulties, and/or inadequate self-help skills were considered most difficult to place, regardless of level of retardation. It should be noted that while the severity of mental retardation, in general, increased problems associated with locating an appropriate placement, the ranking of characteristics did not vary significantly between the three levels.

Table 5

Mean Ratings and Ranking of Resident Characteristics Affecting Community Placement

	Mild		Moderate		Severe/ profound		Total	
Characteristics	mean	rank	mean	rank	mean	rank	mean	rank
Non-ambulatory	1.52	2	1.43	2	1.36	2	1.43	2
Inadequate self-help skills	1.61	3	1.61	4	1.83	8	1.68	4
Limited communication skills	1.90	6	1.76	5	1.54	4	1.73	6
Behavior problems	1.18	1	1.12	1	1.10	1	1.13	1
Inadequate social skills	1.83	5	1.69	6	1.57	5	1.70	5
Under age six	2.13	8	2.04	8	1.77	7	1.97	8
Over age fifty	2.08	7	1.91	7	1.68	6	1.89	7
On-going medical problems (e.g., diabetes, epilepsy, and respiratory complications)	1.67	4	1.54	3	1.44	3	1.55	3

*Data are mean scores based on a three-point rating scale of 1 for "a major, constant problem," 2 for "an occasional problem," and 3 for "rarely a problem."

Problems Causing Community Placement Failures

Problems resulting in community placement failures were considered from two perspectives: the mentally retarded person and the community. Each will be considered independently.

Resident characteristics: As shown in Table 6, physical aggression in nearly any form was judged a major reason for returning a person to a residential facility, regardless of level of retardation. Interestingly, sexual conduct, stubbornness, noisiness, and stereotypic behavior were not considered to present serious problems, at least as they relate to success or failure in the community. In this instance, it will be observed that both rankings and means were similar for all three levels of retardation.

Table 6

Mean Ratings and Ranking of Problems Causing Community Placement Failures: Resident Characteristics

	Mild		Moderate		Severe/ profound		Total	
Characteristics	mean	rank	mean	rank	mean	rank	mean	rank
Physically aggressive *and* dangerous to others	1.30	1.0	1.41	1.0	1.34	1.0	1.35	1
Physically aggressive *but not* dangerous to others	1.46	2.0	1.46	2.0	1.43	2.0	1.45	2
Verbally aggressive	1.89	10.0	1.96	10.0	1.88	8.5	1.91	10
Temper tantrums	1.85	7.5	1.83	8.0	1.76	6.0	1.81	7
Stubborn	2.18	12.0	2.16	13.0	2.09	13.5	2.14	13
Noisy	2.27	14.0	2.23	14.0	2.09	13.5	2.18	14
Hyperactive	1.86	9.0	1.71	4.5	1.73	5.0	1.77	5
Stereotypic behavior	2.24	13.0	2.14	12.0	1.99	11.0	2.12	12
Damages property	1.53	3.0	1.51	3.0	1.48	3.0	1.51	3
Rebellious	1.71	4.0	1.80	6.0	1.82	7.0	1.78	6
Self-abusive	1.82	6.0	1.71	4.5	1.57	4.0	1.70	4
Inappropriate sexual behavior								
a. Masturbation	2.07	11.0	2.07	11.0	2.03	12.0	2.06	11
b. Homosexual activity	1.85	7.5	1.84	9.0	1.88	8.5	1.86	9
c. Heterosexual activity	1.73	5.0	1.81	7.0	1.96	10.0	1.83	8

*Data are mean scores based on a three-point rating scale of 1 for "a major, constant problem," 2 for "an occasional problem," and 3 for "rarely a problem."

Community variables: As shown in Table 7, and as would be anticipated on the basis of previously presented data, major inadequacies in community services included appropriate living settings, behavior management programs, specialized services, and adult programs. Transportation, medical services, educational opportunities, and advocacy were not considered problematic.

In essence, it would appear that all of the various service components critical to effecting an acceptable program of deinstitutionalization, only educational and medical services for moderately and mildly retarded persons are in place. Community living facilities, educational services for the more severely and profoundly mentally retarded individual, adult programming, and programs intended to meet the needs of the more difficult-to-manage individual are seriously lacking.

Table 7

Mean Ratings and Ranking of Problems Causing Community Placement Failures: Community Variables

Problem Area	Mild		Moderate		Severe/ profound		Total	
	mean	rank	mean	rank	mean	rank	mean	rank
Transportation	2.04	6	1.85	5	1.75	6	1.85	6
Medical services	2.29	9	2.21	9	1.99	8	2.16	9
Appropriate homes	1.77	3	1.67	3	1.38	2	1.60	3
Educational programs	2.22	8	2.14	8	1.82	7	2.05	7
Sheltered employment	1.98	5	1.83	4	1.57	4	1.79	4
Recreation/social programs	1.94	4	1.89	6	1.66	5	1.83	5
Specialized services (e.g., PT, OT, speech and counseling)	1.72	2	1.59	2	1.45	3	1.58	2
Behavior management programs	1.45	1	1.21	1	1.32	1	1.32	1
Advocacy or protective services	2.10	7	2.07	7	2.00	9	2.06	8

*Data are mean scores based on a three-point rating scale of 1 for "a major, constant problem," 2 for "an occasional problem," and 3 for "rarely a problem."

Implications

One can summarize the implications of the results of these two surveys quite simply. The population currently being served in PRFs is composed primarily of severely and profoundly mentally retarded, multiply handicapped individuals; and unless all essential programs are developed and implemented in the near future, the current rate of deinstitutionalization will be adversely affected.

References

Bernstein, C. Minutes. *Journal of Psycho-Asthenics*, 1916, *21*, 94-112.

Fernald, W. State programs for the care of the mentally defective. *Journal of Psycho-Asthenics*, 1919, *24*, 114-122.

Howe, S. Cited in *Mental retardation: Past and present*. Washington, D.C.: U.S. Government Printing Office, 1977.

Scheerenberger, R. *Current trends and status of public residential services for the mentally retarded, 1974*. Madison, WI: National Association of Superintendents of Public Residential Facilities for the Mentally Retarded, 1975.

Scheerenberger, R. *Deinstitutionalization and institutional reform*. Springfield, IL: Charles C. Thomas, 1976(a).

Scheerenberger, R. *Current trends and status of public residential services for the mentally retarded, 1976*. Madison, WI: National Association of Superintendents of Public Residential Facilities for the Mentally Retarded, 1976(b).

Scheerenberger, R. Public residential services for the mentally retarded. In N. Ellis (Ed.), *International review of research in mental retardation* (Vol. 9). New York: Academic Press, 1978.

Scheerenberger, R. *Public residential services for the mentally retarded, 1979,* Madison, WI: National Association of Superintendents of Public Residential Facilities for the Mentally Retarded, 1979.

Seguin, E. *Traitement moral, hygiene et e'ducation des idiots et descuetres enfonts arreere's*. Paris: J. B. Bailliere, 1846.

U.S. Department of Commerce. *Statistical abstracts*. Washington, D.C.: U.S. Government Printing Office, 1978.

Recent Growth and Status of Community Residential Alternatives

Robert H. Bruininks
Mary J. Kudla
Florence A. Hauber
Bradley K. Hill
Colleen A. Wieck

University of Minnesota

Government supported and private residential services for mentally retarded and other people with developmental disabilities have existed in the United States for over 100 years (Lakin, 1979; Wolfensberger, 1976). Early institutions tended to be small, almost like boarding schools, with a heavy emphasis on education and rehabilitation. They were run by concerned professionals who, in most cases, believed that retarded people could be taught the skills necessary to function in society and then be returned to community settings (Lakin, 1979; Wolfensberger, 1972).

By the end of the 19th century, segregation through institutionalization, came to be a far more commonly espoused approach to dealing with mentally retarded people. In this period the size of institutions increased, with the view that large institutions could be more efficient than small ones for providing custodial care at minimal cost. Highly influential in creating the social climate which permitted the rapid expansion of large custodial facilities, were the proposals of the eugenicists who linked nearly every social evil to mental retardation.

These multi-purpose facilities provided all services—residential, care, and training—within a single setting. This tendency to consolidate services in one locale served as the primary model for institutional care for the mentally retarded for many decades.

During the last twenty years several major changes have occurred in the delivery of services to mentally retarded people (Mesibov, 1976; Nihara & Nihara, 1975; Nirje, 1976; Wolfensberger, 1972). Evolving social attitudes and changing government policies provided the impetus to reduce the populations of retarded individuals in public residential facilities and to relocate them with their families and in community residential facilities. In 1963, President John F. Kennedy affirmed the importance of decentralized community-based care for retarded citizens in a report to Congress. This commitment was reaffirmed in 1971 by President Richard M. Nixon who announced the national goal of returning one-third of the population of retarded people in institutions to community settings by 1981. The period of the 1970s can be characterized as the decade of deinstitutionalization and growth in community residential services.

Research reported in this manuscript was supported by a grant (54-P-71173/5-04) from the Administration on Developmental Disabilities, Department of Health and Human Services. Portions of this manuscript were printed in earlier articles published in the *American Journal of Mental Deficiency* (1980, Vol. 84, No. 5, 470-478) and in *Mental Retardation* (1980, Vol. 18, No. 3, 125-130). The authors wish to acknowledge the helpful contributions of Charlie Lakin and Susan Certain in the preparation of the manuscript.

History of Community Residential Services

Community residential facilities have changed considerably from "colonies" that were introduced to the United States in the early 1900s. At that time the colony plan called for a number of formerly institutionalized retarded persons to live in supervised groups in large houses and to work either on a farm or in a small, controlled factory (Adams, 1971). Berstein (1927) argued for the colony plan because it offered fewer restrictions, more humane care, was less humiliating than institutional placement, and was economically cost-effective. During the Depression colony care became less economically feasible and its popularity declined. Since that time, cost effectiveness arguments have recurred frequently in support of community care models as less expensive alternatives to the institutional model (Wieck, 1980).

In the 1950s, parents of retarded people organized to protest the deplorable conditions in many state institutions and the lack of community services. The National Association for Retarded Citizens became active in providing and securing community-based programs for retarded citizens who previously were sent to institutions. The parent movement brought to public awareness the plight of retarded citizens and pressured local, state, and federal levels of government to support financially and improve community programs for the mentally retarded.

Sporadic experiments in community residential living have been reported in the literature since the early 1960s. However, community residences began to fully develop as vehicles for deinstitutionalization beginning about 1970. As defined by the National Association of Superintendents of Public Residential Facilities for the Mentally Retarded (1974), deinstitutionalization means:

> (1) prevention of admission by finding and developing alternative community methods of care and training; (2) return to the community of all residents who have been prepared through programs of habilitation and training to function adequately in appropriate local settings; and (3) establishment and maintenance of a responsive residential environment which protects human and civil rights. (pp. 4-5)

These changes in approach toward residential care are expressions of *normalization, least restrictive alternative,* and *developmental models of programming*. As defined by Nirje (1976), normalization means making available to mentally retarded citizens the patterns and conditions of everyday life that are available to persons in the mainstream of society. Wolfensberger (1972) has greatly elaborated on this concept, stressing the importance of culturally normative qualities in training programs, life experiences, and physical environments. The least restrictive doctrine, first defined by court decisions (Halderman v. Pennhurst, 1977; NYARC v. Carey, 1975; Welsch v. Likens, 1974; Wyatt v. Stickney, 1972), emphasizes that people should be served under conditions that maximize opportunities to live and learn in normal settings in society. Similarly, a developmental programming model assumes that the limitations of all retarded people are modifiable regardless of their degree of impairment. These three philosophical concepts—normalization, least restrictive alternative, and developmental models of programming—have led to the generally held view that community residential services should be small, homelike, and stress integration of residents into training, education, leisure, and other areas of life in the typical community.

Previous National Surveys of Community Residential Facilities

Despite the large reduction in population of mentally retarded residents in public residential facilities (Krantz, Bruininks, & Clumpner, 1978; Lakin, 1979;

Scheerenberger, 1978, 1979), very little research has been conducted at the national level to describe the growth and characteristics of alternative community living arrangements or the rate of resident movement into and out of these facilities. Examination of available literature indicates three recent surveys of any national scope.

Between 1972 and 1974, O'Connor (1976) and O'Connor and Sitkei (1975) reported a national survey to identify all facilities which met the following definition:

> . . . any community based residential facility which operates 24 hours a day to provide services to a small group of mentally retarded and/or otherwise developmentally disabled who are presently or potentially capable of functioning in the community with some degree of independence. These living facilities may also be known as group homes, hostels, boarding houses, and halfway houses. (p. 35)

A total of 611 facilities with over 8,000 mentally retarded residents fit the operational definition. Nearly one-half of these 611 facilities were located in six states: Michigan (57), New York (52), Nebraska (48), California (47), Washington (46), and Minnesota (28) (O'Connor, 1976, p. 17). Thirty states reported eight or fewer facilities. Over three-fourths of all community residential facilities in this study had been in existence for five years or less and nearly one-half of them had started within the two years prior to 1972.

Baker, Seltzer, and Seltzer (1974) found 381 facilities that fit their operational definition of a community facility: "opened more than six months, accommodated no more than eighty retarded adults, and regarded itself as an alternative to an institution" (p. 14). Thirty-five percent of the identified residential facilities were providing care to 10 or fewer adults. Approximately 17% of the facilities served five or fewer retarded adults in foster family care. Of the 381 community residential facilities surveyed by Baker and associates in 1973, over one-half had opened within the three years prior to 1973. Only one-fourth had been in operation five years or longer.

The O'Connor (1976) and Baker, Seltzer, and Seltzer (1974) studies reported that approximately equal numbers of males and females resided in community residences. Close to one-half of the residents were between 16 and 20 years of age in the O'Connor study. The average age of residents in the Baker, Seltzer, and Seltzer study was 35 years. O'Connor found that the vast majority of residents in the facilities studied were mentally retarded (89%), while 10% of those residents who were not retarded had other problems, most commonly related to emotional or behavioral disorders. Baker, Seltzer, and Seltzer reported most residents were moderately retarded (42%) or mildly retarded (32%) with severe retardation reported at a much lower frequency (12%). In both national surveys, it was found that over one-half of the residents had previously resided in an institution, while about one-third had moved directly from their own homes.

A Current Profile of Community Residential Facilities

In 1977 a national mail census of community residential facilities was conducted at the University of Minnesota by the Developmental Disabilities Project on Residential Services and Community Adjustment under a grant from the Administration on Developmental Disabilities (Bruininks, Hauber & Kudla, 1979). The purpose of this project was to provide state and federal policy makers with information needed to improve planning, management, and evaluation of residential services for mentally retarded people.

The survey included all facilities and homes throughout the United States that met the following definition of a community residential facility (CFR):

> . . . any community based living quarter(s) which provides 24-hour, 7 days-a-week responsibility for room, board, and supervision of mentally retarded persons as of June 30, 1977 with the exceptions of: (a) single family homes providing services to a relative; (b) nursing homes, boarding homes, and foster homes that are not formally state licensed or contracted as mental retardation service providers; and (c) independent living (apartment) programs which have no staff residing in the same facilities. (Bruininks, Hauber & Kudla, 1979, p. 11)

This category of community residential facilities encompasses a wide range of alternative living arrangements outside the traditional publicly operated institutions. While terms such as community residences, community based facilities or community residential facilities are used loosely in the professional literature and in state regulations, they have no standardized operational meaning across states. These living arrangements vary widely in size, staff composition, age and disability of residents, and in services provided. Since no standard classification system exists from state to state for the categorization of these residential facilities, the Bruininks, Hauber, and Kudla study included all facilities licensed (regulated, certified, approved) by the state to provide residential services to mentally retarded people, except publicly operated institutions.

A complete list of all known eligible facilities serving mentally retarded people was compiled through several sources including: (a) all state Mental Retardation Coordinators; (b) all state Associations for Retarded Citizens; (c) state Developmental Disabilities Councils; (d) administrators of public and private residential facilities; (e) the National Association of Private Residential Facilities; (f) licensing agencies; (g) individuals or agencies listed as contacts in past reports of Developmental Disabilities Office Annual Surveys of Institutions; and (h) the 1973 National Center for Health Statistics Master Facility Inventory of Inpatient Facilities for the Mentally Retarded and a special 1977 update of the earlier listing provided by special request from the agency.

State information was found to be the most reliable, up-to-date source for the registry. Existing national lists such as the National Center for Health Statistics Master Facility Inventory of Inpatient Facilities were found to underestimate the number of community residential facilities. State contacts were made in a systematic fashion according to standard survey research procedures (Bruininks, Hauber, & Kudla, 1979).

The initial mailing was made on August 19, 1977, to 10,271 facilities identified in the national mailing registry. In order to ensure that all facilities on the original list were contacted, three mail follow-up inquiries were sent out and a telephone follow-up was conducted. Due to the large number of administrative systems included in the registry (i.e. single ownerships operating more than one facility), additional facilities were added to the mailing list throughout the survey. The survey was completed on April 28, 1978, with a total number of 11,351 potential facilities and homes participating. Of the total number surveyed, 4,427 facilities met the definition of a community residential facility, 611 facilities did not respond, 350 facilities were duplicate addresses, 2,110 facilities did not meet the operational definition, and 645 facilities were not in business. An additional 2,609 facilities were classifiied as foster or family care homes. In California, based on consultation with state personnel, it was determined that small family care homes were considered part of the residential service system for mentally retarded people. These homes, therefore, were classified as community facilities for the purpose of analysis rather than as foster homes.

In calculating the response rate, the following facilities were excluded: duplicate addresses, facilities not meeting operational definition, facilities out of business, and facilities identified as foster homes. Using the number of facilities that met the definition of a community residential facility, an 87.9% response rate was obtained. Since foster homes differed considerably in organization and management from the other facilities included in the survey, it was decided that information on these programs should be summarized separately. The response rate for foster homes was 76% in the 20 states represented. A complete description of the methodologies employed for these two surveys are reported by Bruininks, Hauber, and Kudla (1979) for community facilities, and Bruininks, Hill, and Thorsheim (1980) for foster homes.

Number of facilities and residents. The 4,427 community residences reported a licensed capacity of 83,688. As of June 30, 1977, a total of 76,250 residents lived within these facilities, of which 62,397 were mentally retarded, resulting in a national mean occupancy rate of 91.1%. Nationwide, approximately 29 of every 100,000 people were living in community based residences for mentally retarded individuals compared to about 70 of every 100,000 people in public residential facilities. The survey of 1,973 specially licensed or contracted foster homes reported 4,999 retarded residents in 20 states. New York family care homes represented 61% of all foster homes included in this survey. The numbers reported from these surveys represent a conservative estimate for community alternative living arrangements. The actual totals would be somewhat higher if adjusted for nonresponse.

Growth of residences. The policy and practice of deinstitutionalization are quite apparent in examining the rapid and substantial growth of community residences in the past several years (Figure 1). The data show that the number of community residences approximately doubled between January, 1973 and June, 1977. Facilities which opened and closed prior to the survey are not included in Figure 1. Therefore, the number of facilities presented is a minimum estimate of annual additions. Based upon the 317 facilities known to have opened during the

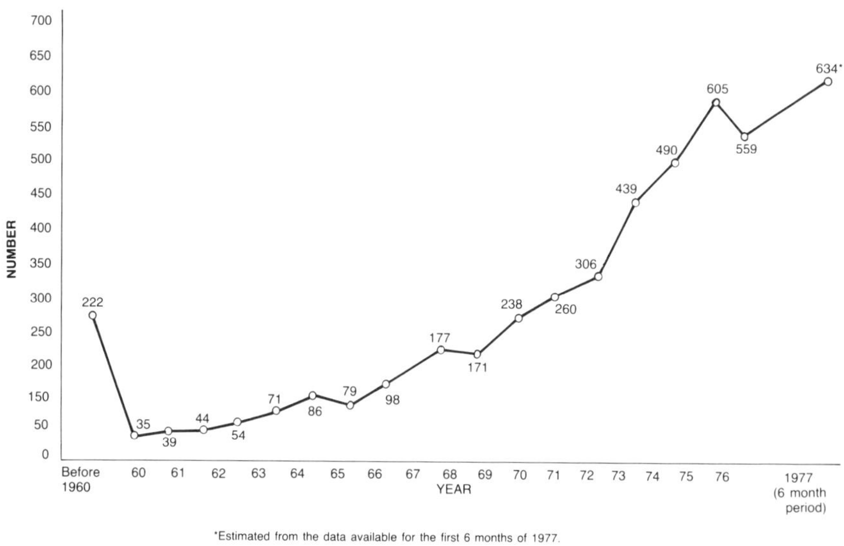

Figure 1. Year of opening for 4,290 community residential facilities (United States, 1977, 97% CRFs Reporting) (Bruininks, Hauber, & Kudla, 1979, p. 58)

first six months of 1977, the total number of facilities for that year is projected as 634. Of the 73% of the foster homes responding to the survey, 70% indicated they had been in operation at least four years.

Size of facility. Size is frequently used as one criterion in evaluating normalization of living environments. As shown in Figure 2, most facilities were small, nearly 73% served 10 or fewer mentally retarded residents, and over 88% of the facilities served 20 or fewer mentally retarded residents. The distribution of mentally retarded residents shows, however, that 28.3% of the total number of mentally retarded residents lived in homes with 10 or fewer people and 43.9% lived in facilities with 20 or fewer people. Over one-half of the mentally retarded residents lived in community based residences which served 31 or more residents. During this same period, foster homes averaged three residents per home.

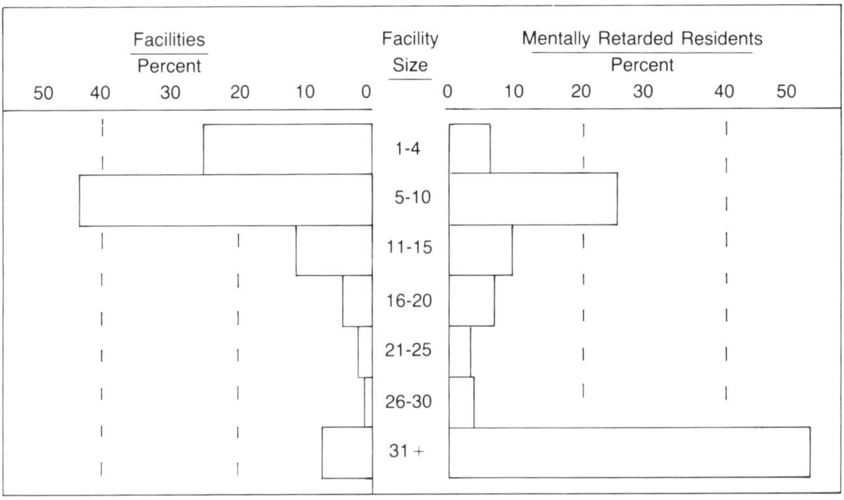

Figure 2. Distribution of Community Residential Facilities and Mentally Retarded Residents by Size of Facility (United States, 1977, 100% CRFs Reporting)

Resident characteristics. Respondents were asked to classify the number of mentally retarded people residing in their facility by sex, age, and level of retardation. The sex distribution shows that there were more males than females: 55.3% male and 44.7% female (Figure 3). Approximately 62% of the mentally retarded residents living in community residential facilities were 22 years or older, and 36% of the residents were school age, that is, between the ages of 5 to 21 years. Foster home residents were primarily adults, 69% were reported over 21 years of age.

Approximately 65% of the mentally retarded residents were classified as borderline, mildly, or moderately retarded, while 32% were considered severely or profoundly retarded. Only 2% could not be classified into one of the levels of retardation by the respondents. Similarly, the level of retardation for foster home residents was reported as 67% borderline, mildly, or moderately retarded, and 33% were considered severely or profoundly retarded.

Resident movement. To assess resident movement during July 1, 1976 to June 30, 1977, respondents indicated the number of mentally retarded residents who were first admissions, readmissions, live releases, and deaths during the previous year.

There were over 16,000 first admissions reported by community residential facilities. This represents one of every four residents living in those facilities. A

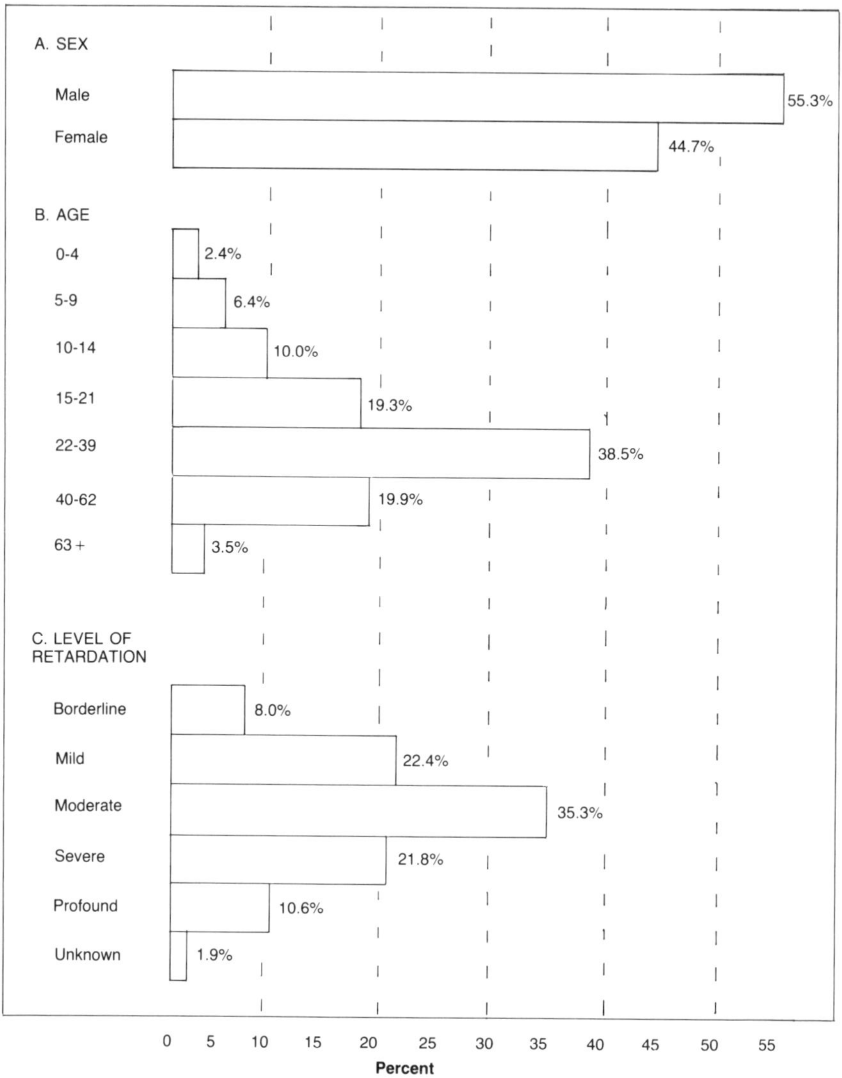

Figure 3. Sex, Age, Level of Retardation of Mentally Retarded Persons in Community Residential Facilities (United States, 1977, 98% CRFs Reporting A, 96% CRFs Reporting B & C)

similar admissions rate was reported by foster homes. However, when the rate of new admissions in community facilities and foster homes is adjusted for the newly opened facilities, the rate of annual first admissions drops to 17% of the total mentally retarded resident population in community residences and 18% of the total mentally retarded population in foster homes. These figures demonstrate the rapid growth of facilities and the sizeable movement of residents in recent years.

The previous placement of first admissions into community residences was also ascertained. Institutions accounted for the largest proportion of previous placements (35%), followed by natural homes (32.4%), other community residential facilities (14.7%), foster homes (9.6%), and all other residential settings (8.3%). Of the newly admitted residents into foster homes, 42% came from public institutions, 32% from other foster homes, and 11% came from their natural homes.

During July 1, 1976 to June 30, 1977 there were approximately 9,300 discharges and 612 deaths reported by community residences. The rates of discharges and deaths for foster homes were similar to the rates in community residences. Over 50% of the community residential facilities reported no movement into or movement out of their facilities during the twelve months covered by the survey. In other words, there were no first admissions, no readmissions, no live releases, and no deaths in one-half of the community residential facilities.

Major Problems and Issues in Community Residential Services

The surveys described in this chapter indicate the relative recency of widespread community residential services in the United States. As of yet, the policy problems and administrative issues associated with this movement have not been extensively researched, although a number of authors have discussed these questions (Bradley, 1978; Braddock, 1977; Bruininks, Kudla, Wieck, & Hauber, 1980). This section summarizes the results of two studies on policy issues and administrative problems in the provision of community residential and related services for mentally retarded and other developmentally disabled people.

In the first sutdy, 2,000 administrators responded to a question regarding major problems in operating and maintaining a community residential facility. These responses produced a number of important implications for improving the planning and management of human services for mentally retarded and other developmentally disabled people. These responses, supported in part by the results of other recent reports (Bruininks, Williams, & Morreau, 1978; General Accounting Office, 1977), imply some need for important changes in management practices and in regulatory and funding policies.

The major problems cited by community residential facility administrators may be grouped into five categories: staffing, funding, services, interagency relationships, and administrative problems (Bruininks, Kudla, Wieck, & Hauber, 1980). The most frequently identified problem was staffing and personnel areas as reported by 85% of the respondents. Recruitment of qualified staff, reduction of turnover, and staff training were clearly the three most pressing areas of difficulty. Also mentioned far less frequently by administrators were wage and hour constraints, staffing patterns, and working conditions.

The second most common obstacle cited by 61% of the respondents was inadequate funding. Maintaining a sufficient average daily resident population, late checks, and outside (county) control of wages and benefits were the most frequently cited problems within the funding category.

The lack of an available continuum of comprehensive services was cited by 46% of the respondents. Within the facility, the development of individualized program plans, inadequate programming, and the lack of program implementation for residents were often considered to be problems. Deficiencies in the range and availability of support services outside the living arrangement in the community were frequently cited, with specific reference to areas such as respite care, transportation, residential alternatives, advocacy, follow-along, and nutrition services.

Problems incurred with interagency relationships ranked fourth in importance. Approximately 22% of the directors mentioned concerns regarding licensing standards, the preponderance of regulations, administrative red tape, and the lack of coordination between local, regional, and state levels of service. Last of all, several administrative problems were mentioned by only 2% of the respondents which included maintenance of the facility relationships with the board of directors, insurance problems, and admission policies.

Respondents from foster homes cited inadequate funding and lack of support from the community as primary problems. Lack of community support included inadequate support services and community attitudes toward mentally retarded people.

In the second study, Bruininks, Williams, and Morreau (1978) used a taxonomy of issues in deinstitutionalization and residential services (cf. Table 1)

Table 1

Issues in Deinstitutionalization and Residential Services

A. Planning for Deinstitutionalization
   1. Use of institutional facilities that are no longer in operation
   2. Training and job placement of displaced institutional staff
   3. Assessing the need for organized development of new residential programs
   4. Coordinating needed community services with residential programs
   5. Prevention and amelioration of developmental disabilities through early diagnosis, referral and treatment
   6. Developing public awareness and acceptance of developmental disabilities

B. Financial Considerations
   1. Providing incentives and support for in-home family care of the developmentally disabled person
   2. Financial resources for starting residential programs
   3. Financial resources for operating residential programs

C. Individualized Program Planning and Evaluation
   1. Evaluating the institutional resident's readiness for community placement
   2. Preparing (training and counseling) institutional residents for community placement
   3. Planning the transfer of individuals from institutions to community residences
   4. Strategies for exchanging information upon transfer of persons from institutions to community placements
   5. Developing individual program plans, including follow-up assessment after placement

D. Regulatory Issues
   1. Licensing and regulation of residential programs
   2. Regulating staffing levels and staff qualifications
   3. Regulating geographic density of residential programs and issues of zoning

E. Legal Considerations
   1. Protection of individual rights
   2. Guardianship laws and services

F. Community Services
   1. Leisure-time and recreation programs
   2. Public transportation services
   3. Health care services
   4. Educational services
   5. Developmental learning/daytime programming
   6. Vocational education/work training
   7. Employment opportunities
   8. Respite care

Source: Bruininks, Williams, & Morreau, 1978, p. 4.

to construct a survey instrument to assess the availability, quality, and need for technical assistance among residential and related programs within a six-state region in the Midwest. Using a 5-point rating scale (1 = lowest rating), the items assessed each of the 27 areas represented in the taxonomy. The questionnaire was sent to 48 representatives of consumer groups, state planners, and state agency personnel.

The ratings of the availability of activities and plans in any area were considered to be a general measure of satisfaction with such activities. In only five of the issue areas did a majority of the respondents believe the availability of plans and activities was adequate. Four of these are among the responsibilities generally undertaken by state agencies: licensing of residential programs, regulation of staff levels and qualifications, guardianship, and educational services. The fifth activity, protection of legal rights, received high ratings of availability and quality in all of the six states in the region surveyed.

The lowest percentage of "adequate" ratings for availability were received by three services provided within a community residential model: incentives and support for care of developmentally disabled people within the family home, the related services of respite care (for which only one person in the region believed availability of services was adequate), and provision of employment activities.

Only 11 of the 28 areas were indicated to be adequate or better in quality by the survey respondents. The issue receiving the highest quality rating across the region was the protection of legal rights of developmentally disabled individuals. The quality of activities and planning in this area was rated well above adequate (3.47), and slightly over half of the respondents (52.5%) believed the availability of protection services was adequate in their states. Regionally, only 30 percent of the respondents expressed a need for program assistance in improving the protection of legal rights for developmentally disabled people.

The mean rating for quality of educational services was ranked second highest (3.42) by the survey respondents. A full 70 percent of the respondents indicated that the quality of educational services for developmentally disabled persons was adequate in their states.

The quality of activities countering restrictive zoning was also rated above adequate (3.26) by the project respondents, although there was great variability in assessment of availability of such efforts in this area and the need for program assistance.

The two issues rated lowest in quality by survey respondents, preparation of institution residents for community placement and public transportation services, were significant in that each is generally considered a requirement for successful community placement. The lowest rating of quality (2.26) was ascribed to the issue of preparation training and counseling of institution residents for community placement. The significance of this assessment becomes clear in view of the fact that the success of a community placement may depend as much on the readiness of a disabled individual to cope with community living as on the readiness of the community to provide needed service to that individual.

The overwhelming majority of the survey respondents (82.5%) indicated that public transportation services for developmentally disabled persons were available to a limited or uneven extent or were not available at all in their state and communities. The mean rating for quality of available transportation services was low (2.35), and a majority of respondents in the region (57.5%) expressed a need for program assistance in the area of public transportation services for developmentally disabled persons.

The findings of this survey indicate that the necessary elements for adequate community based residential and related services are unevenly developed, at least in the Midwest region of the county. Similar patterns of development and problems of implementing services are likely to be found in other parts of the United States.

Trends and Implications for Social Policy

Over the past several years, there has been a significant movement toward providing community residential services for mentally retarded and other developmentally disabled people throughout the United States. The national survey of community residential facilities described here represents an initial effort to gain understanding of community residential services and the impact of deinstitutionalization as a public policy regarding mentally retarded people. Data reported in the national survey described in this chapter documented this expected increase in the development of community based residences (over 4,400 facilities) and foster homes (over 2,600 homes). Over one-half of the community facilities had opened in the three years prior to 1977, with 88% of them serving fewer than 20 residents per facility. Assuming the general patterns of recent years will continue, it is possible to identify several important policy issues.

One of the major factors responsible for the decline of the institutional population is the use of alternative residential placements. In 1979 the most frequent release placement for residents from public institutions were community residences, whereas the natural or adoptive home was the second most frequent release placement (Scheerenberger, 1979). As this national study showed, the most frequent release placement from community facilities was other community residences and the natural or adoptive home was the second most frequent release placement.

Of all the residential alternatives available to mentally retarded people, most states have failed to emphasize adequately the most obvious resource—the person's "natural" home, and similar situations provided by adoptive homes. Existing provisions for subsidy to adoptive and family care parents must be systematically assessed and new program elements developed as needed. In addition, resources to natural parents should be made available to ensure the maintenance and adjustment of mentally retarded persons with their families (Bruininks & Krantz, 1979).

The current trend of declining institutional populations is altering the characteristics of the populations in these facilities. In 1979, over 75% of the residents in public residential facilities were classified as severely or profoundly retarded and 82% were multiply handicapped (Scheerenberger, 1979). Given the degree of impairment of the current institutional population, new community residential facilities and support services (e.g., behavior management, adult programming) must be funded and developed if these citizens are to be adequately served in less restrictive settings.

Examination of data from the survey of community facilities discussed earlier and of recent surveys of public institutions (Krantz, Bruininks, & Clumpner, 1978; Scheerenberger, 1979) suggests strongly that future admissions to community residences from public facilities will be more severely and multiply handicapped than those persons admitted in the past. This factor poses challenges for programming, community services, financing, and residential service models. The continued movement of mentally retarded individuals into community alternatives will undoubtedly affect the level, type, and amount of expenditures for residential care (Wieck, 1980). A second issue concomitant to the shift in populations into the continuum of community residential alternatives is the impact on public schools. In 1977, an estimated 23,000 school-age children lived in community facilities (Bruininks, Hauber, & Kudla, 1979). As greater proportions of severely retarded and multiple handicapped residents enter community settings, the demand on public agencies for appropriate educational and day services will be increased.

A third issue created by recent attempts to rapidly reduce institutional populations is the appropriateness of placing mentally retarded people in nursing homes. In 1977, the National Nursing Home Survey (National Center for Health Statistics, 1979) estimated that 18,900 nursing homes had over 1,300,000 residents. Of the total number of residents, 6.1% or 79,800 were identified with the "chronic condition of impairment" of mental retardation. It should be noted that the results reported in this chapter identified approximately 17,400 fewer mentally retarded residents in community facilities than in nursing homes for the same time period. Nursing homes have been and remain a significantly overlooked factor in residential services for mentally retarded persons, although Scheerenberger (1978) identified nursing homes as a leading placement source. The General Accounting Office report (1977) has also questioned whether the placement of the mentally disabled into nursing homes is deinstitutionalization or simply movement to another setting which is as institutional in its size, structured living environment, and lack of privacy.

Major Barriers

A combination of philosophical, political, organizational and economic factors can account for the trend in providing community residential services to mentally retarded and other developmentally disabled persons. However, several major barriers to successful implementation of deinstitutionalization strategies by state governments have been identified by a number of authors (Braddock, 1977; Bradley, 1978; General Accounting Office, 1977; Gettings, 1977). Among these are:

1. Commitment of states to social services as demonstrated through historical precedence of quality of treatment, per capita expenditures, and utilization of resources. The differences in practice across states also reflect variations in human service delivery systems and the extent to which emphasis has been placed upon development of community based residential services for the mentally retarded persons (Bradley, 1978).
2. Legislative trends that may impede deinstitutionalization efforts are budgetary allocations, organization or reorganization of agencies or programs which may require legislative action (Braddock, 1977).
3. Organizational barriers have generally paralleled the expansion of generic services with complexity, fragmentation, lack of coordination, and a general lack of any interagency cooperation to meet all of the clients' needs in a community based program (Gettings, 1977).
4. Inadequate financing of residential and support services, have been significant barriers for residential providers even though federal funding for mental retardation increased by over 300% between 1970 and 1977 (Gettings, 1977). This problem was graphically pointed out by a recent General Accounting Office report (1977):

> A basic problem at the Federal, State, and local levels is that those agencies primarily responsible for the mentally disabled do not have the

> funds needed to develop adequate...care systems...(nor) the responsibility for...the standards of care in communities. Therefore, they have approached deinstitutionalization by relying on the many social, welfare, and other programs that affect such target groups as the poor, the aged, children, or the disabled, to accomplish deinstitutionalization individually without any central guidance or management. (p. 26)

Concluding Comment

It is often tempting for a recitation of problems to overshadow indications of progress. Clear and dramatic changes have occurred in recent years in the scope, nature, and pattern of community residential services available to retarded and other developmentally disabled people. There is clearly a discernible increase in living arrangements for retarded people that are small and community centered. Despite this growth in small community based facilities, policymakers must remain concerned about inappropriate placements and the quality of care provided by community alternatives. Sustaining this pattern of growth and improving the quality of services, however, may depend upon effectively responding to the many problems cited by administrators of community residential services, and by state agency and consumer group representatives.

References

Adams, M. *Mental retardation and its social dimensions*. New York: Columbia University Press, 1971.

Baker, B. B., Seltzer, G. B., & Seltzer, M. M. *As close as possible*. Cambridge, MA: Behavioral Education Projects, Harvard University, 1974.

Berstein, C. Advantage of colony care of mental defectives. *Psychiatric Quarterly*, 1927, *1*, 419-425.

Braddock, D. *Opening closed doors*. Reston, VA: Council for Exceptional Children, 1977.

Bradley, V. J. *Deinstitutionalization of developmentally disabled persons*. Baltimore: University Park Press, 1978.

Bruininks, R. H., Hauber, F. A., & Kudla, M. J. *National survey of community residential facilities: A profile of facilities and residents in 1977*. Minneapolis: University of Minnesota, Department of Psychoeducational Studies, 1979.

Bruininks, R. H., Hill, B. K., & Thorsheim, M. J. *A profile of foster home services for mentally retarded persons in 1977*. Minneapolis: University of Minnesota, Department of Psychoeducational Studies, 1980.

Bruininks, R. H., & Krantz, G. C. (Eds.). *Family care of developmentally disabled members: Conference proceedings*. Minneapolis: University of Minnesota, Department of Psychoeducational Studies, 1979.

Bruininks, R. H., Kudla, M. J., Wieck, C. A., & Hauber, F. A. Management problems in community residential facilities. *Mental Retardation*, 1980, *18*(3), 125-130.

Bruininks, R. H., Williams, S., & Morreau, L. *Issues and problems in deinstitutionalization in HEW Region V*. Minneapolis: University of Minnesota, Department of Psychoeducational Studies, 1978.

General Accounting Office (GAO), Report to Congress by the Comptroller General of the United States. *Returning the mentally disabled to the community: Government needs to do more*. Washington, DC: U.S. Government Printing Office, 1977.

Gettings, R. N. Hidden impediments to deinstitutionalization. *State Government*, 1977, *50*, 214-219.

Halderman v. Pennhurst. Civil No. 74-1345 (E.D. Pa. Dec., 1977).

Krantz, G. C., Bruininks, R. H., & Clumpner, J. L. *Mentally retarded people in state-operated residential facilities: Year ending June 30, 1978*. Minneapolis: University of Minnesota, Department of Psychoeducational Studies, 1978.

Kudla, M. J. *National resident movement statistics of public and community residential facilities in 1977*. Unpublished master's thesis, University of Wisconsin, 1980.

Lakin, K. C. *Demographic studies of residential facilities for the mentally retarded: An historical review of methodologies and findings*. Minneapolis: University of Minnesota, Department of Psychoeducational Studies, 1979.

Mesibov, G. B. Alternatives to the principle of normalization. *Mental Retardation*, 1976, *14*(5), 30.

National Association for Superintendents of Public Residential Facilities for the Mentally Retarded. *Contemporary issues in residential programming*. Washington, DC: President's Committee on Mental Retardation, 1974.

National Center for Health Statistics. The national nursing home survey: 1977 summary for the United States. *Vital and Health Statistics*. Series 13, No. 43. DHEW Pub. No. (PHS) 79-1974, July, 1979.

New York Association for Retarded Children v. Carey. 393 F. Suppl. 714 (E.D. N.Y., 1975).

Nihira, L., & Nihira, K. Jeopardy in community placement. *American Journal of Mental Deficiency*, 1975, *79*, 538-544.

Nirje, B. The normalization principle and its human management implications. In R. Kugel & A. Shearer (Eds.), *Changing patterns in residential services for the mentally retarded*. Washington, DC: President's Committee on Mental Retardation, 1976.

O'Connor, G. *Home is a good place: A national perspective of community residential facilities for developmentally disabled persons*. (Monograph No. 2). Washington, DC: American Association of Mental Deficiency, 1976.

O'Connor, G., & Sitkei, E. G. Study of a new frontier in community services: Residential facilities for the developmentally disabled. *Mental Retardation*, 1975, *13*, 35-39.

Scheerenberger, R. *Public residential services for the mentally retarded 1977*. Madison, WI: Central Wisconsin Center for the Developmentally Disabled, 1978.

Scheerenberger, R. *Public residential services for the mentally retarded 1979*. Madison, WI: Central Wisconsin Center for the Developmentally Disabled, 1979.

Welsch v. Likens. Civil No. 451, U.S. District Court, District of Minnesota, Fourth Division, 1974.

Wieck, C. A. *The cost of public and community residential care for mentally retarded people in the United States*. Unpublished doctoral dissertation, University of Minnesota, 1980.

Wolfensberger, W. *The principle of normalization in human services*. Toronto: National Institute on Mental Retardation, 1972.

Wolfensberger, W. The origin and nature of our institutional models. In R. Kugel & A. Shearer (Eds.), *Changing patterns in residential services for the mentally retarded*. Washington, DC: President's Committee on Mental Retardation, 1976.

Wyatt v. Stickney. Civil No. 3195-N. U.S. District Court, Middle District of Alabama, North Division, 1972.

Early Perspectives on the Community Adjustment of Mentally Retarded People

K. Charlie Lakin
Robert H. Bruininks
Barbara B. Sigford

University of Minnesota

Social adaptability among mentally retarded persons and the associated problems of its assessment have been persistent concerns among social services providers and researchers for the past 150 years. During this period the provision of services to the mentally retarded has grown from a few isolated efforts to a complex national network of programs. The earliest efforts at providing residential care, for instance, stressed the systematic habilitation of mentally retarded persons to increase their abilities in achieving social and economic independence, so that they might eventually be reintegrated into society. In time, however, professionals adopted a considerably less optimistic view regarding the potential for adaptation on the part of the retarded, and programs once focused on increasing the potential for community integration became dedicated to keeping the retarded out of society through segregation and isolation. Today we have come full circle, and again the goals of programs for the mentally retarded emphasize training in those areas most important in successful functioning in community life. Still, despite the variation over the years in the attitudes of professionals toward retarded people, the concept of social adaptability, or potential for community adjustment, has been central both to defining mental retardation and to conceptualizing approaches to treating persons so categorized.

The social perspective on mental retardation, focusing on each individual's ability to adjust to the demands and responsibilities of community life, has been emphasized in nearly all definitions of mental retardation during the past half century. For example, in 1937 Tredgold defined mental deficiency in adults as:

> . . . a state of incomplete mental development of such a kind and degree that the individual is incapable of adapting himself to the normal environment in such a way as to maintain existence independently of supervision, control or external support (p. 4).

Forty years later the American Association on Mental Deficiency had changed this notion but little:

> Mental retardation refers to significantly subaverage general intellectual functioning existing concurrently with deficits in adaptive behavior, and manifested during the developmental period. . . . Adaptive behavior is defined as the effectiveness or degree with which an individual meets the standards of personal independence and social responsibility expected for age and cultural group (Grossman, 1977, p. 11).

Although the conceptualization of social adaptability contained in contemporary definitions of mental retardation stresses the degree to which persons approximate age-appropriate social behavior, published research in the adjustment of persons released from institutions for the mentally retarded has not generally viewed adjustment in such terms. While some writers have looked at successful adjustment of deinstitutionalized adults as complete (Town & Hill, 1931) or partial (Storrs, 1929) self-sufficiency, others have argued that successful adjustment is the individual's tendency to perform in a setting those adaptive behaviors he/she is capable of performing (Seltzer & Seltzer, 1976). Most frequently, however, community adjustment has been operationally defined as staying out of public institutions for mentally retarded, mentally ill or criminal persons, staying in alternative settings, or avoiding other forms of public supervision and assistance. Very few studies have examined community adjustment as a process (cf. Edgerton, 1967; Edgerton & Bercovici, 1976). For the most part, the term community adjustment remains a nebulous catch-all word for the establishment and maintenance of an adequate harmony in the individual's ability and/or willingness to adapt to life in a community placement and the ability and/or willingness of the caretakers in the community placement to adapt to the retarded person's need of external support. Empiricists may want, and need, a more precise definition, but the writers, in response, can only cite Gregory Bateson's (1972) observation that "the explorer can never know what he is exploring until it has been explored" (p. xvi). While the adjustment of mentally retarded persons to extra-institutional living is being explored, all perspectives, with their varying operational definitions of adjustment, should be welcomed; and all research on the topic should be appraised.

In initially considering the past 60 years of research on the community adjustment of deinstitutionalized mentally retarded persons, the writers were somewhat predisposed to emphasize the most recent research on the topic, mentioning only in passing the early studies of the phenomenon. These "old" studies, however, had much more contemporary relevance than was expected and proved to be another instance of how "as so often happens in science, recently acquired perspectives turn out to be a more precise form of very old perspectives which were left undeveloped" (Bockoven, 1956, p. 138). The thesis of this paper is, therefore, that the contemporary study of community adjustment of deinstitutionalized, mentally retarded persons can profit greatly from examining the earliest research on this topic. The "old" themes to be discussed in this paper are drawn from research published during a 16-year period from 1918 to 1934, the time when the first concentrated efforts took place to measure the effects of deinstitutionalization in this country.

Taking a social rather than clinical perspective on the adjustment of deinstitutionalized persons to community settings, this review will focus, as did the bulk of the research upon which it is based, on the inter-relationships between the social needs of the former institution residents and those features of their environments perceived as most salient in the adjustment process. Very little attention will be given the clinical characteristics of the released residents, since, as will be pointed out, these were seen even then as being considerably less important to adjustment than was the nature of the environment into which they were released.

Social Attitudes and Community Adjustment

Throughout the history of care for persons perceived as mentally abnormal, social attitudes toward such persons have strongly influenced their treatment. Although these attitudes have often permitted insensitive and at times cruel treatment of the mentally handicapped (cf. Foucault, 1973; Wolfensberger, 1976), in retrospect it is important to note that the generally conservative nature of social attitudes has placed an important check on many programs proposed by professionals operating from a clinical conceptualization of abnormality. Many of these professionals, without due respect for the values of the society in which they lived would have, had social attitudes permitted, dealt with the problem in a way which today not only remains contrary to those social attitudes about the treatment of the handicapped, but has since become contrary to professional attitudes as well. This is certainly true in the case of the care provided to the mentally retarded. This interplay between social and professional attitudes concerning the proper treatment of mentally retarded persons can be seen clearly in the writings of professionals and laymen prior to the first formal presentations of data on the community adjustment of persons released from institutions for the mentally retarded.

Beginning in 1840, the U.S. Government, in its decennial census, began a half-century of enumerations of the total number of mentally retarded persons in this country. Among the justifications for this inquiry was what the Director of the Census, Francis Walker, termed the "philanthropic: in order that the humane efforts made by individuals or communities for the protection or relief, and, so far as possible, the restoration to society, of the unfortunate classes, may receive intelligent direction" (U.S. Census Office, 1883, p. 29). The census of "idiotic persons" in 1880 enumerated 77,000 "members of this class," 2,429 of whom were in institutions for "idiots."

The results of this investigation led to the observation by Fredrick Wines, special agent in charge of the census of the "defective, dependent, and delinquent classes" that:

> Provision for the training of idiotic children is of comparatively recent origin and has not yet reached its full development. . . . There is a great unsatisfied demand in the direction, and that the movement for the relief of idiots is in its infancy (U.S. Census Bureau, 1888, p. 28).

To Wines, providing for the "idiotic" meant training in institutions for that "class." At one point, he indicated that:

> Of the 74,466 idiots outside of institutions [specifically for "idiots"], so far as it appears to us, only 809 have received any special training [spent time as an inmate in an institution and following the training had been released] . . . (1888, p. 37).

Of these 809 Wines commented that, "These are certain and positive fruits of the system of public charities in this country" (1888, p. 37).

While the reader is told nothing of the condition or nature of the adjustment of these former institution inmates and might question the implicit logic in calling for greater provision of schools (institutions) for the "idiotic" children while delighting in the "fruits of the system," that is the "restoration to society," this notion is clearly a part of the "philanthropic" spirit of the latter decades of the nineteenth century. By 1880, philanthropy in the United States had moved away from a focus on almsgiving to a posture which its proponents perceived as scientific. This new science had one primary purpose and that was to eliminate pauperism and its threat to the emerging industrial potential of the nation. The goal in regard to all "dependent, defective, and delinquent classes" was to restore them, to whatever degree possible, to the larger society. To achieve this end, training schools were established for the habilitation of the mentally retarded with the assumption that given a proper education, these persons would be capable of adjusting themselves to the demands of their respective communities and even to contribute to the society.

Such enthusiasm, however, was relatively shortlived. Already by the end of the century Wilber (1888) was noting that:

> In the race of life, where an individual who is backward or peculiar attempts to compete with those who are not, the disadvantages are so great that the graduate from the idiot asylum has no chance to succeed. The capacity of the individual is not at fault; but the world is not full of philanthropic people who are willing to take the individual and surround him with the proper guardianship which his case demands (p. 298).

The situation remains unchanged nearly a century later. To some extent those persons released from institutions require "philanthropic people," whether unpaid benefactors or professionals who disperse benevolence by proxy for the other members of society, if they are to adjust to life outside the "sheltering walls of total institutions."

For the most part, however, "professional altruists" and the service system which employed them were slow in evolving in the United States for the mentally retarded. Ironically, this reality was greatly affected by a social activist philosophy beginning around the turn of the century, now termed "Progressivism," which led to a great deal of community-based programming for other groups, but, when coupled with the eugenics movement, left the social engineers of the period convinced that segregation was a logical policy in regard to the mentally retarded. While progressives worked to dissolve the adversarial relationship between the state and other deviant groups by having judges or welfare workers attempt to help and guide rather than punish and institutionalize, with the mentally retarded the situation was different. Not only were they considered by many early professionals as beyond cure, but they were quickly being accepted among the social engineers as a deep-rooted threat to the well-being of the entire society, a threat to the social improvement that the progressives envisioned.

With the eugenics movement the progressives found new and potent reasons to fear and therefore isolate the mentally retarded. In 1912, for example, Edward Devine, in a book entitled *The Family and Social Work,* wrote that the eugenics movement was one "with which social workers may sympathize and in which they should clearly cooperate." Devine foresaw a drastic reduction of "the social burden" if the society could prevent the "feeble-minded, the insane, the incorrigibly criminal, and the hopelessly ineffective" from procreating (1912, pp. 44-45). Isolation and segregation became prominent in the progressive doctrine of social welfare professionals, and mental retardation experts like Fernald and Goddard gained high status in their circles.

While social welfare agencies were developing in the early part of this century, dealing with those classes of deviants they felt were capable of adjusting and advocating isolation for those they felt were not, another model of treatment was beginning to make an impact. This model was educational and represented not a perspective of curing the epidemic of feeble-mindedness, but rather saw adjustment as a continuum along which a person might remain mentally subnormal but still better able to fit into society. It was at least in part this perspective which led to many of the early ungraded or special classes in this country. And it was to test the hypothesis that some degree of adjustment was possible that the first studies of the community adjustment of special class students were conducted.

Two of these follow-up studies were of graduates of New York City's ungraded classes and were reported for the years 1914 (Farrell, 1914) and 1915 (Duggan, 1915).

The 1914 study of 124 graduates (at age 16) who had been out of the special program of the New York City Schools from one to six years found the following status:

Working	54.0%
Cared for at home (some helping)	25.0%
In institution	8.8%
No information	8.9%
Dead	2.3%
Arrested (not necessarily convicted)	5.0%

Commenting on this follow-up Farrell noted the general lack of supervisory after-care for the program graduates and suggested that with better provisions for helping the graduates adjust, the results of the program might be even more positive.

The following year, 1915, another follow-up study of graduates of New York City's ungraded classes was performed. The results of this study were very similar to those of the preceding year. It found graduates:

Cared for at home	24.6%
Employed for wages	54.8%
Employed but out of work at present	8.8%
In institutions for the feeble-minded	3.7%
In other institutions or prison	2.0%
Dead or unknown	4.8%

Along with his discussion of the merits of strong educational programs for the feeble-minded and the need for "after-care" (i.e., persons to help the special program graduate in adjusting to community life), Professor Duggan, who presented these follow-up findings to the New York City Conference on Charities, spoke on the issues of sterilization and segregation frequently advocated during this period. His argument against sterilization showed a more sophisticated knowledge of genetics than was shown by most of his adversaries, and his discussion of segregation showed an equally greater understanding of the contemporary society:

> . . . because of the cost, any comprehensive system of segregating the unfit is remote to say the least. Aside from this economic question, segregation brings to the front the whole idea of personal freedom. The general acceptance by the community of the fact that the parent has unquestioned right to his child will for some time make it impossible for the law to step in and break down this right. Perhaps, it may be stated that in the minds of many, the police power of the state should be extended in order that compulsory segregation should be effected. In any such discussion, however, it must be borne in mind that such extension attacks the cornerstone of Anglo-Saxon common law (1916, pp. 138-139).

Despite the highly publicized comments of the "leaders in the field," which reviews of literature often present as dominating social policy in regard to the mentally retarded, never were policies implemented which attempted to remove systematically persons from the community solely because they were considered to be mentally deficient. Indeed, at times one must infer the posture of society from the degree to which the publicized proposals of experts were not acted upon, but in regard to the institutionalization movement there is a good deal of evidence that legal as well as citizen resistance was evident and strong at the height of the eugenics movement. For example, in 1916 the New York Supreme Court ruled against the application made by authorities of a home of refuge to have a twenty-one year old woman committed to an institution for the "feeble-minded." Numerous habeas corpus releases of residents of the Waverley, Massachusetts, institution were also ordered by that state's Supreme Court prior to 1914 (Fernald, 1919). Such forced releases were also occurring in Maryland (Kanner, 1938).

The writers would like to present one additional note from the period which supports the case that most Americans never considered the place of those persons perceived as feeble-minded to be anywhere but in the midst of the rest of society. The remarks are by Henry Sommerville in an attack on what he disparagingly called the "secular scientific philanthropists." It is a long quotation but is worthy of reading because it captures well what other writers of the period said somewhat less eloquently:

> If the eugenist theories of heredity and feeble-mindedness were put forward only speculatively, they would be interesting and they might be harmless. But they are put forward in support of a practical policy, namely the sterilization of the feeble-minded. Sometimes it is proposed to sterilize by means of vasectomy; sometimes by life-long segregation. The question that is at issue is one of human rights. . . . The sacredness of the individual does not depend on his economic value to society, and the individual does not cease to have human rights because he suffers from mental or physical defects. . . . Whatever eugenists may think, public opinion in this country is not yet inhuman enough to consent to the segregation of all those who are feeble-minded. . . . Moreover, it is comforting to know that segregation of all feeble-minded is impossible because the cost would be prohibitive. . . . Those who are careful of human rights will resist the agitation for the compulsory segregation and sterilization of alleged feeble-minded persons on the eugenist ground that otherwise such persons might get married, and then they might have children who might be feeble-minded and who might therefore become a burden on the community. That kind of outrage on human rights in the name of social benefit is what Christianity has fought since the days of pagan Rome (1917, pp. 216-218).

The point of this rather long discussion of the period immediately preceding the first formal research on the community adjustment of residents formerly in institutions is to demonstrate that there is no evidence of any pervasive feeling among the general populace that mentally retarded persons did not belong in their communities. It is of further interest to note that professional opinion on the care and treatment of retarded people was divided with the lines drawn loosely between educators favoring programs aimed at facilitating assimilation and institution personnel favoring isolation and segregation. In general, however, the eventual discovery that mentally retarded persons could survive outside the institution and do so without detriment to the society, appears to have more greatly surprised those in the professional ranks than it did the layman who, not educated in the clinical aspects of retardation, had always been accustomed to regard "slow," "dumb," or "stupid" persons primarily as citizens.

Early Studies of Community Adjustment of Formerly Institutionalized Mentally Retarded Persons

Prior to the end of the second decade of this century, nearly all superintendents of the nation's institutions were steadfastly maintaining that the vast majority of their residents should remain in the institution so that society could be protected from the feeble-minded. A primary reason for this posture was that they were so preoccupied by their theories of genetic deterioration and the innate social menace of the feeble-minded that they took little time to assess the degree to which the theories were valid. Of course, when they did, they found that the feeble-minded tended to get along in society reasonably well.

Debunking Unfounded Theories

In 1919, Walter Fernald published a study entitled, "After-care study of the patients discharged from Waverley for a period of twenty-five years." It was a classic work in the field of mental retardation for it pretty well closed the door on those strident voices calling for long-term segregation of the feeble-minded. A discussion of this study deserves much more space than is possible to devote to it here. It is to Dr. Fernald's credit that he ever published the work for it challenged all that he had worked for over the previous decade. In fact, Davies (1923, p. 92) later wrote that "Dr. Fernald told the writer [Davies] that he had hesitated for two years to publish the results of this study because it had seemed so much at variance with the then accepted theories of dealing with mental deficiency."

Briefly, the Waverley follow-up study involved the collection of information on 646 of 1537 discharges from the Massachusetts School for the Feeble-Minded at Waverley from 1890 through 1915. Of the 891 discharges during this period not included in the study, 437 actually constituted transfers to other types of custodial facilities, 279 could not be located and 175 had been from other states and were not included within the scope of the study.

Of crucial importance in understanding the effect that this study had on its author and his contemporaries was the fact that for the most part the "discharges" were not residents perceived by the institution staff to be good risks for successful adjustment outside the institution. In fact, Fernald pointed out in his report that the majority were released under protest, that is, against the advice of the institution staff. A sizable number were simply absent without leave, runaways or released under court order. As Fernald freely admitted, "We honestly believed that nearly all of these people should remain in the institution indefinitely" (p. 26).

The methodology of the Waverley study was straight-forward, but represented a major undertaking. First, Fernald sent a letter to known friends and relatives asking for information concerning the discharged persons. In the letter, in which Fernald stated that the School "wanted to know if their stay at the school was of benefit to them," respondents were asked to describe some general facts of former inmates' living conditions as well as whether they would be willing to accept personal visits from one of the institution's social workers. In addition to these arranged interviews, social workers also visited with members of the former residents' community and corroborated information "from several sources in each case" (p. 25).

While the findings of the Waverley study were not nearly as positive as those reported in the follow-up studies of graduates of the New York City ungraded program, they were much more positive than Fernald had ever expected. Briefly, he found among the 470 male "discharges":

Earning a living without supervision	6.0%
Working for wages, supervised at home	18.3%
Living at home, but not earning wages	29.0%
Arrested but not sentenced	4.9%
Sentenced to penal institutions	6.8%
Committed to other institutions	9.1%
Readmitted to Waverley	14.5%
Died	11.5%

Among surviving male "discharges" about two-thirds had demonstrated no dependency on the society or proven delinquency. The findings among the 152 surviving female "discharges" were similar: 60% had remained off the public dole.

Further, Fernald reported, "Of the ninety discharged females, now at liberty, fifty-two are apparently giving no trouble" (p. 28). For the others who behaved "badly" sex offenses were most often reported, but still the fact that could not be overlooked was that only eleven of the 152 women had borne illegitimate children and only thirty-one of the total number had borne any children at all.

The findings in general could not be refuted. To the 27 women who had married only 50 children had been born and "the social worker saw nearly all of these children, and was not sure that any of them were defective" (p. 26). There was relatively little delinquency. The majority of cases were making some contribution to their self-maintenance, and even those who were not were seldom dependent on the state. In short, the rhetoric about the social menace of the feebleminded, their delinquent tendencies and threat to the American gene pool apparently had little basis.

By the time Fernald's follow-up study was published in 1919, he had already begun to increase substantially the discharges from Waverley. Soon most other institutions were following. On the national level between 1910 and 1927 the total number of discharges from public institutions grew four-fold from 1009 to 4165 while the ratio of discharges to first admissions increased from 26% to 46% (Lakin, 1979).

Observations on the Adjustment Process and the Effects of Institutional Living

Fernald's Waverley study was not the only, or even the first, follow-up study made during the years immediately following World War I. There were, in fact, several; and all reached similar conclusions. But in addition to the important general observation that mentally retarded persons were not nearly as dangerous as many professionals had been maintaining, there were many less startling, highly insightful observations made by this group of researchers which ought to be reappraised as the deinstitutionalization movement rekindles interest in the adjustment of mentally retarded persons moving into community-based, residential facilities and other living arrangements. In this section of the paper a number of these will be discussed.

Importance of significant others. The first of these observations was made by Fernald in discussing the outcome of women considered social failures in his follow-up study. Fernald noted that in these cases almost none of the women had friends or relatives willing or able to supervise and aid her adjustment.

On the other hand, a number of women released just as reluctantly and about whom the staff of the institution felt equally sure of failure managed to adapt rather well to the community. About these different outcomes, Fernald concluded that, "Apparently women who had friends capable of understanding them and of properly protecting them did not have illegitimate children and did not become sex offenders" (p. 27). About a more seriously handicapped group of women, of whom ten were seen as maladjusted (most often "noisy and troublesome") and thirteen as well adjusted, Fernald commented that the outcome was not primarily dependent upon the characteristics of the women themselves but that "the character of the home and the intelligence of the family largely determined the result" (p. 28). Similarly, of a group of men who had managed to locate wage-paying work while living either independently or at home, Fernald lauded the positive effects of steady work, good homes, and the beneficent aid of friends and relatives as enabling the former inmates to become productive and adjusted members of society (p. 29).

In another follow-up study of 167 girls (ages 13-19) released from a New Jersey institution from 1928 to 1932, Ellis (1932) was also struck by the importance of significant others to the adjustment process:

> Success on parole at placement is in many instances dependent upon the employer. If she understands the girl, is sympathetic to her needs and desires, if she does not expect too much but on the other hand holds her up to a standard which she is capable of reaching, if she seeks to provide in some way for leisure time activities, if she gives her a good start when she leaves the institution, the girl will in all probability be encouraged to try her hardest for success. Girls who fail in one placement, often succeed in another because of the employer's attitude rather than their own difficulties (p. 43).

Passing as normal. A second feature of adjustment noted among those conducting follow-up studies of former residents of Waverley was the strong desire of these persons to pass as normal, to hide the fact that they had once been institutionalized or were mentally deficient. Discussing the adaptation to the community of a hundred "boys" (young men actually) who had left the institution on trial, Matthews (1922) reported,

> Now that they have what they call a "chance," they exert every effort to suppress their unfortunate traits and habits. . . . They try not to let their fellow workmen know that they have been in the school or that there is anything going on that they do not understand. Some of the more intelligent ones get the reputation of being reserved because of their quiet withdrawal when the subject of discussion is beyond their comprehension (p. 339).

It might also be noted here that a recognition of the stigma associated with being perceived as mentally subnormal has been documented for well over a century. Perhaps the most "official" recognition came with the 1860 census where data collected regarding the total number of "idiotic" persons in the United States were largely discounted because of the "sensitiveness to public exposure which widely exists among persons who look upon mental alienation in a false light, regarding it as humiliating, and often a special dispensation of Divine Providence, rather than as one of the numerous diseases which afflict the human race" (Kennedy, 1864).

Negative effects of institutions. It is often assumed that a large scale movement toward community placement of mentally retarded persons did not begin until the 1960's because there was a general failure on the part of those responsible for the care of mentally retarded persons to recognize the dehumanizing effects that these large facilities had on their residents. There is ample evidence, however, that these effects were well recognized by at least some of those persons involved in the daily operation of these facilities over 50 years ago. For example, Bernstein wrote in 1927 that:

> We found that the general effect of institutional life is to institutionalize the inmates; that after several years of continuous existence in an institution—even the best—a large majority of individuals thus cared for require correction of many habits of life contracted through association with large numbers and constant supervision, resulting in their losing or never gaining self-reliance or initiative. . . . As we see the situation of 1,000 or more inmates, not only are many of the inmates sitting around in a most inactive and listless state and gradually deteriorating . . . but there is also a very considerable number who are greatly disturbed and troublesome. In the case of the latter a large amount of energy is going to waste, or worse, even to destruction, not only of physical property but also of bodies and minds . . . (p. 425).

So impressed was Bernstein with the negative effects of institutional life that in 1934 he bluntly stated that "Any boy or girl that goes out into a home and has a place to eat and sleep in a decent environment, even if there is no money, is better off than the boy or girl who stays in the institution" (p. 52).

In 1934, Edgar Doll, after observing the system of housing 3,000 handicapped persons in private homes in the vicinity of state institutions in Gheel, Belgium, noted that:

> The community aspect of mental deficiency rouses a very interesting question of the possibility of providing in the community for those feeble-minded who do not require institutional care and custody. Institutional care is expensive, and this method of segregation is in many ways contrary to the happiness and usefulness of these people. . . . This plan [of Gheel, Belgium] is both more economical and more satisfactory to the patient and his family than is ordinary institutional segregation. The patient has the advantage of adequate medical care and social supervision, as well as the advantages of family life and personal freedom consistent with his disabilities and limitations (pp. 42-43).

Why did institutional settings have such a negative effect on their residents? One reason, noted Doll and Longwell (1934), was that, "Programs of institutional training are usually designed to prepare the patient for life in the institution rather than for return to society" (p. 450). A primary factor in this process was what Doll (1934) called "regimentation" and explained it saying:

> The institution may not assume all the risks that the family might be willing to hazard, and therefore controls the patient more solicitously in many respects than the family may have done by setting up a more rigorous system of environmental opportunity and restraints than provided by the family (p. 144).

Given these highly negative aspects of institutional life and the concomitant social-psychological process Doll called "institutionalization," most institutions, by the early 1930's, were, to some extent, actively involved in getting residents back into the community. For the most part, however, the alternatives for return to the community were only those that could be developed by the institution itself and the alternatives open to the institution were greatly restricted by this fact. For the most part those persons discharged from the institution fell into the higher IQ range. In 1922, for example, 56.5% of the 2964 discharged were classed as "morons" (IQ between 50 and 75) while by 1937, 77.3% of the 5801 discharged were so classed (Lakin, 1979). In addition, the number of persons not formally discharged but residing outside the public institutions, excluding those in "colonies," grew from about 4,000 in 1922 to over 14,000 in 1937. Counting those in colony care the number residing outside the institutions in 1937 would have been considerably larger although no census of the number of persons in colony care was ever conducted.

In the period from 1918-1934 several reports of follow-up studies of formerly institutionalized mentally retarded persons were published in a range of professional journals. Alongside these were studies of mentally retarded children identified in clinic and school settings. Any one who takes the time to read through them will recognize that what are now regarded as limitations of public institutions, what are perceived to be more positive attributes of smaller, community-based facilities and what factors are most important in the adjustment of mentally retarded persons to community living were recognized, at least by some writers —primarily persons involved in institutional care—within 15 years of Fernald's landmark study in 1919. Indeed to the degree which they were able, many persons were actively involved in finding and utilizing alternatives to institutional placement. Unfortunately, however, seldom were these alternatives part of a larger state plan for residential services for the mentally retarded. Clearly, communities which were still providing education for only a small minority of their handicapped children could not yet be seen as ready to accept the burden of community supervision.

Relative unimportance of individual characteristics to adjustment. Actually the first published follow-up of persons released from institutions for the mentally retarded was written by Wallace (1918). It would appear that there were at least two factors making the impact of Fernald's study considerably greater than Wallace's. The first was, of course, Fernald's stature in the field, especially as an advocate of programs for the social control of the mentally retarded. The second factor was the poor prognosis of Fernald's "discharges" as compared with Wallace's group which was made up of parolees of whom a considerably higher level of adjustment was expected. Wallace described his follow-up as a "Study of our experience with 85 parole cases from the institution [Wrentham State School, Massachusetts] over a period of three years" (p. 60). Of the 85 cases only 13 (15%) had been returned to the institution from parole. Wallace analyzed a number of factors which he thought might affect the ability of the parolees to stay in the community. The findings as reported by Wallace were:

1. We find little relationship if any between the length of time spent in the institution and success of parole.
2. No relation between occupation and success of parole.
3. No relation between history and success of parole (even when this included anti-social behavior prior to admission).
4. Little relation, if any, between mental age and success of parole.
5. We do find, however, a close relationship between temperamental conditions and success of parole.
6. We also find a close relationship between character of supervision and success of parole. (p. 79)

Unfortunately Wallace's findings were presented in outline form, and it is impossible to judge exactly what he meant by temperamental conditions and character of supervision. It would appear, however, that these were subjective judgments of the social workers conducting the follow-up. Success of parole referred to avoiding return to the institution.

Another follow-up study during this period reached similar conclusions about the relative unimportance of individual variables in the adjustment process. After presenting a list of factors which they found to have little or no power to predict successful adjustment of parolees from a New York institution, Potter and McCollister (1926) concluded:

> It is probably unwise to generalize on the basis of statistics where the problem is such a human one as this study represents. . . . No one factor by itself, family, environment, mental age level, or personality make-up is a criterion on which to base a social prognosis. The patient must be considered as a whole after a careful analysis of his own individual assets and liabilities in relation to specific environmental situations (pp. 178-179).

Effect of placement on adaptation. The year following Fernald's publication of the Waverley follow-up, Bernstein (1920) outlined the colony care and parole system of the Rome Asylum in New York. What is most important to note about the Rome Asylum colonies is that certain of these were the first to be, in effect, community-based, residential programs in which residents lived but left each day for work outside the facility. In addition, it should be noted that Bernstein, the superintendent at Rome, perceived these community-based colonies as training centers for a more independent life. Bernstein's comments speak directly to the variable effect of placement settings on the adjustment of residents.

> During the past ten years I have seen many boys and girls thus (through colony care or parole) rehabilitated, and the fact that a few fail on first trial or even repeatedly is no sure proof that we are mistaken in our judgment of their ability to live outside the institution. Often I have seen these failures succeed almost immediately when placed in another environment, and continue to succeed from thence on. . . . Most of us normal individuals have at one time or another been at the point of failure, and probably would have failed had indulgent parents and friends not given us a chance to try again and yet again until we actually found ourselves (pp. 27-28).

The interaction between the characteristics of the placement environment and the characteristics of individuals, however, was perceived early as complex and difficult to fathom without careful case study. As Raymond (1923) noted:

> We find that many a respectable home, with all physical comforts, where suitable recreation is available proves the wrong one for a particular girl. The reaction of the personalities of the members of the family upon her may prove quite unwholesome or even disastrous. A careful study of the personality of a particular girl in the relationships of the daily life of a particular family may reveal the cause of her failure to adjust (p. 107).

In short, as noted by Popenoe (1927), "It is not the amount of intellect, but the personality make-up . . . together, of course, with the surroundings in which the patient is placed" (p. 97) which determined whether a placement would be successful.

Another perspective on the effects of the placement environment on the adjustment of its residents was offered by Hubbell (1934) in a case study description of the placement of former inmates from Newark State School in New York into boarding homes for children. Of the 11 cases presented (ranging in age from 5-15 years and in IQ from 47-85), Hubbell reported that eight were displaying excellent adjustment, two fair, and one had been returned to the institution (for frequent masturbation). The author devoted some space to the subtle aspects of foster placements, noting that four of the children had been unsuccessful in foster homes immediately before being sent to the institution, but in the new home were all doing well. In addition, Hubbell made note of a problem in boarding former residents with care workers from the institution, a common practice at the time he was writing:

> We frequently see the statement made that patients could be more profitably placed with trusted former employees [of the institution], but our experience does not bear this out, and we have come to the conclusion that the best homes are with those who have never had any contact with the state institution. There is bound to be a certain amount of institutional discipline maintained by ex-employees which is not conducive to a normal life for children (p. 485).

Since placements were recognized as not all being equally beneficial to their residents, it seemed to some worthwhile to attempt to specify characteristics of good and poor environments so that potential placement settings could be rated. This quantification of quality proved as difficult 50 years ago as it is for those attempting it today.

Assessment of treatment environments. The first attempt to characterize extra-institutional "treatment environments" during the period was done by York in

1929 in an unpublished report on the status of parolees presented to a weekly study group at the Rome School. In this study all parolees were placed in farm settings with employment on the farm. York attempted to divide the homes in which working placements were made into three categories: "superior," "medium" and "poor." To York a "superior" home was one "located on a state road, near a large community, thoroughly modern in all equipment, housing and recreation, at no time isolated, employer financially successful, family intelligent." A typical "medium" home was "located off the state road, within possible reach of a smaller village, church, occasional movie or community entertainment, farm medium size, complete set of buildings and farm equipment, limited mechanical equipment, small dairy, machine or hand milked, fishing, trapping, other recreation on the farm itself." The "poor" home was typified as "located away off the main road, hills, poor buildings, especially the home, oil lights, poor heating, bedding, food, planning of work, no recreation on farm, little off" (cited in Stebbins, 1931, pp. 50-51).

The results of York's classification system must have been somewhat discouraging. Of the nine placements of parolees made to work environments considered superior, all eventually ran away and were classed as failures. The reason attributed to this finding according to York was the parolees' "inability to keep up to the pace, get along with the hired help, assimilate advantages of work and home as well as recreation offered, in other words, environment out of proportion to capacity" (cited in Stebbins, 1931, pp. 51).

Among the "medium" parole environments, York found that of the 159 placements, 116 (73%) remained successfully until released from parole. Forty-three placements were judged as failures with the parolees being returned to the institution or running away. The reasons given by York for the failures were "poor judgment in placing, emotional disturbances, inability to get along with children, hired men, neighbors, machinery, desire of too much freedom and conditioned institutional habits unyielding" (p. 51).

As notable as was the failure rate among the "superior" environments was the success rate of the 32 placements in "poor" homes. Of these, only nine (28%) were failures (all runaways) making the average failure rate among "poor" environments lower than the rate for the 200 placements as a whole (30.5%). Speculating on the reason for failure, York noted a "desire for more companionship" and "better general conditions," but speculations on the notable rate of success were not reported.

Undaunted, the Rome group continued its attempt to develop a systematic method for judging home environments for the placement of parolees from the State School. The eventual end product of this process was a "Parole Employer's Score Card" (Stebbins, 1931), but in the process considerable vacillation occurred among the developers as to what such a score card should measure. As has been seen, at the time of the York study the emphasis was primarily objective, i.e., environments were rated primarily according to location, home conditions, working conditions, opportunities for recreation, and so forth. In all there were eight domains, all quite objective upon which the environment was rated. Subsequently a ninth was added measuring subjectively "Attitude of Employers." While the "Subjective Elements" attitude was originally only one-ninth of the total rating by 1931, after the "Parole Employer's Rating Scale" had been field tested, the "Subjective Elements" had been expanded to five items and weighted so that one-half the environmental score was derived from subjective analysis of personality, family harmony, recreational interests, habits and understanding of the employing family.

The focus of the "Score Card" was practical, as was almost all research related to adjustment during this period, conducted as it was by people involved in actual programming. It appears therefore that the "Score Card" once developed to the satisfaction of its authors was not further validated by them. It was, however, used in follow-up case studies of four girls in 1932 who had an inexplicable jump of three years in their measured mental ages within a year of being paroled from an institution (Camp & Waite, 1932). The Parole Employer's Score Card was used to assess the quality of the environment which the authors assumed to be responsible for the change. In general, it was found that the homes received above average ratings on the objective elements of the scale (location, quality of housing, family composition, type of work and recreational contacts) and "definitely superior" ratings on the subjective elements. In addition to the high interpersonal quality of the placement environments of the four girls, the authors also noted the systematic way in which progressively greater responsibilities were given to the girls.

Overconcentration of community placements. One problem related to the quality of community placements and caused by the lack of a residential service system other than that which could be developed by the institutions themselves was that colonies and parole placements tended to become congregated around the institutions themselves creating "ghettos" of mentally retarded persons. This "diluting of the [normal] population" worried Bernstein (1931). Discussing a town of 500 to 600 persons in which what he felt were too many placements of mentally retarded persons, he observed that "we have found that we must not dilute the population more than five percent. We are putting too many fools in some towns—that is doubling the number [5%]" (p. 68). The effects of overconcentration were not only to affect the normal life of the community, but also to impede the chances for normal experiences on the part of the retarded persons placed in the community.

Other Major Studies

Institution releases. Four additional follow-up studies of persons released from institutions were reported during this period. All had large samples, but none of the four attempted to measure the qualitative factors related to adjustment in the community, and none produced any startling new facts. These studies will only be briefly mentioned here. In 1922 Hoakley reported on a questionnaire study of the placement success of 1417 parolees released from public institutions in the preceding year. Hoakley found that of the 34 states returning his questionnaire, 18 had initiated parole programs and that 94% of the males and 87% of the females placed on parole in these programs had successfully remained in the community for a one-year period. In 1929 Storrs followed up on females discharged from Letchworth Village in New York. Of the 616 former residents, he found 72% had been successful in maintaining at least partial self-sufficiency while only 4% had been so unsuccessful so as to be readmitted to the institution.

At the same meeting of the American Association for the Study of the Feebleminded, Foley (1929) presented data from a similar follow-up of discharges. His study involved 636 of approximately 3091 patients discharged from Rome State School between 1904 and 1924, half of whom had since died. Of the group studied, Foley found that 12% of the males and 17% of the females had been recommitted to various institutions while 79% of the males "followed various occupations with greater or less success" and 62% of the females were employed.

Utilizing the same population as Foley but restricted in the length of time since discharge, Town and Hill (1931) also followed a group released from Rome State

School. They, however, applied extremely rigorous standards for successful adjustment: 1) ability to support oneself completely; 2) ability to regulate one's life without assistance, either financial or supervisory; 3) ability to live within the law to the extent of arrest or commitment. Of the 136 discharges in their study only eight (6%, exactly the figure found by Fernald) met all three criteria following release. While the fact that this study took place during the depression cannot be overlooked, to a large extent it demonstrated the vulnerability of the mentally retarded persons studied. Total independence, especially during "hard times," was a difficult goal to attain. Town and Hill also did a rather thorough examination of factors which may have been important in the complete adjustment of the eight "successful" cases. They found no consistent pattern among factors such as length of time residing in the institution, behavior in the institution or the type of community placement.

By the time these studies had been published, two points were relatively clear. One was that the number of persons released from institutions who could be judged as adjusting to community life was highly dependent on how one operationally defined adjustment (Town & Hill, 1931) and who was making the judgment (Little & Johnson, 1931). The other point was that straight statistical counts of the number of persons released from institutions who had succeeded or failed at establishing some degree of adjustment to community life had served their purpose, but that it was now time to examine the adjustment process more carefully. Noted Foley (1929) at the conclusion of his report,

> The most desirable progress in the future concerning parole and discharge will come neither by adherence to the idea that these are wholly desirable or undesirable socially but rather by better information as to what actually happens under different systems of administration [i.e., how those being studied live in the different types of placement] (pp. 203-204).

Mentally retarded persons never institutionalized. The late 1920's and early 1930's also produced a number of studies of mentally retarded persons who had never been placed in institutions. Three of these will be briefly described here because their findings relate directly to the general consideration of community adjustment.

Kinder and Rutherford (1927) studied the environmental conditions in which their mentally retarded subjects lived subsequent to an examination in a psychiatric clinic. The adjustment of these children was then followed up four to five years later and compared with an independent evaluation of the environment in which the children lived. Concluded the authors, "The data of this study have placed the emphasis in social maladjustment rather more upon the individual's environment than upon the factor of mental retardation" (p. 833).

Hay and Kappenburg (1931) rated mentally retarded children referred to a clinic into one of five levels of adjustment within three domains: home, friends, school. They also amplified the factors examined to include IQ, economic status of family, age, time since seen in clinic, sex, behavior disorders and home environment (emotional tone of home and parental attitudes). On follow-up only the ratings of behavior disorders and home environment across domains predicted later adjustment, and of these the latter was more predictive.

Shimburg and Reichenburg (1933) made a somewhat different discovery in their follow-up of 189 "mentally subnormal" children. These children who had reached the age of 18 and had been seen in a clinic at least four years prior were rated according to the following criteria of adjustment:

> *Successful* when the subject was working regularly and had caused no trouble in the community subsequent to examination. . . .
>
> *Doubtful* when the subject had been a disturbing element in the community, had an unstable work record, but had committed no actual court delinquency. . . .
>
> *Failure* when the subject had been a constant disturbance in the community, had worked irregularly, had a court record, or had done so poorly that he had to be committed to an institution for the defective or delinquent (p. 456).

Of the 189 cases, 41 were classed as failure, 47 as doubtful, and 101 as successful.

In addition to the adjustment classification of subjects, a wide range of variables concerning the youth and their environments was considered (family economic status, personality traits of the youth, the degree to which clinic suggestions had been acted upon, type of supervision). Of all the factors examined the authors concluded that personality, supervision and carrying out clinic recommendations were the most important variables in successful adjustment: "Sixty-six percent of those with good personality traits (based on a psychiatric interview, psychological testing *and* interviews with parents and school personnel) succeeded as against 13% of those whose personality traits were a handicap. . . . When the children with good personality traits were well-supervised, the percentage of successes was raised to 88%" (pp. 461-462). The authors went on to note that

> . . . the background of the individual—his heredity, home conditions [economic], physical make-up, race, siblings, and so forth—seemed to have little relationship to success and failure except in individual cases. . . . In the specific details of treatment, no one course of action seemed to be a panacea for all ills. How imperative is the need for careful individual study of each case becomes clear as we read the records. In successes or failures, it is often, if not always impossible to tell what "turned the trick." An infinite number of factors are involved in each pattern (p. 462).

In light of the findings that only 21% of the group had failed, the authors took some time to reflect on the work of Town and Hill cited previously. The criterion of absolute independence employed in their study as a condition of success was more than one should expect from someone considered mentally retarded. Supervision "was the stumbling block. Only a very small percentage of the feebleminded can attain the highest standard of adjustment to community life" (p. 460). One might add that those who can achieve this standard, fit no acknowledged definition of mental retardation developed in the past 50 years.

Impediments to the Establishment of Alternative Settings

If so much was recognized about institutional life and the adjustment of former residents to community life within fifteen years of Fernald's study, why were community alternatives so relatively little used during the period up until the 1960's? The central problem was clearly that while most institutions were making some attempt to find alternatives for those mentally retarded persons considered able to adjust on the outside, there were very few organized programs outside the institutions. There were no funds waiting to be spent, relatively few "services" to be tapped, and in some states there were serious legal problems to be overcome. For example, in Pennsylvania it was ruled that persons admitted to state institutions could be "maintained only on property owned by the state *and* officially designated for that purpose," effectively eliminating the possibility for predischarge extra-institutional care (Sandy, 1926, p. 193). In short, although the benefits seemed apparent, release programs were piecemeal, fraught with serious economic and legal problems and run directly by institutions themselves. Beyond the limited programs that the institutions were able to set up, there was little organized assistance available to mentally retarded persons who were discharged except, of course, those friends and informal benefactors who took an interest in the individual mentally retarded person.

Bernstein, a most foresightful thinker of this period, if today's values can stand as a measure, exemplifies the dilemma. His colonies from the Rome Asylum grew steadily in number and diversity between 1912 and 1935. But during this period they were almost always for those who were "productive," not because they were the only ones seen worthy of release, but primarily because sponsorship, to whatever extent necessary, had to come from the funds appropriated to the institution. Since funds for community placements were not provided, early colonies and those persons placed on parole needed to be relatively self-sufficient, or at least cost no more than they would remaining in the institution. In 1934, Hubbell noted this problem saying that if his family care program were to be extended "it would probably be necessary to have an appropriation from the legislature. . . . [Up until now] money has been obtained from various funds which cannot be counted upon indefinitely in the future" (pp. 487-488).

Doll and Longwell (1937) noted, "Every superintendent appreciates that certain patients could safely be returned to their families or restored to the community if the public would support such a program or if adequate services were available for the community supervision of the feeble-minded to which patients could be referred" (p. 451).

By the mid-1930's there was another major factor at work which impeded institution staffs from providing for the further development of those community care options that had grown rapidly during the twenties and early thirties. That factor was the interaction of constant financial appropriations with an institutional population which was progressively more seriously retarded, a reality caused by the release patterns of the period and not by changes in admissions. From 1922 through 1942 the national, average cost of maintaining a person in an institution remained virtually unchanged. The cost in 1922 was $310 and in 1942 the cost was $315 (in 1967 dollars, $606 and $646 respectively; Lakin, 1979).

During this same period the ratio of patients to staff remained nearly constant. There were 6.6 patients per staff member in 1922 and 6.7 in 1942 (Lakin, 1979). In effect then the institutions were progressively called upon to deal with a more seriously handicapped population with the same resources, and this it appears eventually changed both the nature and spirit of these facilities.

Little (1923) perceptively foresaw this coming:

> What our institutions will be 25 years from now is an interesting conjecture. With the special or ungraded class coming more and more into use and offering training to all backward children who have homes; with the special institution for the defective delinquent, whatever she or he may be; with a parole and colony system taking our highest grade cases away from the institutions, it would appear that the State institution for mental defectives will be largely filled with idiots, and a sprinkling of defectives who are without homes. Before that time comes, however, I sincerely hope to be very far removed from this problem (p. 65).

Pense (1946) later documented Little's worst expectations in Little's home state, New York:

> There has been a decrease in the proportion of patients with higher intellectual endowment in the institutional population. . . . Over a ten-year period the

> percentage of morons was reduced from 53.9% in 1934, to 40.7% in 1943, with an equalizing increase of idiots and imbeciles, most of whom require . . . infirmary care. For obvious reasons efforts to adjust the feeble-minded to the community have been more successful with the moron than with the lower mentality patients. This tends to increase the institutional residue of low grade cases (p. 455).

In short the continued progress of the early attempts to release persons capable of adjusting to the community would have required, given the more seriously handicapped population, progressively more heavily supervised and expensive placement alternatives. This was not forthcoming. In fact the depression was in the eyes of some (e.g., Matthews, 1934) seriously affecting those programs already operating although Bernstein considered this more a crisis of spirit than of economics. People were simply "getting into a rut," he said (1934, p. 51).

Bernstein's observation not withstanding, programs of community placement fell into a period of stagnation by the late 1930's due to circumstances for the most part beyond the control of those persons who had actively initiated such programs in the preceding two decades. During the period of fiscal conservatism prior to Roosevelt's election and continuing to maintain an insignificant place next to the larger work programs during the depression, almost no community-based agencies and programs, as we know them today, developed until after World War II. Nothing shows more clearly how weak conceptualization is without fiscal allocation.

In retrospect there seems to be a terrible irony in the fact that the same fiscal conservatism which protected those mentally retarded persons in the community from falling under the watchful eye of probation officers under the forced registration and supervision systems suggested during the first one-third of the century, came eventually to affect the number of persons who could have been helped to return successfully to the community once having been institutionalized. But at any rate very little new happened in the conceptualization of community adjustment from the early 1930's until the early 1960's. The rate of discharges to first admissions remained remarkably stable from 1927 to 1963, consistently falling between 45 to 60 discharges per 100 first admissions (Lakin, 1979). For the system to change it would require that community adjustment be reconceptualized as "adjustment *of* the community" as well. This would come largely in the 1970's in the form of community-based residential services funded by a number of federal and state sources with an array of supportive social, vocational and educational services never dreamed of fifty years earlier.

Summary and Conclusion

In the early 1960's a number of factors were visibly reshaping the system of residential services for mentally handicapped persons. But subtle changes had begun prior to that time, so that by 1960 it was generally recognized that institutions had gotten far too large and already the average population of public residential facilities had begun to decrease (Lakin, 1979). Among the more obvious events which continued to affect the residential services provided to mentally retarded persons during this period was the publication of a large number of studies reporting higher mortality rates (Spitz & Wolf, 1947; Tarjan, Wright, Dingman & Sabagh, 1959), lower measured intelligence (Centerwall & Center wall, 1960; Kugel & Regue, 1961), lower verbal abilities (Lyle, 1960; Sievers & Essa, 1961), and more frequently disordered personalities (Farrell, 1956; Goldfarb, 1943, 1945; Slobody & Scanlon, 1959) among institution populations when compared with similar non-institutionalized populations, as well as powerful descriptions of the realities of life in total institutions (Barton, 1959; Goffman, 1961) which convincingly argued that the heart of the problem was the institution itself. In addition came moral and political pleas such as President Kennedy's (1963) call "to reduce over a number of years, and by hundreds of thousands, the persons confined to these institutions" and "to retain in and return to the community the mentally ill and mentally retarded," and the legal and fiscal support to begin realizing such goals through the Community Mental Health Act of 1963. Also occurring in the 1950's and 1960's were strong demands for rights rather than charity on the part of the handicapped and their advocates, demands given a powerful moral force by the fact that many of the handicapped were casualties of World War II. Programs which demonstrated the nation's commitment to the handicapped in areas of educational, vocational and social services grew tremendously during this period.

More recently there has been increased state funding for alternatives to institutions and massive federal funding through Medicaid and Medicare for reimbursing services provided in skilled nursing homes (SNFs) and intermediate care facilities (ICFs) and Supplemental Security Income and Title XX of the Social Security Act. Of all the factors discussed above, the more recent economic incentives have been, of course, those most directly responsible for the major changes seen in the residential service system in the past decade. Many problems in the "community placement" of mentally retarded persons derive directly from this fact. As a Minnesota state legislative subcommittee, holding hearings on residential facilities, recently noted, "Decisions made to date have been based strictly on monies without consideration given to persons involved" (Developmental Disabilities Planning Office, 1979, p. 1).

A number of powerful political, legal, theoretical and economic forces have been operating to shape the movement of mentally retarded persons into community-based facilities not just in recent years, but in the past as well, when that movement was relatively much slower. Today, in contrast to a half century ago, many of these factors favor the opportunity for mentally retarded persons to live ideally with, but at minimum nearby, nonhandicapped citizens.

Still, assuming that the human problems of assimilation for persons who, because of mental retardation, require some degree of social support are not substantially different now than they were 50 or 60 years ago, the writers have returned to the earliest research on deinstitutionalization for guidance in considering the study of community adjustment today. Among the observations made in this research were that:

1. the routinization of the lives of institution residents had an "institutionalizing" effect and this process had detrimental effects on an individual's potential for independent living;
2. the same negative effects of institutionalization could be produced in extra-institutional settings when institutional patterns of discipline were maintained;
3. with help most released institution residents could make an adequate adjustment to community living;
4. if "successful" adjustment required a complete, unaided independence, then few released residents would be able to succeed;
5. the quality of supervision and guidance given released residents was directly related to successful adjustment;

6. supportive employers, family, foster parents and friends were essential to the adjustment process;
7. movement of institution residents back into the community was an ideal directly tied to the number of persons and facilities willing and able to provide supervision and training, and the degree to which this ideal was supported by government agencies, laws and court decisions;
8. major demographic factors (e.g., age, mental age, sex) were of relatively little importance to successful placement;
9. the social behavior of released residents was generally important to adjustment although its importance varied according to the attitudes of those providing supervision;
10. placement success involved the interaction of personal characteristics of released residents and the expectations for individuals by their caretakers;
11. the interpersonal aspects of placement settings were more important to adjustment than were physical features such as location, privacy, availability of entertainment and commercial establishments, number of residents, or physical appeal of the home;
12. former institution residents felt stigmatized by having been previously identified as retarded and concealing this fact from those with whom they associated in the community was part of the adjustment process;
13. overconcentration of community placements was not beneficial to either the retarded persons or the community; and
14. research regarding the placement of former institution residents in the community should attempt to describe the process of adaptation rather than focusing only on the outcome after an elapsed period of time. Case studies were one method proposed to study the process.

Finally, it was recognized during this period that the definition of adjustment employed and the perspective of the persons assessing it were crucial to the findings of any research program. Although most of the research during this period considered adjustment as more than merely avoiding reinstitutionalization, the perspective taken on adjustment was certainly a more narrow one than was taken by others writing at this time about other groups within the society. For example, a 1938 Educational Policies Commission statement proposed objectives for education which depicted the adjusted citizen as one who 1) achieved some degree of self-realization; 2) developed positive human relationships; 3) achieved economic efficiency; and 4) performed his/her civic responsibilities. While often so abstract that they defied the definitional clarity required for research, these particular domains of adjustment have recently been modified and reproposed as having considerable potential utility in structuring the assessment of quality of social adjustment realized by mentally retarded persons being reintegrated into the community (Bruininks & Bruininks, in press). Similarly, many of the issues in the community adjustment of mentally retarded persons outlined half a century ago are highly applicable to the study of community adjustment today and should not be overlooked as research questions are formulated and studies are designed.

Since Wallace's (1918) follow-up of persons released from Wrentham State School in Massachusetts, over 200 studies have reported on the adjustment of former residents of institutions. (Major reviews of this research have been written by Windle [1962], McCarver & Craig [1974] and Heal, Sigelman & Switzky [1976].) During these six decades the group dominating the field of mental retardation changed from medical professionals to behavioral scientists. This later group altered considerably the way in which research on community adjustment was conceptualized and conducted. In the years which have passed since those studies mentioned in this paper were conducted, research became characterized more and more as a search for those client characteristics which best predicted community adjustment. For the most part this search has been in vain for, as was well noted by the researchers mentioned in this review, adjustment was not dependent solely on the characteristics of the retarded individual. In the past 15 years there has been a clear move away from prognostic studies. A number of studies have focused on the service system; and they, not surprisingly, have generally found it inadequate for the many needs of its clients. But far more valuable it would seem are those studies which do not attempt to distill the complex forces of life into overly simplified categories. While much current writing on the topic of community adjustment, including that which is found in this volume, shows an awareness of the complexity of the adaptation process, returning to the earliest research confirms that this complexity has long been recognized, and that a good place to start a review of research on community adjustment is to start at the very beginning.

References

Barton, R. *Institutional neurosis*. Bristol, Eng: Wright, 1959.

Bateson, G. *Steps to an ecology of the mind*. New York: Chandler Publishing Co., 1972.

Bernstein, C. Colony and extramural care for the feeble-minded. *Mental Hygiene*, 1920, *4*, 1-28.

Bernstein, C. Advantages of colony care for mental defectives. *Psychiatric Quarterly*, 1927, *1*, 419-425.

Bernstein, C. Discussion. *Journal of Psycho-asthenics*, 1934, *39*, 107-117.

Bockoven, J. S. Moral treatment in American psychiatry. *Journal of Nervous and Mental Disease*, 1956, *124*, 167-194, 292-321.

Bruininks, R. H. & Bruininks, V. L. Deinstitutionalization and social integration for developmentally disabled people. In B. Bates (Ed.), *Current knowledge bases about mainstreaming*. Minneapolis: National Support Project, University of Minnesota, in press.

Camp, B. M. & Waite, T. E. Report of four cases of "mental defectives" on parole. *Journal of Psycho-asthenics*, 1932, *37*, 381-392.

Centerwall, S. A. & Centerwall, W. R. A study of children with mongolism reared in the home compared to those reared away from the home. *Pediatrics*, 1960, *25*, 678-685.

Davies, S. P. *Social control of the feeble-minded*. Utica, NY: State Hospitals Press, 1923.

Developmental Disabilities Planning Office. *Barriers to deinstitutionalization: Update*. St. Paul: Minnesota State Planning Agency, 1979.

Devine, E. T. *The family and social work*. New York: Frontier Press, 1912.

Doll, E. A. Social adjustment of the mentally subnormal. *Journal of Educational Research*, 1934, *28*, 36-43.

Doll, E. A. The institution as a foster parent. *Journal of Psycho-asthenics*, 1937, *42*, 143-148.

Doll, E. A. & Longwell, S. G. Social competence of the feeble-minded under extra-mural care. *Psychiatric Quarterly*, 1937, *11*, 450-464.

Duggan, S. P. Methods for the treatment of mental defectives of the border-line type. In *Proceedings of the Seventh New York City Conference of Charities and Correction, 1916*. New York: Vail-Ballou, 1916.

Edgerton, R. B. *The cloak of competence: Stigma in the lives of the mentally retarded.* Berkeley: University of California Press, 1967.

Edgerton, R. B. & Bercovici, S. M. The cloak of competence: Years later. *American Journal of Mental Deficiency,* 1976, *80*(5), 485-497.

Educational Policies Commission. *The purposes of education in American democracy.* Washington, DC: National Education Association, 1938.

Ellis, W. J. Institutional education and training for community release. A study of mentally deficient girls paroled from the North Jersey Training School in Totowa. *Journal of Psycho-asthenics,* 1933, *38,* 35-46.

Farrell, M. J. The adverse effects of early institutionalization of mentally subnormal children. *AMA Journal of Diseases of Childhood,* 1956, *91,* 278-281.

Fernald, W. E. After-care study of the patients discharged from Waverley for a period of twenty-five years. *Ungraded,* 1919, *5,* 25-31.

Foley, R. W. A study of patients discharged from the Rome State School for a twenty year period ending Dec. 31, 1924. *Journal of Psycho-asthenics,* 1929, *34,* 180-207.

Foucault, M. *Madness and civilization.* New York: Vintage, 1973.

Goffman, E. *Asylums.* Garden City, NY: Doubleday, 1961.

Goldfarb, W. The effects of early institutional care on adolescent personality. *Journal of Experimental Education,* 1943, *12,* 106-129.

Goldfarb, W. Psychological privation in infancy and subsequent adjustment. *American Journal of Orthopsychiatry,* 1945, *15,* 247-255.

Hay, L. & Kappenburg, B. The social adjustment of children of low intelligence. *Smith College Studies in Social Work,* 1931, *2,* 146-174.

Heal, L. W., Sigelman, C. K., & Switzky, H. N. Community residential alternatives for the mentally retarded. In N. R. Ellis (Ed.), *International review of research in mental retardation* (Vol. 9). New York: Academic Press, 1976.

Hoakley, Z. P. Extrainstitutional care for the feeble-minded. *Journal of Psycho-asthenics,* 1922, *27,* 117-137.

Hubbell, H. G. Colonization as a therapeutic measure. *Psychiatric Quarterly,* 1934, *8,* 476-488.

Kanner, L. Habeas corpus releases of feeble-minded persons and their consequences: A follow-up study. *American Journal of Psychiatry,* 1938, *94,* 1013-1033.

(Kennedy, J. C.) U.S. Census Office. *Population of the United States in 1860.* Washington, DC: U.S. Government Printing Office, 1864.

Kennedy, J. F. Message from the President of the United States. *House Documents, 1963,* Eighty-eighth Congress (Number 58). Washington, DC: U.S. Government Printing Office, 1963.

Kinder, E. F. & Rutherford, E. J. Social adjustment of retarded children. *Mental Hygiene,* 1927, *11,* 811-833.

Kugel, R. B. & Regue, D. A. A comparison of mongoloid children. *Journal of the American Medical Association,* 1961, *175,* 959.

Lakin, K. C. *Demographic studies of residential facilities for the mentally retarded: An historical review of methodologies and findings.* Minneapolis: Department of Psychoeducational Studies, University of Minnesota, 1979.

Little, A. N. & Johnson, B. S. A study of the social and economic adjustments of one hundred thirteen discharged parolees from Laconia State Hospital. *Journal of Psychoasthenics,* 1932, *37,* 233-248.

Little, C. S. Random remarks on state institutions. *Journal of Psycho-asthenics,* 1923, *28,* 59-65.

Lyle, J. G. The effect of an institution environment upon the verbal development of imbecile children. *Journal of Mental Deficiency Research,* 1960, *4,* 1-13.

Matthews, M. A. One hundred institutionally trained mental defectives in community under supervision. *Mental Hygiene,* 1922, *6,* 332-342.

Matthews, M. A. Some effects of the depression on social work with the feeble-minded. *Journal of Psycho-asthenics,* 1934, *39,* 46-50.

McCarver, R. B. & Craig, E. M. Placement of the retarded in the community. In N. R. Ellis (Ed.), *International review of research in mental retardation* (Vol. 7). New York: Academic Press, 1974.

Pense, A. W. Trends in institutional care for the mentally defective. *American Journal of Mental Deficiency,* 1946, *50,* 453-457.

Popenoe, P. Success on parole after sterilization. *Journal of Psycho-asthenics,* 1927, *32,* 86-103.

Potter, H. W. & McCollister, C. L. A resume of parole work at Letchworth Village. *Journal of Psycho-asthenics,* 1926, *31,* 165-188.

Raymond, A. Observations on the placement and supervision of mental defectives in the community. *Journal of Psycho-asthenics,* 1923, *28,* 100-118.

Sandy, W. C. Community responsibility and mental deficiency. *Journal of Psycho-asthenics,* 1926, *31,* 189-194.

Schroeder, P. L. & Bartelme, P. A mental health program as a juvenile court method of supervising the feeble-minded. *Journal of Psycho-asthenics,* 1928, *33,* 37-58.

Seltzer, G. B. & Seltzer, M. M. *The Community Adjustment Scale.* Cambridge, MA: Behavioral Education Projects, 1976.

Shimburg, M. E. & Reichenberg, W. The success and failure of subnormal problem children in the community. *Mental Hygiene,* 1933, *17,* 451-465.

Sievers, D. J. & Essa, S. H. Language development in institutionalized and community mentally retarded children. *American Journal of Mental Deficiency,* 1961, *66,* 413-420.

Slobody, L. B. & Scanlon, J. B. Consequences of early institutionalization in mental retardation. *American Journal of Mental Deficiency,* 1959, *63,* 971-974.

Somerville, H. Eugenics and the feeble-minded. *Catholic World,* 1917, *105,* 209-218.

Spitz, R. A. & Wolf, K. M. Anaclitic depression: An inquiry into the genesis of psychiatric conditions in early childhood. In *Psycho-analytic studies of childhood* (Vol. 2). New York: International Universities Press, 1947.

Stebbins, I. F. An evaluation of homes for parole placement of mental defectives. *Journal of Psycho-asthenics,* 1931, *36,* 50-67.

Storrs, H. C. A report on an investigation made of cases discharged from Letchworth Village. *Journal of Psycho-asthenics,* 1929, *34,* 220-232.

Tarjan, G., Wright, S. W., Dingman, H. F., & Sabagh, G. The natural history of mental deficiency in a state hospital: II. Mentally deficient children admitted to a state hospital prior to their sixth birthday. *American Journal of Diseases of Childhood,* 1959, *98,* 370-378.

Town, C. H. & Hill, G. A. *How the feeble-minded live in the community.* Buffalo, NY: Children's Aid Society, 1930.

Tredgold, A. F. *A textbook of mental deficiency* (6th ed.) Baltimore: Wood, 1937.

U.S. Census Office. *Compendium of the tenth census.* Washington, DC: U.S. Government Printing Office, 1883.

Wallace, G. L. Parole of the feeble-minded. *Journal of Psycho-asthenics,* 1918, *23,* 60-81.

Wilbur, H. B. Institutions for the feeble-minded. In *Proceedings of the Fifteenth National Conference of Charities and Correction.* Buffalo, NY: NCCC, 1888.

Windle, C. Prognosis of mental subnormals. *American Journal of Mental Deficiency,* 1962, *66* (Monograph Supplement).

(Wines, F. H.) U.S. Census Bureau. *Report on the defective, dependent, and delinquent classes of the population of the United States.* Washington, DC: U.S. Government Printing Office, 1888.

Wolfensberger, W. *The origin and nature of our institutional models.* Syracuse, NY: Human Policy Press, 1975.

A Conceptual Approach to Deinstitutionalization of the Mentally Retarded: A Perspective From the Experience of the Mentally Ill

Leona L. Bachrach

Maryland Psychiatric Research Center
University of Maryland School of Medicine

Deinstitutionalization of services for the mentally retarded, one manifestation of the social reform momentum that has for several decades prevailed in the nation, has a counterpart in the development of new programs for the chronically mentally ill. There have been remarkable parallels in the aims and purposes of deinstitutionalization for both of these mentally disabled populations. It is noteworthy, however, that surprisingly little systematic exchange has taken place between program planners of both disciplines, even though such sharing has considerable potential for producing positive results.

Researchers in mental retardation have explored a number of areas that are of major concern to the planners of services for the chronically mentally ill in this era of deinstitutionalization. There is now a body of literature in the field of retardation that is rich with techniques for assessing both client needs and client satisfaction. Similarly, new directions in the programming of services for the retarded have yielded a variety of effective rehabilitation protocols. Planners of programs for the chronically mentally ill are only now beginning to focus in depth on these practical and basic concerns. They can potentially avoid considerable trial and error by careful study of the procedures developed in the field of mental retardation.

On the other hand, the massive depopulation of institutions for the mentally ill, which both predates and outnumbers that of the retarded, can now be viewed with something approaching historical detachment. The mental health literature contains numerous analyses of the sociopolitical dimensions of deinstitutionalization. And many of the planning and implementation difficulties that are currently surfacing in the literature on deinstitutionalization of the retarded have a *deja vu* quality for readers who have confronted the same kinds of issues in planning programs for the chronically mentally ill.

Deinstitutionalization of the mentally ill, in short, now has a history of sufficient length to allow planners and caregivers to understand something of the etiology of and prognosis for the numerous problems that have characterized the movement. The aim of this discussion is to demonstrate that those insights gleaned from a sociological analysis of deinstitutionalization of the mentally ill can be profitably applied to program planning for the mentally retarded.

In no way is this conceptual work to be construed as an effort to minimize the differences between these two groups of mentally disabled persons. There are certainly major distinctions between the mentally ill and the mentally retarded, and it appears that viewing the two populations as if they were one and the same has at times served the needs of neither. Fincher (1977) indicates that

> . . . public perceptions of the mentally ill and the retarded are the same: that mental retardation is seen by many people as a form of mental illness . . . [and] the two are often confused. Both groups arouse contempt, fear and unease in those who associate with them, and both are often seen as threatening and potentially dangerous.

Thus, it is not surprising that an item in the *New York Times* reports that the success of a program for hiring mentally retarded individuals in noncompetitive municipal jobs has been slowed because agency supervisors "mix them [the mentally retarded] up with those who are emotionally disturbed" (Gupte, 1977). In the strong words of the Liaison Task Panel on Mental Retardation of the President's Commission on Mental Health, the confusion between mental illness and mental retardation "has had unfortunate consequences for retarded people and their families. It has led to public misunderstandings and has fostered inappropriate professional services and administrative models" (President's Commission, 1978a).

On the other hand, it is possible to look at the social processes that uniformly affect these populations without doing violence to either group's individuality. Since deinstitutionalization is very much a sociological event, with certain attributes that characterize the process itself regardless of what particular persons undergo it, it is possible to distill some of its conceptual elements.

There is one additional preliminary concern to address before embarking on this conceptual exercise, and that is acknowledgment of the sizable number of persons who are both mentally retarded and mentally ill. Some of these individuals are treated within the mental health service system and others within the mental retardation service system. Undoubtedly, some are not treated at all. The Liaison Task Panel on Retardation of the President's Commission on Mental Health devotes the bulk of its report to the needs of these people (President's Commission, 1978a).

As for those mentally retarded persons treated in the mental health system, by far the majority are found in state mental hospitals. Of the estimated 171,000 residents of state mental hospitals in 1976, 18,266, or 10.7%, had a primary diagnosis of mental retardation. Persons diagnosed as mentally retarded had somewhat less prominence among additions to, as opposed to residents in, state mental hospitals. In 1976, there were 11,765 additions with a diagnosis of mental retardation, and this number accounted for only 2.8% of total additions to state mental hospitals (Division of Biometry, 1978a).

Except for this group who are both retarded and mentally ill, these two populations have been, for the most part, separated physically, although now with the movement toward community placement they may be coming together geographically in increasing numbers. Separate as they are, however, problems in planning for deinstitutionalization for both of them converge at a number of points. Buzz words like fragmentation, coordination, tracking, least restrictive setting, accountability, normalization and many more appear in both popular and professional literature regarding both populations.

The literature reveals that a number of common factors affect the deinstitutionalization of both of these groups. First, both populations include individuals with a wide range of disabilities and service needs. In sharp contrast to the breadth of these needs, planning of services has often tended toward pragmatic simplicity instead of relevance. Second, for both populations there appears to be roughly an inverse relationship between degree of impairment and appropriateness of deinstitutionalized program plans. Third, planning of services for both populations takes place against a backdrop of stigma that is extremely difficult to penetrate. Fourth, fragmentation of services and authority is a serious problem in both instances. This makes integration and coordination essential dimensions of planning for both populations. And fifth, in the bodies of literature covering both groups, there is a great deal of semantic confusion. Two particular sources of perplexity are the words "community" and "deinstitutionalization."

Semantic Concerns

Panzetta (1971) aptly writes that "Certain words have a way of taking on meanings never intended. Words of a high level of abstraction are like that." With specific regard to the word "community," he continues: "It can be applied in a variety of situations and so is versatile as a one-word concept. But it also is prone to multiple connotative meanings and so can be easily misunderstood."

Unfortunately, the word "community" has come to be used so loosely in the literature concerning the mentally disabled that it has lost its original meaning and has become synonymous with "noninstitution." The difficulty is that many persons have, by some faulty logic, confused the word "community" with the characteristic of *gemeinschaft*, which refers to community of spirit. But merely calling something a community-based facility does not automatically invest it with *gemeinschaft*.

In reality, the mentally disabled in the "community" are found in a wide variety of settings—including the family home, halfway houses, apartment hotels, foster homes and board and care homes—with varying degrees of *gemeinschaft*. Over one-quarter of a million mentally disabled persons (including both mentally ill and mentally retarded individuals) are in nursing homes (Division of Biometry, 1978b). Because the word "community" has been used indiscriminately to refer to all of these places, it has been stripped of any uniform meaning that it might have had, save that as the opposite of an institution. And that is the definition of community which unfortunately, remains: outside the institution.

Semantic confusion similarly surrounds the use of the word "deinstitutionalization" itself. Sometimes, in fact, those associated with the care of the mentally disabled become quite upset with the word and express a wish to do away with it—as if getting rid of the word will somehow also make the problems that it implies disappear. In one sense, however, there may be a special advantage in using this particular word, for it suggests the breakdown of traditional (or "institutional," in the sociological sense) ways of dealing with problems associated with the care of the mentally disabled. Although admittedly cumbersome, the word itself is really neutral. It carries no value judgments as to whether these old ways of dealing with the mentally disabled are good, bad, adequate or indifferent; it merely indicates social *change*. It is up to caregivers, researchers and planners to evaluate that social change.

Neither avoiding nor endorsing a word in itself affects the evaluation process. But preoccupation with semantics *can* potentially detract from and stall evaluation, and it is important to guard against this. However the word "deinstitutionalization" is perceived, it appears that the inherent moral worth of the movement is widely accepted as an appropriate and proper development. This is so in spite of variations in understanding of how complete deinstitutionalization, in theory, should be. Questions of whether large institutions should be totally eliminated or whether they should be kept for specified purposes—and, if the latter, what role they should play in the spectrum of service delivery facilities—are still not resolved. Nonetheless, most members of the helping professions appear to agree that community care has true potential for being a good thing for most, if not all, mentally disabled persons.

But this belief has at times biased investigators and has interfered with their evaluation of the consequences of deinstitutionalization. It must be acknowledged that despite some notable successes over the past couple of decades in deinstitutionalization efforts, the movement has been plagued by a variety of problems.

The Task Panel on Deinstitutionalization, Rehabilitation and Long-Term Care of the President's Commission on Mental Health describes this situation in very certain language by stating that deinstitutionalization has "fallen short of its goal." The Task Panel report continues:

> Unfortunately, deinstitutionalization has too often occurred without adequate planning. . . . All too commonly, no one reviews the requirements of disabled persons to assess whether hospitalization or community care is more appropriate to their level of functioning. . . . It is not uncommon for these patients to be released [from institutions], without adequate aftercare planning, to community settings that are hostile and lack the flexibility to meet their needs (President's Commission, 1978b).

Defining Deinstitutionalization

That deinstitutionalization is a complex phenomenon with many facets is frequently overlooked in practice. It should be apparent that deinstitutionalization is variously perceived. The educational psychologist in the state school, for example, is bound to have a perspective that differs materially from that of the public school teacher who is trying, with grossly inadequate funds, to mainstream retarded children. Any working definition of deinstitutionalization must be sufficiently abstract to accommodate differences in individual experience.

For purposes of this analysis, deinstitutionalization may be defined as a process involving two elements: the eschewal (or shunning, or avoidance) of traditional institutional settings for the care of the mentally disabled, and the concurrent expansion of community-based facilities for the care of these individuals. The major point in this definition is that it is erroneous to look at deinstitutionalization unidimensionally as if it referred only to persons released from institutions. It is, in fact, a much broader event that affects even persons who have never been hospitalized.

There are at least three separate but closely interrelated aspects of deinstitutionalization. Deinstitutionalization is a process. It is also a fact. And it is also a philosophy.

Process

Those who view deinstitutionalization simplistically tend to perceive it as a single migratory experience—that of moving clients out of the institution and into the community. But deinstitutionalization is more complex than this. It is *a dynamic and continuing series of adjustments involving constant accommodation of all components of the service delivery system.* Ideally, at least, with deinstitutionalization clients are expected to move about freely from facility to facility or even in and out of the service delivery system. Conceptually, deinstitutionalization holds that utilization is determined by each client's needs in a kind of free market model: as service needs change, so will patterns of care vary.

In fact, the dynamic nature of deinstitutionalization for the mentally ill is evidenced in changes that have affected the resident population of large state hospitals. At one time quite recently, the bulk of the chronically mentally ill were admitted to state mental hospitals where they usually stayed for the rest of their lives. This was a relatively static population pool; it was affected primarily by new admissions and deaths. Today, this large population pool is in flux, and five population subgroups have emerged, two in the community and three in the hospital. They include: 1) released state hospital patients living in the community; 2) other chronically mentally ill persons in the community who, as a direct result of current deinstitutionalization policies, have never been hospitalized but probably would have been admitted to state hospitals in the past; 3) old long-stay patients —i.e., veteran residents of state hospitals who remain there despite deinstitutionalization efforts; 4) new long-stay patients—i.e., recent state hospital admissions who are likely to remain hospitalized indefinitely; and 5) short-stay patients—i.e., recent state hospital admissions who will soon be discharged. Documentation for these patient subgroups is provided elsewhere (Bachrach, 1978). There is some exchange among these subgroups, particularly the first and the last, and this movement is responsible for what has come to be known as the revolving-door phenomenon.

Although the directions and relative magnitudes of population shifts are, obviously, not precisely parallel for the mentally ill and the retarded, there is enough similarity to permit distillation at a higher level of abstraction. Thus, deinstitutionalization may be seen as a complicated, multifaceted process that continues dynamically to alter patterns of service delivery. Planning for deinstitutionalization should ideally accommodate a variety of clients possessing vastly different residential histories, not only those who are discharged from institutions. Each population subgroup represents, in its own way, fallout from the deinstitutionalization movement. In reality, however, the planning of deinstitutionalized services for the mentally disabled has been spread so thin that it has not adequately met the needs of any of these subgroups.

This conceptualization of deinstitutionalization as a process, based on the experience of the mentally ill, is strikingly reinforced in a statement concerning the mentally retarded:

> To deinstitutionalize persons does not mean to simply move them out of state hospitals into community placements. It refers to more than the collection of buildings commonly called "institutions." Instead, deinstitutionalization deals with the process of opening up less routinized and more varied behaviors for both individuals and settings, no matter *what* the facility or *where* it is (Pappas, Smead, Miller & Tracy, 1976).

Fact

In addition to its being a process, deinstitutionalization is also a fact with measurable dimensions. That the phenomenon really is occurring is reflected in nationwide statistics concerning the depopulation of large institutions. For the mentally ill, there has been a marked decrease in the resident population of the nation's state hospitals. This population peaked in 1955 at 558,992. Ten years later it stood at 475,202 and 20 years later at 193,436. Thus, the resident population of these facilities showed a decrease of 15% over one decade and a striking decrease of 65% over two decades (Division of Biometry, 1979).

Deinstitutionalization of the mentally retarded is also reflected in institutional depopulation statistics, although there are notable differences in numerical trends between them and the mentally ill. The resident population in public facilities for the retarded peaked 12 years later than that in state hospitals for the mentally ill. In 1967, the peak year, the resident population in institutions for the mentally retarded stood at 193,183 (Butterfield, 1976) and at 148,752 a decade later (Krantz, Bruininks & Clumpner, 1978)—a decrease of 23% in ten years.

These differences in timing in the depopulation of institutions for the mentally ill and the retarded reflect variations in the conditions giving impetus to the deinstitutionalization movement for both populations—a point that will be elaborated in the discussion that follows.

Philosophy

In addition to its being a process and a fact, deinstitutionalization has an intellectual foundation—i.e., a philosophy. The philosophy of deinstitutionalization proceeds from at least three fundamental assumptions concerning the care of the mentally disabled. First, there is an assumption that community care is a good thing—that *community-based care is preferable to institutional care for most, if not all, clients*. A second underlying assumption is that *communities not only can, but also are willing to, assume responsibility and leadership in the care of the mentally disabled*. And a third assumption regarding deinstitutionalization is that *the functions performed by institutions can be performed equally well, if not better, by community-based facilities*.

These three philosophical assumptions taken together lead to an understanding of the *goal* of deinstitutionalization. Deinstitutionalization has assumed no less a task than that of "humanizing" the care of the mentally disabled—of reversing the dehumanizing influences that are widely understood as accompaniments of institutional residence. In this sense, deinstitutionalization shares a great deal with other social efforts to enhance the life of individuals. Like other civil rights protests, deinstitutionalization is ideologically committed to improving the lot of persons perceived as helpless in gaining access to life's entitlements. It is a movement dedicated to the dignity of individuals.

If anything, this ideological commitment to social reform has had even more impact on deinstitutionalization of the mentally retarded than on that of the mentally ill. A number of factors in addition to the social reform ideology are credited with giving rise to the deinstitutionalization of the mentally ill. These include the introduction of antipsychotic medications to control the symptoms of mental illness and the development of crisis intervention techniques in psychiatry (Smith & Hart, 1975; Talbott, 1978).

By contrast, it appears that the civil rights thrust has been almost singlehandedly responsible for deinstitutionalization of the mentally retarded (Silverman, 1979). At least, other contributing factors are given scant attention in the literature. Roos (1975) classifies the major civil rights issues for the mentally retarded into three categories: the right to education, the right to treatment and the freedom from peonage. To these may be added the right to care and residence in the least restrictive setting (Thurlow et al, 1978).

Deinstitutionalization for both populations has occurred largely during an era when a more generalized political philosophy of social reform, stressing society's responsibility to help the individual, has predominated. But the movement owes much to more conservative forces. Acceptance of the progressive philosophy of deinstitutionalization is facilitated by its attractiveness to those who are interested in fiscal reform—a situation making for strange bedfellows among its proponents.

Since the movement began, deinstitutionalization has been widely believed to be cheaper than institutionalization. At least in the early phases of a social movement, the accuracy of this kind of belief is much less important than its acceptance, even though disillusionment may eventually settle in. The fact that people *do* believe in the money-saving powers of deinstitutionalization is one of the things that has made the movement acceptable to many who might otherwise oppose it.

In addition to the presumption of cost savings in community-based care, there has been a desire on the part of state legislatures to reduce their own budgets by "shift[ing] the cost and responsibility of the formerly institutionalized to a different level of government" (Cramer, 1978). With the closing of large institutions, many disabled persons have relied on federal public assistance funds for support. It is not difficult for states to justify reduced fiscal responsibility in the light of what is regarded so widely within the helping professions as a more humane system of care.

In short, the fact that the philosophy of deinstitutionalization has been allied with more than one political stream has accounted in large part for the rapid spread of the movement. Progressive reformers and fiscal conservatives alike have found something to support in the movement. Recent developments on the American economic scene have, however, generated suspicion that the wedding of these different views is coming to an end and that the ideological commitment to deinstitutionalization is being diluted. The philosophical basis for deinstitutionalization is fragile and subject to the fickleness of political winds, particularly in times of inflationary stress. Thus, for example, an article in the *Washington Post* states that "The explosive growth of government social welfare programs that has dominated domestic politics for the past quarter-century has come to an end," and it quotes the Dean of Columbia University's School of Social Work as saying that this represents the "end of an era" in social programming (Rich, 1979).

Some of this ideological shift has to do with the fact that the fiscal superiority of deinstitutionalization has never really been firmly established. It is now generally agreed that providing high-quality care for the metally disabled is not cheap, no matter how the locus is shifted. Deinstitutionalization has not proved to be the overall money-saving solution that had been anticipated. Not only is the cost of community-based care high, but beyond a certain point in resident population reduction, the per capita cost of running an institution must, obviously, increase. The savings that were supposed to accompany the depopulation of institutions simply have not materialized on a nationwide basis. To illustrate this point, suit was recently filed by two patients and the Mental Health Association of California against Governor Brown. The plaintiffs point out the high economic costs of community care and claim that the state's increase of $25 million over last year's budget for this purpose is "woefully inadequate" and that it "barely keeps up with inflation." And the Governor is being held responsible for the "unnecessary confinement" of thousands of patients in institutional facilities (Kotkin, 1979).

Implications

What does this all mean? The perspective that deinstitutionalization is a process and a philosophy as well as a fact permits better understanding of some of the problems associated with the movement. Were deinstitutionalization merely concerned with the exchange of settings for client care, many of the problems known to exist would not have arisen. The community would have simply replaced the institution as the locus of care, and resultant problems would have been of a logistical nature, easily negotiated and resolved. The fact is, however, that deinstitutionalization has, since its inception, confronted obstacles every step of the way. Fiscal disappointments are only one reality. There are numerous other issues associated with deinstitutionalization, and experience has shown that these problems are sometimes very difficult to resolve. The issues that surround deinstitutionalization for the mentally ill have been discussed at length in the literature (Bachrach, 1976), and a taxonomy of them is provided in Table 1. Examination of the professional and popular literature on mental retardation reveals very substantial concordance (Bruininks, Williams & Morreau, 1978; Thurlow et al., 1978) despite those variations in timing that have differentially characterized the movement for both populations.

Thus, what Gettings (1977) writes of fragmentation of services for the mentally retarded (Issue II-B, Table 1) might easily have been written about programs for the mentally ill:

> Each federal agency with an actual or potential impact on deinstitutionalization of the mentally retarded tends to develop its operational policies with limited regard to their impact upon ancillary programs operated by other federal and state agencies and with little or no sensitivity to the overall impact of the federal government's efforts at the state and local levels.

Similarly, two newspaper articles (Kihss, 1978; Weiner, 1976) report, respectively, that the Civil Service Employees Association is protesting the movement of mentally retarded clients from a government facility on Governor's Island, New York, to a privately operated medical rehabilitation program (Issue IV-C); and that suburban residents are resisting the presence of a halfway house for the mentally retarded in their neighborhood (Issue IV-A). Once again, these articles are practically indistinguishable from similar ones about the chronically mentally ill.

Problems surrounding implementation of the 1975 Education for All Handicapped Children Law (PL 94-142) are given extensive attention in the literature (Issue VII; Anonymous, 1977; Diehl, 1979; Gettings, 1977; Huey, 1978; Krucoff, 1978; McCaffrey & Higgins, 1977; Silverman, 1979). In this connection, the issue of precipitate implementation (Issue IX-A) is also notable, as demonstrated in the following report:

> The law has created as many problems as solutions, bringing friction between local school districts and Washington, between parents and schools and sometimes between teachers and teachers, to say nothing of the effects on children. When President Ford signed this legislation . . . he complained about its boundless ambition. "Unfortunately, this bill promises more than the federal government can deliver." He signed it, nevertheless, and the good intentions became a promissory note that is proving very hard to make good (Omang, 1979).

Other writers on deinstitutionalization of the mentally retarded discuss still other issues included in the taxonomy in Table 1. In short, there is good reason to conclude that whether or not one views the deinstitutionalization problems of these two populations as separate and distinct depends on one's level of conceptualization. Despite the very real clinical differences in kinds of impairment and the possibility that concentrating on the needs of one group may be in some way detrimental to the other, there is a level of abstraction at which the issues in deinstitutionalization of the mentally ill and the mentally retarded come together. One approach to understanding these issues is through a functional analysis of the kind frequently employed in sociological inquiries.

Table 1

A Taxonomy of Issues in Deinstitutionalization[a]

I. Issues related to the selection of patients for community care
   A. Chronically ill patients
   B. Patients inadequately prepared for life in the community
   C. Disadvantaged and minority groups

II. Issues related to the treatment course of patients in the community
   A. Inadequate range of treatment services
   B. Fragmentation and lack of coordination in treatment services
   C. Inaccessibility of treatment services
   D. Questionable quality of care in community services

III. Issues related to the quality of life of patients in the community
   A. Inadequate community support systems
   B. Residential facilities and living arrangements

IV. Issues related to the greater community
   A. Community resistance and opposition to mentally ill individuals
   B. Efforts on communities to which patients are released
   C. Ecological impact on hospital staff
   D. Ecological impact on hospital community
   E. Effects on patient's family

V. Issues related to manpower
   A. Training and retraining of staff for community work
   B. Maldistribution of personnel
   C. Role-blurring
   D. Attitudes of staff toward working with chronically mentally ill

VI. Financial and fiscal issues

VII. Legal and quasi-legal issues

VIII. Informational issues and accountability
   A. Necessity for evaluation studies
   B. Difficulties in locating and following patients in the community
   C. Inadequacy of existing follow-up studies

IX. Additional issues resulting directly from process of deinstitutionalization
   A. Timing: precipitate implementation of new programs
   B. Inadequate attention to patients' desires
   C. Problems related to providing adequate services in hospitals during phase-out
   D. Failure to establish liaison between hospitals and community-based facilities
   E. Disenchantment with the deinstitutionalization movement: resistance to further change

[a]Adapted from L. L. Bachrach, *Deinstitutionalization: An analytical review and sociological perspective.* Rockville, MD: National Institute of Mental Health, 1976.

Functional Analysis

It was previously noted that one underlying philosophical assumption of the deinstitutionalization movement is the premise that the functions performed by the institution can be performed equally well, if not better, by community-based facilities. What, exactly, are these functions? A review of the literature suggests that the range of functions performed by institutions for the mentally ill is surprisingly complex and is far more extensive than might at first glance be supposed (Bachrach, 1976). An attempt to isolate the functions of mental hospitals as identified in the literature yields a list of 21 separate items as shown in Table 2. This listing includes only those functions explicitly stated in the literature. Were it to be expanded by including additional functions that are implicit, it would doubtless be even longer. It is very probable that the functions of institutions for the mentally retarded very closely, if not precisely, parallel those shown in Table 2. Some of these functions apply exclusively to clients and some to other elements of society. It is safe to say that some were not originally intended but have evolved as the system of institutional care has grown in the nation.

The listing in Table 2 includes the widely acknowledged function of providing long-term treatment for disabled individuals, as well as the function of asylum which is frequently understood as an important aspect of institutional care. But the listing goes further than this to include a whole series of additional functions less readily perceived or acknowledged—such as rendering relief to the client's family, providing a sort of hiding place outside of the community for some of its less attractive members, or providing an economic base for the community in which the institution is located.

An important observation emerges when the listing of institutional functions in Table 2 is compared with the issues in deinstitutionalization provided in Table 1. The issues fall into two major groupings vis-a-vis the functions. Either the issue has at least one referent among the functions listed, or else the issue has come into being as a direct consequence of the deinstitutionalization movement itself. Thus, for example, Issue IV-E in Table 1, "effects on patient's family," has the functional referent of "relieving the patient's family from disruptive social inter-action." And Issue III-B, "residential facilities and living arrangements," has the functional referent of "providing a residential environment for the mentally ill."

It seems clear that efforts to reduce the stature of, or to eliminate, institutions have too often overlooked, or neglected, to stress the necessity for alternatives for the full range of functions noted. Not even the central functions of treatment and asylum have been assured for deinstitutionalized individuals, not to mention the various other functions that have an impact on other elements of society. It is inevitable that any movement that so ignores the cultural makeup of society will encounter severe opposition. And it has.

It is also apparent that the zeal and dedication that have motivated deinstitutionalization have left in their wake a series of dysfunctional elements resulting directly from rapid, sometimes heedless, implementation of incomplete program plans. Planning for deinstitutionalization has, unfortunately, often proceeded in a sort of functional vacuum. It has certainly failed to address the needs of the diverse patient population subgroups described earlier as comprising the universe of mentally disabled persons.

Table 2

Functions of Mental Hospitals[a]

Providing long-term treatment for chronically disturbed individuals
Providing crisis intervention for patients undergoing acute stress
Providing for patient respite from mounting pressures
Removing the patient from his usual environment and from whatever pathological influences that environment may have
Protecting the patient from exploitation by others
Providing a residential environment for the mentally ill
Providing constant and continuous monitoring and review of the patient's course of illness
Providing a social structure within which the role of the mentally disturbed individual is clearly defined
Providing the mentally ill individual with an alternative to due process of law
Providing the patient with a place to which he may escape from the greater society
Providing a means by which society can segregate some of its deviants
Relieving the patient's family and community from disruptive social interaction
Protecting the society from the acts of dangerous individuals
Supplying an ostensibly relatively inexpensive form of patient care
Providing an economic base and employment for a community or a portion of a community
Providing job security and other job perquisites for numbers of employed persons
Providing a tax base for local communities
Providing for mental health professionals a funnel for the removal of unattractive and often poor patients
Diverting attention from the need for local planning and expenditures by creating an illusion that the mentally ill are being adequately treated elsewhere
Providing a place for research on mental illness
Providing a place for the training of mental health professionals

[a]Adapted from L. L. Bachrach, *Deinstitutionalization: An analytical review and sociological perspective.* Rockville, MD: National Institute of Mental Health, 1976.

Effective Planning: Some Considerations

What is seen, then, is in reality that the philosophy, the process and the fact of deinstitutionalization have been in some degree disjunctive, and it is necessary now to consider what, if anything, may be done to improve the situation. Recent literature on the mentally ill does, in fact, indicate increasing awareness of the complexities of deinstitutionalization planning, and this is a hopeful sign. Recognition of the full range of functions associated with institutions is becoming more prevalent. And this recognition is often accompanied by pleas for more realistic and more sensitive planning so that whole groups of people are not automatically excluded from the planning process.

What steps must be taken to stem past planning deficits and to assure effective program designs for the future? For one, considerable effort must be devoted to the clarification of concepts. Not only must the semantic difficulties discussed earlier be dealt with realistically, but other areas of vagueness must be identified and, where possible, eliminated.

Descriptions of facilities for the care of the mentally disabled continue to be particularly fuzzy and bothersome to program planners. One frequently reads of the necessity for a "range of facilities" for the care of the mentally disabled, and this, although it is accepted terminology, is very misleading. It implies a straight line or continuum along which different kinds of facilities can potentially be located. But each specific facility for the care of the disabled can theoretically be classified according to a host of other variables that transcend facility type—such as kinds of services provided, treatment philosophy, emotional climate, level of autonomy accorded clients, relationships to external agencies and staffing policies. Intagliata (1979) expresses this simply but effectively with regard to residential facilities: "The strategy of comparing across residential types implies that there is more variation between different types of settings than within a given setting type," even though studies have shown, to the contrary, that "there is great variation within treatment types."

If, in addition to the residential function discussed by Intagliata, a facility also has a service function, the situation is even more difficult to conceptualize along a continuum. Butler and Bjaanes (1978) present a taxonomy of characteristics of facilities serving the mentally disabled. This taxonomy, summarized in Table 3, includes intrafacility, extrafacility and type-of-care variables. Any halfway house, apartment house, board and care home, family home or institution can be characterized differentially along these and other dimensions. The picture that emerges is thus one of extreme complexity, and one begins to get the notion that facilities for the mentally disabled are better conceptualized within a matrix than along a continuum. It is not enough to specify a kind of facility by name; one must also specify those characteristics that cut across facility types and that have relevance to the treatment and well-being of the client population. Once again, semantics interfere with perceptions of the complexity of the phenomena with which one is concerned.

Closely related to, and indeed part of, the need for more precision in the use of concepts is the need for careful definition of target populations. It is increasingly acknowledged that one of the first steps in implementing successful deinstitutionalization programs must be the specific delineation of who—what clients—are to be treated in the community. A corollary consideration is: Are there some clients who cannot be regarded as "good risks" or as appropriate candidates for community care? And, if there are, where and how shall they be treated? The answers to these questions are not simple and depend on the specific community involved and on the special resources that it has. The answers depend on timing, as well. Some communities are at any given time better equipped—in terms of available services, manpower and attitudes—to handle the mentally disabled than are others. But the fact that a community does not demonstrate readiness for deinstitutionalization does not necessarily indicate a permanent state of affairs. Lack of readiness may be a temporary phenomenon accompanying the careful and judicious design of program plans. Or it may be virtually permanent if the community foresees no way of providing alternatives for institutional functions. Isolated rural communities may be particularly hard-pressed to supply these alternatives (Bachrach, 1977.)

The element of timing is confounded by the fact that there is necessarily a time lag between assessment of service needs and implementation of program plans. In deinstitutionalization, planning certainly tends to focus on communities as they are today instead of as they will be tomorrow. But a community's needs change constantly. In 1968, when depopulation of facilities for the retarded was just beginning, Jaslow wrote:

> We cannot simply develop a number of programs for the mentally retarded in a community, and expect that these shiny new programs will then automatically fit together in a dynamic structure. It is difficult enough for the community to plan concretely for all the needs of the retarded in the beginning. Philosophies change. And if planning for the present is difficult, planning for the future seems nearly impossible. Yet it must be done.

Table 3

Characteristics of Facilities Serving the Mentally Disabled[a]

I. Intrafacility
   A. Client population
   B. Staff
   C. Programmatic (vocational, educational, social)
   D. Behavioral environment
   E. Size
   F. Physical plant
   G. Other

II. Extrafacility (including attitudes, availability of recreational resources, transportation and sheltered employment)
   A. Community at large
   B. Immediate neighborhood
   C. Other

III. Type of care
   A. Therapeutic
   B. Maintaining
   C. Custodial

[a]Adapted from E. W. Butler & A. T. Bjaanes, Activities and use of time by retarded persons. In G. P. Sackett (Ed.), *Observing behavior: Theory and applications in mental retardation.* Baltimore: University Park Press, 1978.

If a given community cannot provide high-quality, community-based care for all of its mentally disabled residents, this should not necessarily be construed as failure in the mission of humanizing care. One may eventually conclude that at least some part of the institution's role in the spectrum of services for the mentally disabled is too difficult to replace in alternative settings in all communities, and that the institution's role should be enhanced through new and innovative programming and not downgraded. Researchers are still at the point of hypothesis-testing; they must remember that it is not, after all, where clients are treated that should be of primary concern, but rather how relevant to their needs specific programs are.

In fact, increased tolerance of the role of the institution is showing up in writings concerning both the mentally ill (Bachrach, in press) and the mentally retarded. Dokecki, Anderson and Strain (1977) write that a broad civil libertarian understanding of the charge of deinstitutionalization of the mentally retarded implies that the process may to some degree "be accomplished within the institution as well as beyond its walls and jurisdiction." Just as there are certain mentally ill persons "who will somehow always be guided back to the mental hospital" (Rachlin, 1976), so is there a group of mentally retarded individuals who "cannot fit into community programs or into family situations. This group is large enough to create pressure for more institutional construction" (Jaslow & Spagna, 1977).

This emphasis on appropriate and equitable programs for the range of mentally disabled persons, and not on places *per se*, is important. It is reflected in recent literature that stresses the rehabilitation component in deinstitutionalization planning. For those clients for whom a rehabilitation approach is indicated, it can provide a most humane framework for programming. Of course, it must be acknowledged that not every mentally disabled person is an appropriate candidate for rehabilitation. Lamb (in press) holds that rehabilitation as a goal for the mentally ill has been oversold in that "A portion of our patients will never be able to accomplish it." Similar statements have been made on behalf of the retarded (Baily, 1978; Fisher, 1978). Silverman (1979) is particularly concerned with those retarded clients who are forced into mainstreaming situations, and he concludes that the "Civil and human rights of some [retarded] children require that they not be forced to be normal, that they be accepted and supported as the different people that they are" (p. 68).

It is important that we not base our expectations for all mentally disabled individuals on educational, vocational and social goals derived from studies of the least disabled—studies that have little to do with the most severely impaired clients' range of possibilities. There is an urgent need to develop special outcome evaluation techniques that permit measurement of program success for those clients whose progress, when it occurs, is so imperceptible that it cannot be assessed by the conventional criteria employed in rehabilitation programs.

Deinstitutionalization planning can, then, potentially proceed in a number of ways, some of them more, some less, sensitive to the needs of individual clients. The least sensitive planning which is not properly described as planning at all, although it has often passed as such, makes little effort to match clients and settings. It is, instead, wholesale placement of clients without consideration for individual needs. Such placement may occur either in an institution or in the community, and it leads to what has popularly been referred to as "dumping." Effective planning begins to take place when an effort is made to match clients and settings. The simplest kind of matching involved studying a client's level of functioning and attempting to place him in the setting most compatible with that level. Most placements in deinstitutionalization have, until now, been of these two kinds— either dumping or planned placements in settings deemed to be consistent with a client's level of functioning.

But deinstitutionalization is most sensitive and humane if it carries the process one step further so as to enhance, where appropriate, a client's skill development. In a "skills-training" (Anthony, 1977) or rehabilitation approach, placements are based on the client's potential rather than on his current level of functioning. The client's capabilities—and not his disabilities—are emphasized.

Conclusions

Many of the most serious problems in deinstitutionalization arise from conceptual oversights and confusion. Non-institution is confused with community in the sense of *gemeinschaft*. And change of locus is confused with improved treatment. Merely changing the locus of care does not in itself ensure fulfillment of the goal of humanizing services. It is necessary to couple changed location with programs based on sensitivity to the needs of individual clients. Deinstitutionalization is destined to "fail miserably if residents are simply depopulated from institutions into communities which now lack vital supportive programs" (Braddock, 1977).

For both mentally ill and mentally retarded persons, the successful deinstitutionalization program proceeds from concepts with clearly understood referents and from a precise statement of program goals. It is one in which there is a focused effort to fill in gaps in services (James, 1978). And it is one that strives to meet the special needs of the mentally disabled in *all* settings, those in institutions as well as those in the community. A quotation from Thiele, Paul and Neufeld (1977) epitomizes those principles of effective deinstitutionalization that the present discussion has sought to elaborate:

> The institutionalization process . . . is deeply entrenched in the culture of caregiving systems. The purpose of programming for deinstitutionalization is not to stop institutionalization. It is, rather, to minimize the negative impact of institutions and institutional practices. Stated positively, deinstitutionalization is an attempt to revitalize the potential of service-delivery systems for responding appropriately and efficiently to the needs of persons that those systems are established to serve.

References

Anonymous. Mainstreaming. *Currents*, 1977, *2*, 9-14.

Anthony, W. A. Psychological rehabilitation: A concept in need of a method. *American Psychologist*, 1977, *32*, 658-662.

Bachrach, L. L. *Deinstitutionalization: An analytical review and sociological perspective*. Rockville, MD: National Institute of Mental Health, 1976.

Bachrach, L. L. Deinstitutionalization of mental health services in rural areas. *Hospital and Community Psychiatry*, 1977, *23*, 669-672.

Bachrach, L. L. A conceptual approach to deinstitutionalization. *Hospital and Community Psychiatry*, 1978, *29*, 573-578.

Bachrach, L. L. Planning mental health services for chronic patients. *Hospital and Community Psychiatry*, in press.

Bailey, S. Mental center standards need changing, say experts. *Birmingham (Alabama) News*, November 30, 1978.

Braddock, D. A national deinstitutionalization study. *State Government*, 1977, *50*, 220-226.

Bruininks, R. H., Williams, S. M., & Morreau, L. E. *Issues and problems in deinstitutionalization in Region V* (Information and Technical Assistance Project on Deinstitutionalization, Project Report No. 2). Minneapolis: Department of Psychoeducational Studies, University of Minnesota, 1978.

Butler, E. W. & Bjaanes, A. T. Activities and use of time by retarded persons in community facilities. In G. P. Sacket (Ed.), *Observing behavior: Theory and applications in mental retardation*. Baltimore: University Park Press, 1978.

Butterfield, E. Some basic changes in residential facilities. In R. B. Kugel & A. Shearer (Eds.), *Changing patterns in residential services for the mentally retarded*. Washington: President's Committee on Mental Retardation, 1976.

Cramer, P. K. *Report on the current state of deinstitutionalization: Period of retrenchment*. Philadelphia: Health & Welfare Council, Inc., 1978.

Diehl, J. Educating handicapped puts pressure on P. G. schools. *Washington Post*, January 29, 1979.

Division of Biometry and Epidemiology. *Additions and resident patients at end of year, state and county mental hospitals, by age and diagnosis, by state, United States 1976*. Rockville, MD: National Institute of Mental Health, 1978 (a).

Division of Biometry and Epidemiology. *Nursing home residents with mental disorders or senility, United States 1977* (Memorandum No. 41). Rockville, MD: National Institute of Mental Health, 1978 (b).

Division of Biometry and Epidemiology. *Data sheet on state and county mental hospital patients*. Rockville, MD: National Institute of Mental Health, 1979. (mimeo)

Dokecki, P. R., Anderson, B. A., & Strain, P. S. Stigmatization and labeling. In J. L. Paul, D. J. Stedman, & G. R. Neufeld (Eds.), *Deinstitutionalization: Program and policy development*. Syracuse, NY: Syracuse University Press, 1977.

Fincher, R. *An examination of the notion of difference, and its implications for community survival courses for the deinstitutionalized mentally ill and mentally retarded*. Princeton, NJ: Princeton University, 1977. (mimeo)

Fisher, B. Psychologist says many at Partlow untrainable. *Tuscaloosa (Alabama) News*, November 29, 1978.

Gettings, R. M. Hidden impediments to deinstitutionalization. *State Government*, 1977, *50*, 214-219.

Gupte, P. Program provides city jobs for mentally retarded. *New York Times*, January 31, 1977.

Huey, K. Conference report: Placing the mentally retarded: Where shall they live? *Hospital and Community Psychiatry*, 1978, *29*. 596-602.

Intagliata, J. A qualitative look at community adjustment in family care homes. Presented at University of Minnesota Conference on Community Adjustment, Minneapolis, March 15, 1979.

James, J. F. Principles in developing a community support system. *Hospital and Community Psychiatry*, 1978, *29*, 34-35.

Jaslow, R. I. A modern plan for modern services to the mentally retarded. *Clinical Pediatrics*, 1968, *7*, 80-82.

Jaslow, R. I. & Spagna, M. B. Gaps in a comprehensive system of services for the mentally retarded. *Mental Retardation*, 1977, *15*, 6-9.

Kihss, P. Plan to shift retarded from Gouverneur defended. *New York Times*, May 4, 1978.

Kotkin, J. Governor Brown is sued over confinement of mental patients. *Washington Post*, February 14, 1979.

Krantz, G. C., Bruininks, R. H., & Clumpner, J. L. *Mentally retarded people in state-operated residential facilities: Year ending June 30, 1978* (Developmental Disabilities Project on Residential Services and Community Adjustment, Project Report No. 4). Minneapolis: Department of Psychoeducational Studies, University of Minnesota, 1978.

Krucoff, C. Schools locating disabled children. *Washington Post Maryland Weekly*, January 18, 1977, 1, 3.

Lamb, H. R. Roots of neglect of the long-term mentally ill. *Psychiatry*, in press.

McCaffrey, M. & Higgins, S. T. Education of handicapped children: A state government perspective. *State Government*, 1977, *50*, 249-254.

Omang, J. Entry of handicapped children into schools brings problems. *Washington Post*, January 14, 1979.

Panzetta, A. F. The concept of community. *Archives of General Pschiatry*, 1971, *25*, 291-297.

Pappas, V., Smead, V., Miller, T., & Tracy, M. *Deinstitutionalization: An ecological response*. Bloomington, IN: Indiana University Developmental Training Center, 1976.

President's Commission on Mental Health. Report of the Liaison Task Panel on Mental Retardation. In *Task panel reports submitted to the President's Commission on Mental Health* (Vol. 4). Washington, DC: President's Commission on Mental Health, 1978 (a).

President's Commission on Mental Health. Report of the Task Panel on Deinstitutionalization, Rebahilitation and Long-Term Care. In *Task panel reports submitted to the President's Commission on Mental Health* (Vol. 2). Washington, DC: President's Commission on Mental Health, 1978 (b).

Rachlin, S. The case against closing state hospitals. In P. I. Ahmed & S. C. Plog (Eds.), *State mental hospitals*. New York: Plenum Publishing Corp., 1976.

Rich, S. Figures show end of era in social-program growth. *Washington Post*, February 14, 1979.

Roos, S. The future of residential services for the mentally retarded in the United States: A Delphi study. Arlington, TX: 1975. (unpublished manuscript)

Silverman, M. Beyond the mainstream: The special needs of the chronic child patient. *American Journal of Orthopsychiatry*, 1979, *49*, 62-68.

Smith, W. G. & Hart, D. W. Community mental health: A noble failure? *Hospital and Community Psychiatry*, 1975, *26*, 581-583.

Talbott, J. A. *The death of the asylum: A critical study of state hospital management, services and care*. New York: Grune & Stratton, 1978.

Thiele, R. I., Paul, J. L., & Neufeld, G. R. Institutionalization: A perspective for deinstitutionalization program development. In J. L. Paul, D. J. Stedman, & G. R. Neufeld (Eds.), *Deinstitutionalization: Program and policy development*. Syracuse, NY: Syracuse University Press, 1977.

Thurlow, M. L., Bruininks, R. H., Williams, W. M., & Morreau, L. E. *Deinstitutionalization and residential services: A literature survey* (Information and Technical Assistance Project on Deinstitutionalization, Project Report No. 1). Minneapolis: Department of Psychoeducational Studies, University of Minnesota, 1978.

Weiner, H. Columbia residents fight to block halfway house for retarded. *Washington Post*, October 28, 1976.

II. Issues in Research on Deinstitutionalization and Community Adjustment

A Qualitative Approach to the Study of Community Adjustment

Steven J. Taylor
Robert Bogdan

Syracuse University

In 1976, we published "The Judged, Not the Judges: An Insider's View of Mental Retardation," an article describing the findings of some of our research involving indepth interviewing with mentally retarded persons (Bogdan & Taylor, 1976). That article presented one man's first person account of being defined as mentally retarded. We received mixed reactions from that article. Some reviewers and colleagues praised the article for revealing how a retarded person views himself and his experiences in the world. Others, ignoring the thrust of our article, questioned whether we had in fact merely presented the story of an unfortunate young man who happened to have been misdiagnosed as mentally retarded. And still others, while commenting that the article made for interesting reading, regarded our work as somehow less than scientific or rigorous. "Real" research, these commentators stated, involves large samples, precise sampling strategies, measurement devices, and statistical analysis. What these latter colleagues failed to understand was that, regardless of the merits of that particular article, our research was based on a long-standing and widely used sociological and anthropological approach known as qualitative research methods.

The origins of qualitative research can be traced to the 19th and early 20th centuries when field research came into its own in European and American anthropology. Presumably, anthropologists, unlike most other researchers, were unable to use methods such as demographic analysis and survey questionnaires to study so-called primitive societies. Further, they were unfamiliar with the everyday lives of the people they wished to study and therefore could not take anything for granted in their research.

The use of qualitative methods first became popular in American sociology in the studies of the "Chicago School" some time after the turn of the century. While interest in qualitative research waned throughout the 1940's and 1950's with the growth in prominence of quantitative methods, the 1960's and 1970's have witnessed a reemergence in the use of qualitative methods. The number of published studies based on these methods has steadily increased, and there are now volumes of collected essays (Filstead, 1970; McCall & Simmons, 1969) and monographs (Bogdan & Taylor, 1975; Bruyn, 1966; Glaser & Strauss, 1967) on how to collect and interpret qualitative data. And in the field of mental retardation, the qualitative studies of Edgerton (1967), Edgerton and Bercovici (1976), and Goffman (1961, 1963) have become widely known and respected.

Yet there remains widespread misunderstanding of qualitative research methods. As Rist (1977) notes, quantitative methods are more widely published, taught, accepted, and rewarded in research circles and are generally equated with the "scientific method." For this reason, as suggested above, there has been a tendency to judge qualitative studies by the same criteria used to judge quantitative studies. Many researchers view methods such as participant observation, indepth interviewing, and analysis of personal documents from a vantage point reflecting their training in statistics and formal research design. These researchers may raise criticisms which are difficult for qualitative researchers to answer, simply because the criticisms revolve around standards which qualitative researchers do not apply to their efforts.

In this paper, we address the applicability of qualitative research methods to the study of community adjustment, or more precisely the experience of persons leaving public institutions for the mentally retarded, and answer some of the questions commonly directed toward qualitative research. The next section offers a brief description of qualitative methods and deals with conceptual issues related to the study of community adjustment. Then we discuss the issues of validity, reliability, subjectivity, generalizability, and methodology, respectively. The concluding section of this paper presents some suggested qualitative studies in the field of mental retardation and deinstitutionalization.

Qualitative Research and Community Experience

As in any school of thought, different qualitative researchers define qualitative research differently. Some associate qualitative research with specific research tools such as participant observation, indepth interviewing, and analysis of personal documents. *Participant observation* refers to research characterized by a period of social interaction between the researcher and subjects, in the milieu of the latter, during which data are unobtrusively and systematically collected. *Indepth interviewing* refers to intensive unstructured interviewing in which the subject provides a first-person account of the whole or part of his or her life, or the subject's reflection on a specific event or topic. *Personal documents* are materials in which people reveal in their own words their views of their lives or a part of them, or some other aspect about themselves. Diaries are the most commonly studied type of personal documents. For us, qualitative research is not a set of tools or specific research procedures, but rather a general approach to and way of thinking about the empirical world. Thus, while we have used the specific methods of participant observation, indepth interviewing, and document analysis in our own research, qualitative research is not defined by these tools.

Qualitative research may be characterized as inductive, holistic, and oriented to people's subjective experience. By *inductive,* we mean that qualitative researchers develop their concepts and analytical categories from the data themselves, rather than from preconceived, structured operational definitions (Filstead, 1970). In qualitative studies, researchers follow a flexible and open-ended research design. They begin their studies with only vaguely formulated research questions and, indeed, may even attempt to suspend or "bracket" their assumptions and common sense understandings about the subject matter of inquiry. For example, Goffman (1961), in his classic study *Asylums,* developed the concept of "total institutions" to describe such seemingly disparate settings as mental hospitals, monasteries, concentration camps, and boarding schools. In effect, Goffman had to suspend what he already "knew" about these settings (i.e., that they are dramatically different) in order to reveal their common elements.

Whether or not persons released from public institutions for the mentally retarded have been integrated into the community is a matter to be investigated and not assumed. We cannot assume that we are studying the community experiences of the mentally retarded when we study settings referred to as "group homes," "halfway houses," "board and care homes," and "community-based facilities." Bercovici's research and our own experience indicate that many deinstitutionalized persons have simply been transferred from one form of total institution to another. Bercovici (this volume) writes, ". . . many dehospitalized mentally retarded persons are not, and do not perceive themselves to be, living in the normal community, contrary to the assumptions that are generally held." In short, the researcher who predefines community according to administrative categories may not be studying the community at all. The qualitative researcher avoids this pitfall by setting aside preconceptions and relying on careful description and inductive analysis.

Quantitative analysis may be characterized as component analysis; qualitative analysis may be characterized as holistic analysis. In qualitative research, the subject of the study is not reduced to variables or isolated components, but is viewed instead as part of a whole. The qualitative researcher studies subjects in the context of their past and the situations in which they find themselves.

Operational definitions of community adjustment based on a specific variable or set of variables are bound to be arbitrary and misleading. Researchers have defined and measured community adjustment in terms of the individual's happiness, return or non-return to the institution (Gollay, 1977), adaptive behavior (Taylor, 1976), and staff accounts of the individual's adjustment (Nihira & Nihira, 1975). Each of these definitions can be shown to be misleading, simply because it reduces a complex process into a one-sided variable. Happiness is an illusive concept for which we lack an appropriate standard (Is anyone happy?). Further, retarded persons, for a host of understandable reasons, tend to give overly positive evaluations of their caretakers and facilities (Taylor, 1977; Bercovici, this volume). One's tenure in the community—return or non-return to the institution—may have nothing to do with an individual's adjustment, but may be governed by a set of contingencies beyond the individual's control—the financial situation of the caretaker, licensing procedures, availability of day programs, institutional policies, and so on. Adaptive behavior may or may not signify adjustment to community living and normal routines and rhythms of life. As Goffman (1961) very clearly demonstrates, some behaviors which are considered strange or abnormal in the wider society represent *successful* adjustment to life in total institutions. Thus, the skills required for successful adjustment in some nonpublic institutions may be inconsistent with those generally associated with adaptive behavior. Similarly, staff accounts of a person's adjustment may measure nothing more than the person's conformity to facility practices and routines—whatever these happen to be.

The qualitative researcher studies the individual's experiences in everyday situations to learn how he or she is adjusting in life outside of the public institution. In our interviews with Ed Murphy, a 26-year-old former institution resident, he related a story of going to the movies on a date. He described his nervousness and his inept handling of tickets. His story revealed the obvious—people do not learn how to act at movie theaters in institutions. New experiences are always difficult. By observing and listening to the experiences of formerly institutionalized persons, we learn about the process of adjusting to life in the community.

Central to qualitative research, as we define it, is an interest in people's own views and perspectives on their lives. The qualitative researcher views human behavior—what people say and do—as a product of how people interpret their world. The task of the qualitative researcher is to capture this process of interpretation. This requires what Weber (1968) called *verstehen*—empathetic understanding or the ability to reproduce in one's own mind the feelings, motives, and thoughts behind the actions of others. In order to grasp the meanings of a person's behavior, one must attempt to view things from that person's point of view.

Any behavior is understandable when viewed from the person's frame of reference (Goffman, 1961). Our assumption is that people's subjective states—feelings, motives, perspectives, definitions—guide their behavior. Just because people's subjective states may not be directly accessible to us—as in the case of non-verbal retarded persons, this does not mean that they have no subjective states.

One aspect of our work that differentiates it from most other research in mental retardation is that we do not assume that mental retardation exists. That is to say, mental retardation is a social construction, metaphor, and administrative category. The retarded person plays a social role determined by societal beliefs and stereotypes. While the *concept* of mental retardation may be useful for certain purposes, it can erect a barrier to understanding how persons experience their world. For example, if one views mental retardation as a pathological condition, one will interpret behavior such as rocking and headbanging as inherent in mental retardation rather than as a natural and normal response to certain kinds of environments. Thus, we suspend our *beliefs* about mental retardation to better understand the retarded person.

Validity

The term "validity" means the general correspondence between what the researcher intends to study and what he or she actually studies. When quantitative researchers speak of validity, they usually mean the fit between their concepts, such as intelligence, and their indicators, such as IQ. When qualitative researchers speak of validity, they have in mind the meaningfulness of their research; that is, the fit between their findings and what actually happens in the world. Quantitative researchers have tended to emphasize reliability, or consistency and replicability, in their studies while qualitative researchers have emphasized validity, or meaningfulness, in their research.

For qualitative researchers, the validity of a study depends on whether the researcher has utilized methods which provide first-hand knowledge of the phenomenon under inquiry as it exists in the world. If researchers wish to study validly the empirical world, they must observe directly the empirical world in such a way that does not alter the nature of that world. One's study is valid to the extent that one has examined how people think and act in the settings and situations in which they normally find themselves.

Qualitative researchers are aware that they may have untoward effects on their subjects by virtue of their presence, but they attempt to minimize or control these effects. In their studies, qualitative researchers interact with subjects in a natural, unobtrusive, and nonthreatening manner. As Jack Douglas (1976) argues, the more controlled and obtrusive one's research, the greater the likelihood that one will end up studying the effects of one's own methods. Since participant observers are interested in how people act and think in their own settings, they attempt to "blend into the woodwork," or to act in a way such that the activities which occur in their presence do not differ significantly from those that occur in their absence. Similarly, since interviewers in this type of research are interested in how people think about their lives, experiences, and situations, they model their interviews after a conversation rather than a formal question and answer session between a researcher and a respondent.

Researchers can never eliminate all their effects on subjects. They can, however, understand their effects on subjects through an intimate knowledge of a setting and use this understanding to generate additional insights into the nature of social life. Deutscher (1973) advises researchers to "discount" their data, that is, to interpret them in context. One often finds that subjects attempt to manage one's impressions of them and their activities, especially during the initial stages of the research (cf. Douglas, 1976). In a study of a "state school" for the mentally retarded, for example, one of the authors found that attendants routinely evade, lie to, and misinform researchers, outsiders, and even supervisors (Taylor, 1977). One can use such knowledge of how subjects react to outsiders to develop new understandings of settings and the people within them. In their reaction to outsiders, people reveal as much as in their reactions to insiders, provided, of course, one knows the difference.

Reliability

In quantitative research, reliability refers to the consistency of results produced by observations made by different researchers or the same researcher over time. Some qualitative researchers claim validity on their side but apologize for the limited reliability of their studies. Others reject reliability as a meaningful standard by which to judge research. Still others, while they admit the importance of reliability, believe that the concept has been overemphasized in social science research. Deutscher (1973), for instance, writes, "We concentrate on consistency without much concern about whether we are consistently right or wrong. As a consequence we may have been learning a great deal about how to pursue an incorrect course with a maximum of precision" (p. 41).

Since researchers vary according to their backgrounds and interests, it should not be surprising that different researchers studying the same settings and subjects might produce different, though not necessarily inaccurate or contradictory findings. Researchers may vary widely according to their academic or professional fields—psychology, sociology, medicine, social work, special education, and so on. One's discipline and training necessarily relate to the questions one brings to an area of study. In a study of a group home, for example, the social worker or planner might be interested in the setting's financial and administrative arrangements; the clinician might direct attention to programmatic aspects of the home; the sociologist might wish to study the social structure of the home or the stigma experienced by the residents in interacting with the local community. Social workers, clinicians, and sociologists will pursue their interests in different ways, spending more time in some places than others or speaking more with certain persons than others. They will collect different types of data and reach different conclusions. Similarly, one's theoretical perspective within a given field will structure one's study. Two researchers studying a single setting may come up with different data and produce different findings, with both studies being reliable. One would only question the reliability of one or both studies if they yielded incompatible results.

One should also not be surprised to find that a single researcher may obtain different or even contradictory data at different times. Some attribute changes in a researcher's observations over time to the unreliability of that researcher's procedures. Most qualitative researchers, in contrast, assume that since people may say and do different things at different times and in different situations, it is only natural for the researcher to obtain apparently contradictory data. As indicated, qualitative researchers direct their attention to the contexts in which data are collected. What first appears inconsistent may not be inconsistent at all when viewed in context. In the institutional study mentioned earlier, the observer found that attendants offer contradictory views on the intellectual capacities of the residents under their charge. For instance, one attendant stated on one occasion, "They're not as dumb as they look," and on another, "These here are all low grades." The observer learned over time that attendants emphasized residents' deficiencies when they were called upon to provide them with training or therapy, but that they deemphasized these deficiencies when they were called on to justify their punishment of residents (e.g., "They know better than to do something like that."). Contradictions often disappear when data are examined in the proper context.

In qualitative studies, researchers are concerned with the accuracy and comprehensiveness of their observations and interviews. Qualitative researchers tend to view reliability as the fit between what they record as data and what actually occurs in the setting under study, rather than the literal consistency of different observations. Qualitative researchers attempt to record everything that occurs during an interview or observation session. In participant observation, researchers complete detailed field notes after every encounter with subjects. Observers often record as many as thirty pages of field notes for a single hour of observation. In short, a qualitative study is based not on off-the-cuff impressions or shorthand summaries of observation sessions, but on an indepth analysis of meticulously recorded and detailed field notes or interview transcripts.

Qualitative researchers may also conduct their research in teams as opposed to total isolation. In many studies, qualitative researchers rely on others to read their field notes, interview transcripts, or other types of data and to provide them with feedback on the comprehensiveness and accuracy of what they have recorded. Douglas (1976) advocates team research as a replacement to the "lone ranger approach" as a way of "keeping the research honest" or providing a check on the researcher's objectivity. When qualitative researchers do not work in teams, they typically have a colleague or mentor read through and critique their materials and data.

Subjectivity

In qualitative studies, researchers are usually interested in understanding people's subjective states, what are referred to as their perspectives, world views, cognitive maps, common sense understandings, definitions of the situation, and so on. Those who are new to qualitative methods often confuse the researcher's interest in people's subjective states with the researcher's own subjectivity or bias. Some, in fact, question the ability of the qualitative researcher to be objective in the field.

As noted, qualitative researchers guard against their own bias by recording detailed field notes and sometimes by working in teams. There are other ways in which these researchers attempt to control their own preconceived notions and subjective bias. For one, qualitative researchers go out of their way to record their own personal feelings, prejudices, evaluations, and even hypotheses. Participant observers, in their field notes, often use the notation "O.C." for "Observer's Comment" to distinguish their evaluations and interpretations from descriptive data. Similarly, in other types of qualitative studies, researchers typically maintain a log of their impressions, ideas, and feelings. As their studies progress, qualitative researchers refer back to these comments to examine whether they have merely seen what they wanted to see. During their analysis, qualitative researchers constantly hold up their hypotheses and ideas to their data in an effort to check their own subjectivity. Some even conduct frequency counts of data bearing on their hypotheses to provide evidence for their conclusions (cf. Becker, Geer, & Hughes, 1968).

Qualitative researchers also examine their own subjective states as a source of understanding the setting and subjects under study. In a sense, the participant observer or open-ended interviewer treats himself or herself as one of the subjects of the study. The researcher is a carrier of the culture of which he or she is a part. Through a critical examination of one's own perspective, one often obtains insights into the perspectives of others. For example, one may reflect on one's own stereotypes of the mentally retarded as a way of understanding others' stereotypes.

Qualitative researchers, since they generally participate in the setting under study, often find themselves in the same situations as their subjects. In the state school study, the observer found himself avoiding interaction with residents who were covered with food or excrement during his observations. This provided insights into attendants' perspectives on and interaction with the residents under their care. In qualitative research, then, one forces oneself to examine critically one's own subjective views, both as a means of controlling one's bias and of achieving a better understanding of the subject matter under inquiry.

Generalizability

Social scientists are concerned with the generalizability of their research findings beyond their specific research subjects and settings. In traditional studies, researchers employ standardized selection procedures designed to assure the representativeness of the populations under study. In qualitative studies, however, researchers generally choose their subjects on the basis of availability or their own specific interests. They seldom use random or stratified sampling techniques. In fact, many qualitative studies are case studies; researchers confine themselves to one or a small number of settings and subjects.

Some qualitative researchers lament the limited representativeness of their study populations. They would prefer to work from a larger and more representative data base, but simply lack the time and resources to conduct an indepth study of more than a few subjects. These researchers reluctantly sacrifice breadth for depth, in other words, representative findings for a detailed understanding of a single set of research subjects. They may be willing to make this sacrifice because they view their studies as a first in an area.

Many qualitative researchers hold up their studies as exploratory in nature. They regard the question of generalizability as one to be answered by other studies. They make no claims of representativeness or generalizability. These researchers may also cite other evidence to demonstrate the generalizability of their findings. For instance, they may draw on other studies to expand their findings or they may conduct a larger number of less intense mini-studies to show the non-idiosyncratic nature of their work.

Other qualitative researchers are less bothered by the apparent unrepresentativeness of their study samples. These researchers may attempt to formulate universal statements which apply to all of their subjects. For instance, in a study of ex-residents of public institutions, the researcher might look for common adjustment problems confronting all of the people. Edgerton (1967) used the concept of stigma to describe the problem faced by all retarded persons in managing relations with others.

Qualitative researchers sometimes employ a conscious procedure called analytic induction in their quest to identify universal patterns and processes in their data (cf. Becker, 1963; McCall & Simmons, 1969; Robinson, 1951; Turner, 1953). Becker (1963) used an approach similar to analytic induction in his classic study of marijuana smokers based on open-ended interviews. Becker's study began with indepth interviews among the small number of marijuana smokers. As his study progressed, he began to develop a theory of how or the process by which people become marijuana smokers. As he continued his interviews, he modified his theory to fit each and every new case, refining the details of the process along the way. Becker proceeded in this manner until he no longer came across cases which his theory did not fit. At the conclusion of his study, Becker had identified the essential steps in becoming a marijuana user. In using analytic induction, researchers generally choose subjects in such a way as to maximize the variation in their samples. Throughout one's research, one looks for subjects who are different from those one has already interviewed or observed in an effort to cover all sectors of a population. This procedure enables researchers to identify universal patterns among their subjects or, where appropriate, typologies reflecting the range of differences among them.

Finally, still other qualitative social scientists approach the issue of generalizability from a point of view reflecting their interest in understanding general social processes as opposed to a predefined substantive type of setting (e.g., an institution or group home). These researchers start with the assumption that human behavior is not simply random or idiosyncratic. They therefore concern themselves not with the question of whether their findings are generalizable, but rather the question of to what other settings and subjects are they generalizable. Goffman's (1961) *Asylums* was based on a first-hand study of a single type of setting—mental hospital. Yet Goffman generalized his findings to apply to a broader type of settings—total institutions. Similarly, findings of studies of various kinds of group living situations—communes, fraternities, sororities—may lend insight into the nature of group homes for the retarded. Or studies of any people adjusting to new situations—people living in a foreign country, ex-prisoners of war returning home, or prison inmates released on parole—may be generalizable to persons released from institutions for the retarded. According to some qualitative researchers, every subject or setting is a laboratory in which some general aspect of human behavior can best be studied because there it is best illuminated. Since the researcher cannot always, if ever, determine which aspect of human behavior will appear in bold relief in a setting before the study, he or she leaves open the question of generalizability until the latter stages of research.

Some qualitative researchers use a sample selection logic designed to examine whether and to what extent findings revealed in one type of setting apply to other types of setting. Glaser and Strauss (1967) use the phrase "theoretical sampling" to refer to a procedure whereby researchers consciously attempt to develop, refine, and expand theory and concepts by juxtaposing different types of settings. Through this procedure, researchers seek not to test their findings, but to broaden their applicability. These researchers select their subjects and settings on the basis of whether these subjects and settings will yield additional insights into the phenomena under consideration.

Methodology

Quantitative approaches to data collection and analysis have become standardized to a large extent. Instruments have been developed; analytical procedures refined; computer programs written; and conventions established. At most universities, texts and course sequences guide the novice through the steps of becoming a quantitative researcher. In qualitative research, approaches and procedures have not become standardized. On the contrary, most field workers learn their methods through an apprenticeship relationship with an experienced researcher. Theirs has been an oral tradition.

As stated in a preceding section, a qualitative study is not an impressionistic, off-the-cuff analysis of a setting or subjects based on a few visits or interviews. It is a careful piece of systematic research conducted with demanding, though not necessarily highly standardized, procedures. Most qualitative researchers spend a year or more in the field. Increasingly, field workers are being trained in graduate seminars. As qualitative methods become more accepted in universities, the oral tradition is being captured and recorded in written form. The number of texts and readers on qualitative methods has rapidly increased over the past decade (Bogdan & Taylor, 1975; McCall & Simmons, 1969; Schatzman & Strauss, 1973). Over the past few years, several qualitative researchers have published manuscripts which challenge the traditional assumptions and methods of field workers (Douglas, 1976; Johnson, 1975).

To reiterate, qualitative methods have not been as refined and systematized as other research approaches. This is in part an historical artifact which is changing and in part a reflection of the nature of the methods themselves. Qualitative researchers place an emphasis on openness and flexibility in their research design. The researcher is modeled after a craftsperson. There are guidelines to be followed but not rules. The methods serve the researcher.

There are universal criteria for judging any piece of research. They are rooted in the conventions that define science. In qualitative methods, as in quantitative, good research is judged by the extent to which it represents a disciplined inquiry into the phenomenon under consideration, that is, the extent to which it is guided by a theoretical perspective, a set of explicit assumptions about the empirical world, and rigorous procedures. While qualitative procedures have not been standardized, qualitative studies, like other studies, can be judged by the way they have been conducted and by the use of findings they produce.

Suggested Areas Of Research

Thus far in this paper we have provided an overview of a qualitative approach to studying people released from institutions for the retarded. We have also discussed how qualitative researchers think about validity, reliability, subjectivity, generalizability, and methodology. We conclude with a discussion of potentially fruitful areas of research on community adjustment.

Edgerton and his colleagues began an important trend in research by attempting to capture the day-to-day experiences of people leaving institutions. We definitely need many more studies of this type. We do not have a wealth of good qualitative research on the lives of ex-institutionalized persons. Further, Edgerton's research did not examine the range of living arrangements among retarded persons outside the institution. Nor did Edgerton devote attention to young persons or to persons labeled severely and profoundly retarded or multiply disabled.

Clearly, we need more indepth accounts and life histories of retarded people as they experience the world and try to make sense out of that experience. We must also enlarge the range of people we study to include the young and the old, minority group members, and the more severely disabled. In regard to this latter group, we must be rigorous in our attempts to develop techniques to understand the subjective states of those we have traditionally considered as being impossible to understand. If we have not understood the severely disabled person, it is because we have not really attempted to do so. The problem is ours and not theirs.

There is also a need to study the different circumstances under which retarded people live. We need to study various living units, their structures and their distinctive cultures (Bercovici, this volume). We must be imaginative in how we conceptualize these studies. Thus, researchers should not only try to understand how community settings are different from institutions but also how they compare to normal settings like boarding homes, fraternity houses, communes, and families. We need to develop more precise and sophisticated concepts than "group home" and "institution."

Too much of the research on community adjustment has focused on the retarded person to the exclusion of others in the situation. A qualitative approach directs attention to the need to study settings and subjects holistically. We know relatively little about the staff of community settings and professionals in the community. How do they define their work? How do they see the retarded? How do they interact with their clients? Similarly, we have little understanding of how others—relatives, neighbors, shopkeepers, the police, and generic service providers—think about and interact with persons defined as retarded.

Other research challenges involve the level on which we study community adjustment and deinstitutionalization. Deinstitutionalization is a social phenomenon involving the government at all levels, the judicial system, the economic system, and the mass media. These "institutions" are as much a proper focus of deinstitutionalization research as the individual retarded person. Through qualitative research, we can study the legal and legislative process, we can carefully observe decision-making and the influence of various groups on the political process. By studying the media, we can understand how stereotypes about the retarded and other persons with disabilities are transmitted to and shape the opinion of the general public.

Finally, as researchers, we must study ourselves—our beliefs, prejudices, and assumptions. We must begin to view ourselves as carriers of our common culture and attempt to transcend the conceptual schemes and world views that prevent us from understanding the world of previously institutionalized persons—as they experience it.

We do not mean to suggest that qualitative research is the only way to study community adjustment and deinstitutionalization. Every research approach has its strengths and its weaknesses. And every research approach does well by its own standards of judgment and poorly by the standards of judgment of others (Rist, 1977). Particular research approaches are best suited for particular research questions. Up until recently, researchers have not asked the kinds of questions which qualitative research can answer. It is time to fill in the gaps in our knowledge about persons defined as mentally retarded and their experiences in the world by asking new questions and adopting new research approaches.

References

Becker, H. S. *Outsiders*. New York: Free Press, 1963.

Becker, H. S., Geer, B., & Hughes, E. *Making the grade*. New York: Wiley, 1968.

Bogdan, R. & Taylor, S. *Introduction to qualitative research methods*. New York: John Wiley, 1975.

Bogdan, R. & Taylor, S. The judged, not the judges: An insider's view of mental retardation. *American Psychologist,* 1976, *31*(1), 47-52.

Bruyn, S. T. *The human perspective in sociology*. Englewood Cliffs, NJ: Prentice-Hall, 1966.

Deutscher, I. *What we say/what we do*. Glenview, IL: Scott, Foresman & Co., 1973.

Douglas, J. *Investigative social research*. Beverly Hills, CA: Sage Publications, 1976.

Edgerton, R. *The cloak of competence*. Berkeley: University of California Press, 1967.

Edgerton, R. & Bercovici, S. The cloak of competence: Years later. *American Journal of Mental Deficiency,* 1976, *80*(5), 485-97.

Filstead, W. (Ed.). *Qualitative methodology*. Chicago: Markham, 1970.

Glaser, R. & Strauss, A. *The discovery of grounded theory*. Chicago: Aldine, 1967.

Goffman, E. *Asylums*. New York: Anchor Books, 1961.

Goffman, E. *Stigma*. Englewood Cliffs, NJ: Prentice-Hall, 1963.

Gollay, E. Deinstitutionalized mentally retarded people: A closer look. *Education and Training of the Mentally Retarded,* 1977, *12,* 137-144.

Johnson, J. *Doing field research*. New York: Free Press, 1975.

Lofland, J. *Analyzing social settings*. Belmont, CA: Wadsworth, 1973.

McCall, G. & Simmons, J. (Eds.). *Issues in participant observation*. Reading, PA: Addison-Wesley, 1969.

Nihara, L. & Nihira, K. Normalized behavior in community placement. *Mental Retardation,* 1975, *13*(2), 9-13.

Rist, R. On the relations among educational research paradigm: From disdain to detente. *Anthropology and Education,* 1977, *8*(2), 42-50.

Robinson, W. S. The logical structure of analytic induction. *American Sociological Review,* 1951, *16,* 812-818.

Schatzman, L. & Strauss, A. *Field research*. Englewood Cliffs, NJ: Prentice-Hall, 1973.

Taylor, J. R. Comparison of the adaptive behavior of retarded individuals successfully and unsuccessfully placed in group living homes. *Journal of Special Education for the Mentally Retarded,* 1976, *11,* 56-64.

Taylor, S. J. The custodians: Attendants and their work at state institutions for the mentally retarded. Unpublished doctoral dissertation, Syracuse University, 1977.

Turner, R. H. The quest for universals in sociological research. *American Sociological Review,* 1953, *18,* 604-611.

Weber, M. *Economy and society* (G. Roth & C. Wittich, Eds.). New York: Bedminster, 1968.

Community Adaptation and the Impact of Deinstitutionalization

Marsha Mailick Seltzer
Boston University

Clarence C. Sherwood
Boston University

Gary B. Seltzer
Pawtucket Memorial Hospital

Sylvia Sherwood
Hebrew Rehabilitation Center for Aged

A large body of literature is available that focuses on the assessment of the community adaptation of retarded adults following their deinstitutionalization. (For reviews of this literature, see Gollay & Friedman, 1966; Jones & Jones, 1976; McCarver & Craig, 1974; Seltzer & Seltzer, 1978.) While this body of literature has made an important contribution to the description of the functional performance of deinstitutionalized retarded persons, it is believed that a reconceptualization of the concept of ''adaptation'' can add considerably to the field, both through a reinterpretation of findings from previous studies and from the kind of crucial knowledge that can be gained from future studies. Specifically, the purpose of this paper is to present an expanded and somewhat new conceptualization of community adaptation in the context of a research methodology that provides a basis for the investigation of the causal relationship between deinstitutionalization and community adaptation.

Briefly, this new conceptualization of community adaptation has three important features. First, adaptation is broader than just the performance of activities of daily living. Because adaptation connotes complex behavioral components, the definition of adaptation being suggested here also includes as integral components the measurement of behavior problems and the extent to which the person under study is satisfied with his or her community lifestyle. Second, as defined here, the concept of adaptation is not synonymous with ''normal behavior.'' From this perspective, a retarded person does not have to behave in a ''normal'' way in order to be seen as having adapted to some degree to community life. Instead, adaptation is defined in terms of the extent to which a person has made *improvements* in his or her behavior, that the behavior is closer to normal than it was. Third, because the concept of adaptation implies the behavior of a person in an environmental context, adaptation is not viewed exclusively in terms of the behavior of the retarded person. Instead, the person's behavior should be assessed in the context of the environment in which the person functions. The person adapts to something; behavior does not occur in an environmental vacuum.

The Measurement of Community Adaptation

As discussed above, adaptation should consist of improvements in a variety of complex behavioral areas, and as such, the range of the behaviors included for measurement should be comprehensive. At a minimum, community adaptation should consist of improvements in the following three dimensions. First, community adaptation should consist of improvements in clients' *performance of community living skills*, such as self-help, housekeeping, cooking, shopping skills. It is this aspect that is most commonly included in conceptualizations of community adaptation. Second, reductions in *behavior problems* should be seen as evidence of community adaptation. As a retarded individual becomes less self-abusive, displays less stereotypic behavior, is less aggressive, and his/her behavior becomes more socially appropriate, this person is seen as better adapted. Finally, it is insufficient to conclude that community adaptation consists only of improved performance of community living skills and reduced behavior problems. Also important is the extent to which the individual is more *satisfied with his or her lifestyle in the community* than in the institution with respect to many aspects, including the physical environment, social relationships, degree of autonomy. Thus, an individual can be said to have adapted to the extent that he or she improves in performance, manifests fewer behavior problems, and/or increases in satisfaction. The importance of viewing adaptation as improvement in functioning is further discussed below.

Community Adaptation as Improved Functioning

Past conceptualizations of community adaptation have used "normal" functioning as a standard against which to assess the adaptation of retarded persons. Those individuals who do not function "normally" are not considered to be adaptive. This perspective equates skill performance with adaptation and results in the inevitable rating of nearly all persons diagnosed as severely and profoundly retarded as not adaptive, given their poor performance of skills. Since the deinstitutionalized populations of the present—and even more so of the future—consist of more individuals who are severely retarded and multiply handicapped than in the past, it is highly probable that the measure of adaptive behavior most commonly used will assess them to be non-adaptive, irrespective of any improvements they might make in their performance.

The conceptualization of community adaptation as improved functioning, along with an associated measurement strategy, has several important features. First, it begins with a rejection of the approach of evaluating a retarded person's performance in relation to non-retarded performance and is committed to enabling a severely or profoundly retarded person to be considered adaptive even though his or her skills are limited. Second, it involves the repeated measurement of community living skills, behavior problems, and satisfaction. A person is adaptive to the extent to which his or her behavior improves over time.[1] Level of performance is too redundant with level of retardation to be of real interest, especially with severely and profoundly retarded individuals. It is not the absolute level of a person's performance at any one point in time that should be of interest, but rather the extent to which a person makes improvements over time. In this way, a severely retarded person who increases his or her level of performance over time is considered to be adapting to the community more favorably than is a mildly retarded person who makes no improvements whatsoever. Although the mildly retarded person's absolute level of performance is higher, the extent of improvement displayed by the severely retarded person is considered in the proposed conceptualization to be more adaptive.

To summarize, the proposed conceptual and operational definitions of community adaptation center around the notion of *improved not absolute* level of performance, which will make it possible for individuals who function on all levels

[1]Methodologically sound techniques of estimating improvements are proposed below (see footnote 3).

of retardation to be considered adaptive. As such, this strategy calls for prospective studies, in which individuals are assessed repeatedly at regular intervals, with improvement (or the lack of it) being observed over time; this model of repeated assessment is proposed to replace both retrospective analyses and one-shot assessments, neither of which is satisfactorily reliable or valid.

Community Adaptation in an Environmental Context: The Impact of Deinstitutionalization on Community Adaptation

The model presented above for assessing community adaptation can profitably be used in the investigation of the impact of deinstitutionalization on community adaptation. Such research would require that behavioral ability, maladaptive behaviors and personal satisfaction be measured prior to deinstitutionalization and again following some period of residence outside the institution. Deinstitutionalization can be said to have an impact to the extent that community adaptation is found to be a *consequence* of the move from one environment to another (from the institutional setting to the community residence). In this way, community adaptation can be investigated with respect to an environmental context. In order to legitimately substantiate an hypothesized causal relationship between deinstitutionalization (change in environment) and community adaptation, methodologies must be developed that directly investigate the impact of the deinstitutionalization program.

The impact of deinstitutionalization can be defined as being the difference between how the deinstitutionalized clients have fared in the community and *how they would have fared at that same point in time* had they remained in the institution. Unfortunately, even the more sophisticated projects which have studied the deinstitutionalization of retarded persons have generally taken the form of follow-up investigations rather than impact research. Changes in clients are traced (often retrospectively), but there is little effort to provide "controlled" comparisons. However, *changes over time, even when measured prospectively, are not synonymous with impact*. In order to draw conclusions about impact one must first have a basis to say that the observed changes *would not have taken place* without the particular intervention (in this case, movement from an institution to a community living arrangement).

The quality of the research on deinstitutionalization and the number of alternative community-based programs have grown considerably over the past six or seven years, but as yet, no research has investigated the impact of deinstitutionalization. In the early 1970s, program descriptions were published that described a single group home or deinstitutionalization program. By the mid-1970s, more systematic investigations were completed in which community residences were described empirically and classified according to a multi-dimensional taxonomic system (Baker, Seltzer & Seltzer, 1977). More recently, a number of investigations have followed-up deinstitutionalized persons and described their lifestyle in community living arrangements (Gollay & Friedman, 1976; Jones & Jones, 1976; Seltzer & Seltzer, 1978). These studies have demonstrated that it is possible for deinstitutionalized retarded persons to "make it" in a community setting. This, by itself, is an important finding. However, since deinstitutionalization has not, to date, been studied within an impact model design, it is not known to what extent deinstitutionalization affects the behavior patterns and life satisfaction of those persons who are returned to life in a community setting.[2] There have been

[2]Perhaps of greater importance, we have no knowledge concerning which types of community environment best meet the needs of different types of individuals. A discussion of a model for the investigation of this very important issue is presented below.

descriptive research and clinical support for the idea that deinstitutionalization makes a difference; it is now time to conduct impact evaluation to investigate whether or not deinstitutionalization results in improved community adaptation.

It is important to re-emphasize that changed behavior in clients alone is not evidence of the impact of deinstitutionalization; it must be demonstrated that the change in behavior was *caused* by the change in environment before it is possible to say that deinstitutionalization has had an impact. Some change in behavior will occur naturally over time as individuals develop and mature; thus, change should not be confused with impact. In fact, *no change* may someday be shown to be a positive result of deinstitutionalization. For example, it is possible for deinstitutionalization to enable persons to sustain skills already learned that would have deteriorated had they remained in the institutional setting. If it were established that there is behavioral regression associated with being placed in an institution and that such a regression did not take place or was arrested by a community placement, there would be reason to conclude that deinstitutionalization had an impact on the clients even though no improvements occurred in their behavior. The central methodological issue, then, is how one estimates what the behavior of the deinstitutionalized clients would have been had they remained in the institution.[3] This has not yet been attempted with respect to the deinstitutionalization of retarded persons.

Deinstitutionalization can thus have an impact on clients who do not adapt; clients who deteriorate *less* as a result of deinstitutionalization are evidence of the impact of that intervention at the same time that these clients do not make any improvements at all.

Although the position taken in this paper is that the impact of deinstitutionalization should be investigated rather than assumed, there is *no* implication intended that if research indicates deinstitutionalization has no impact that it should be discontinued. Deinstitutionalization is important and justifiable on humanitarian grounds alone. However, if deinstitutionalization is found not to have an impact on the clients' behavior, it is important that professionals refrain from asserting its value on programmatic grounds and instead advocate for its continuation on humanitarian grounds. If deinstitutionalization has no impact on a person's behavior, the person cannot be said to be better adapted; yet the quality of that person's life may still be improved, given the improved qualities of the environment, such as increased cleanliness and personalization, and stimulation. Furthermore, should research findings consistently show no impact, the need to focus on developing new forms of supportive community environments which might in fact result in positive impact would be highlighted.

To summarize, the investigation of the impact, or effect, of deinstitutionalization on the community adaptation of retarded persons can only be accomplished with controlled experimental methodology in which the post-release performance of the subjects is compared with estimates of what their performance would have

[3]One method of providing these estimates is by the use of a control group, that is, individuals who remain in the institution who are very similar to those who are deinstitutionalized. In order to control for threats to internal validity, the two groups must be as much alike as possible. The traditional and preferred method of generating equivalent groups is randomization (Campbell & Stanley, 1963). However, when randomization is not possible, an alternative procedure can be used that constructs statistically and clinically equivalent groups. The procedure was developed at the Department of Social Gerontological Research of the Hebrew Rehabilitation Center for Aged (HRCA) in Boston, Massachusetts. It has been applied and tested several times by HRCA and found to be successful (Sherwood, Greer, Morris, & Sherwood, 1973; Sherwood, Morris, & Sherwood, 1975; Sherwood, Greer, Morris, Mor, & Associates, 1978).

been had they remained in the institution. In the absence of such research, the effect of deinstitutionalization cannot be determined. As the populations being released from institutions increasingly consist of the "hard to place" (including retarded persons who are medically fragile, multiply handicapped or elderly, those with severe behavior problems, and the more severely and profoundly retarded), an analysis of the effect of deinstitutionalization on these types of individuals becomes more and more important. Because the needs presented by these types of persons are very complex, it cannot be casually assumed that deinstitutionalization will produce the uniformly positive effects hoped for; careful investigation of the impact of deinstitutionalization is, therefore, a political, ethical, and clinical necessity in the field of retardation at the present time.

The Impact of Differential Community Environments on Community Adaptation

As the trend toward deinstitutionalization has gained strength, there has been an increasing amount of interest focused on the community residential settings to which deinstitutionalized residents have moved. Descriptive and analytic discussions are available in the literature concerning community residential environments, the types of programs that have developed, and their distribution nationwide (Baker, Seltzer, & Seltzer, 1977; O'Connor, 1976). The literature is replete with ideological and theoretical discussions concerning the optimal structure and programmatic components of community residences (Fritz, Wolfensberger, & Knowlton, 1971; Wolfensberger, 1969, 1971, 1972; Wolfensberger & Glenn, 1975). The normalization principle has thus normatively guided the development of community residences, despite the fact that almost no data are available that indicate the effect of specific environmental features on residents. The few studies that have attempted to relate characteristics of the environment to client performance (e.g., Seltzer & Seltzer, 1978) generally find that better performing individuals tend to be found in the "better" community residence environments. The impact of the environment on the individual is one explanation for this finding. However, another plausible explanation is *selection* —better performing individuals are placed in better environments, and were probably performing better before the environment had the chance to make any impact on them. Thus, it would be a major error in interpretation to infer from these studies any knowledge about the *impact* of community residential environments on residents. If selection and other threats to internal validity are not controlled for by the study methodology, the question of whether the environment had an impact on the clients' performance—that is, whether their performance would be different if the environment were different—remains unanswered.

A major assumption guiding all deinstitutionalization efforts is that changes in released residents' community adaptation will be a consequence of the differences between their residential environments in the institution and their residential environments in the community. It is expected that the greater the difference between the institutional ward and the community residence, the greater will be the improvements made by residents with respect to their community adaptation. However, there are no data available to support this expectation. It is, therefore, proposed that future research on community adaptation include the experimental investigation of the assumption that the amount of change in community adaptation will be a direct function of the amount of environmental differences between the institution and community residence.

Furthermore, it is proposed here that a strategy for the assessment of environments be developed that would enable the environments to be rated individually for each person. Most measures of the environment (e.g., Wolfensberger & Glenn, 1975) are oriented to the fixed features of the environment; that is, the setting as a whole gets a single score. This assessment strategy assumes that all clients who live in a setting are affected by that environment in a uniform manner. Such an assumption is unrealistic, especially insofar as environments are intentionally designed to individualize the program for each client. Therefore, the strategy proposed here for the measurement of environments calls for individualized environmental assessment. With this approach it is theoretically possible to generate different environmental change scores for persons who move together from the same institutional ward to the same community residence since the features of the environment that are salient for one individual may be very different from those which are salient to another.

In the suggested analysis, the independent variable would be "degree of difference between the institutional ward environment and community residence environment" and the dependent variable would be "community adaptation." It is crucial that the individuals who are classified in the various levels of the independent variable are equivalent with respect to other variables in order to protect against threats to internal validity; this equivalence can be accomplished either by randomization or by alternative procedures, for example, through multivariate clustering. Subjects would be assessed with respect to the dependent variable at least twice, enabling the direct investigation of the assumption that changes in community adaptation are a function of changes in the environment.

Summary and Conclusions

In this discussion, a proposed model for future research on community adaptation was presented. It included the following key features:

1. The measurement of community adaptation not in relation to normal behavior but in terms of improvements made by retarded persons over time, thereby enabling even severely and profoundly retarded persons to be considered adaptive;
2. The use of multiple measures of community adaptation that could include in addition to performance of community living skills, assessment of reduction in clients' behavior problems, and measures of their feelings of satisfaction with their community lifestyles;
3. The use of individualized measures of the environment so that the environmental features salient for each person can be assessed; and
4. The use of impact methodology, in order to provide a methodologically sound understanding of the effects of deinstitutionalization and differential community environments on community adaptation.

In an era of shrinking economic resources, potential community backlash against community-based programs, and increased severity of the disability of the population receiving services, it seems crucial that the field of retardation directly investigate the basic assumptions that have guided the rapid development of innovative services that has occurred during the 1970s.

References

Baker, B. L., Seltzer, G. B., & Seltzer, M. M. *As close as possible: Community residences for retarded adults.* Boston: Little, Brown & Co., 1977.

Campbell, D. G. & Stanley, J. *Experimental and quasi-experimental designs for research.* Chicago: Rand McNally, 1963.

Fritz, M., Wolfensberger, W., & Knowlton, M. *An apartment living plan to promote integration and normalization of mentally retarded adults*. Downsview, Ontario: Canadian Association for the Mentally Retarded, 1971.

Gollay, E., & Friedman, R. *A study of the community adjustment of deinstitutionalized mentally retarded persons*. Cambridge, MA: Abt Associates, 1976.

Jones, K. J., & Jones, P. P. *The measurement of community placement success and its associated costs*. Waltham, MA: Brandeis University, 1976.

McCarver, R., & Craig, E. Placement of retarded in the community: Prognosis and outcome. In N. R. Ellis (Ed.), *International review of research in mental retardation* (Vol. 7). New York: Academic Press, 1974.

O'Connor, G. *Home is a good place: A national perspective of community residential facilities for developmentally disabled persons*. Washington, DC: American Association on Mental Deficiency, 1976.

Seltzer, M. M., & Seltzer, G. B. *Context for competence: A study of retarded adults living and working in the community*. Cambridge, MA: Educational Projects, Inc., 1978.

Sherwood, S., Greer, D. S., Morris, J. N., Mor, V., & Associates. *The Highland Heights story*. Boston: Hebrew Rehabilitation Center for Aged, 1978.

Sherwood, S., Greer, D. S., Morris, J. N., & Sherwood, C. C. *The Highland Heights experiment: A final report*. Washington, DC: U.S. Government Printing Office, 1973.

Sherwood, C. C., Morris, J. N., & Sherwood, S. A multivariate non-randomized matching technique for studying the impact of social interventions. In E. Struening & M. Guttentage (Eds.), *Handbook of evaluation research*. Berkeley, CA: Sage Publications, 1975.

Wolfensberger, W. A new approach to decision making in human management services. In R. B. Kugel & W. Wolfensberger (Eds.), *Changing patterns in residential services for the mentally retarded*. Washington, DC: President's Committee on Mental Retardation, 1969.

Wolfensberger, W. Will there always be an institution? II: The impact of new service models. *Mental Retardation*, 1971, *9*(6), 31-38.

Wolfensberger, W. *Normalization: The principle of normalization in human services*. Toronto: National Institute on Mental Retardation, 1972.

Wolfensberger, W., & Glenn, L. *PASS: A method for the quantitative evaluation of human services*. Toronto: National Institute on Mental Retardation, 1975.

Some Conceptual and Methodological Issues in Studying the Community Adjustment of Deinstitutionalized Mentally Retarded People

Elinor Gollay

Gollay Associates
Santa Fe, New Mexico

There are many lessons to be learned from conducting an extensive and complex research project, particularly when the research is largely exploratory in nature. Such a study was conducted by Abt Associates Inc., under contract to the Bureau of Education for the Handicapped, U.S. Office of Education. The primary purpose of the project was to identify those factors that affect the community adjustment of deinstitutionalized mentally retarded individuals. This research yielded numerous valuable results, many of which have been reported elsewhere and will not be repeated here.[1] In this paper two topics will be covered that have not been addressed as fully or explicitly elsewhere: first, some of the key findings reflecting the differences in the community experiences of individuals who are severely or profoundly retarded as compared with the experiences of less retarded individuals will be summarized; and second, some of the key conceptual and methodological issues that faced the project will be critically analyzed in order to point toward possible future directions for further research.

The project was divided into five major phases. The first phase involved conceptualizing the study, reviewing related literature, and designing the various data gathering instruments. Phase two involved sending a mail questionnaire to approximately 250 institutions known to serve mentally retarded persons to obtain information about their release patterns. During the next phase, ten institutions were selected for in-depth site visits. These institutions then became the ''releasing institutions'' for identifying the deinstitutionalized mentally retarded individuals who became the focus for the remainder of the study. During the next project phase interviews were conducted with 440 individuals. These individuals had been released from nine institutions in nine states spread across the country. The individuals had all lived in the institution for at least two years prior to their release, were generally between the ages of 6 and 40 at the time of their release, and had been released to a community setting rather than to another institutional setting (nursing homes were excluded). During the final phase of the project the data obtained were coded, computerized, and analyzed.

Data collection procedures for the deinstitutionalized individuals consisted of four main points: an interview with the ''family'' of the retarded persons (i.e., the residential caretaker—natural parents, foster parents, group home managers, semi-independent living supervisors, or other knowledgeable person for people

[1]See in particular *Coming back: The community experiences of deinstitutionalized mentally retarded people* (Cambridge; MA: Abt Publications, 1978). For more details about the project on which both the book and this paper are based, see the six volumes of the project final report, available from Bureau of Education for the Handicapped (Contract #OEC-0-74-9183).

living independently); an interview with the retarded person; the family respondent's scoring of the individual on the AAMD Adaptive Behavior Scale; and the interviewer's final comment sheet rating the environment and family qualities. In addition, some information was obtained on each person from institutional records.

The Community Experiences of Severely/Profoundly Retarded People

Previously, much of the information gathered in the Abt Associates study has been presented with particular emphasis on the differences between people who remained in the community and people who returned to the institution. This section, however, will focus on the key differences between the community experiences of people who were classified as having different degrees of retardation (mild, moderate, and severe/profound), and is based upon descriptive data collected in the study.

Characteristics of Severely Retarded People Entering the Community

The study obtained information on the level of retardation of 414 of the total 440 individuals in the sample. Of this group, approximately 41% were mildly retarded. In general the more seriously retarded people were younger and were more likely to have disabilities in addition to their retardation. These characteristics of the sample are shown in Tables 1, 2 and 3.

Table 1

Age and Level of Retardation

Age	Level of Retardation							
	Mild		Moderate		Severe		Total	
	N (169)	%	N (134)	%	N (106)	%	N (409)	%
Children	23	14	20	15	31	29	74	18
Adults	146	86	114	85	75	71	335	82

Note: All tables from *Coming back* by E. Gollay, R. Freedman, M. Wyngaarden & N. R. Kurtz (Cambridge, MA: Abt Publications, 1978). Reprinted by permission.

Table 2

Number of Additional Disabilities by Level of Retardation

	Level of Retardation							
Number of	Mild		Moderate		Severe		Total	
Disabilities	N (171)	%	N (137)	%	N (106)	%	N (414)	%
None	78	46	65	47	31	29	174	42
One or more	93	54	72	53	75	71	240	58

Table 3
Type of Additional Disability by Level of Retardation

Type of Disability	Mild N (171)	%	Moderate N (137)	%	Severe N (106)	%	Total N (414)	%
Blindness	12	7	7	5	11	10	30	7
Deafness	11	6	9	7	13	12	33	8
Mobility limitation	16	9	14	10	22	21	52	13
Speech impairment	31	18	44	32	57	54	132	32
Epilepsy	21	12	15	11	14	13	50	12
Psychological problems	28	16	16	12	10	7	54	13

The institutional experiences of the more severely retarded group differed from those of their less retarded counterparts. In general, both the children in the sample and the severely retarded individuals as a whole were twice as likely to have participated in *no* specific day placement in the institution prior to their release. This lower level of participation is reflected in the perceptions of the families of the more severely retarded individuals. In general, these families were considerably less satisfied with the prerelease preparation that the individual had received than were families of the less retarded population. Families of children were generally as satisfied as families of adults, indicating that any dissatisfaction was related to the level of retardation of the subjects and not their age. The differences in the number of day placements of the subjects by level of retardation is presented in Table 4.

Table 4
Number of Day Placements by Level of Retardation

Number of Programs	Mild N (165)	%	Moderate N (137)	%	Severe N (106)	%	Total N (408)	%
None	26	15	38	28	51	48	115	28
One	95	56	81	59	42	40	218	53
Two or more	44	29	18	13	13	12	75	19

Community Experiences of Deinstitutionalized Severely/Profoundly Retarded People

According to the descriptive data collected in this study, there were no important differences in the characteristics of the communities into which the severely/profoundly retarded people were placed. However, once placed, the more severely retarded people had experiences in the community which were noticeably different from the less retarded people. Most of this is likely to be a function of the age distribution of subjects since children were more likely than severely retarded people to be placed with their natural families.

Type of community placement was quite similar for the severely retarded subjects and mild and moderately retarded subjects. For severely retarded people, as with all other levels of retardation, the most common placement within the sample was the group home. This type of placement was made with over half the sample. There were a few people labeled as severely retarded in foster homes and even some in semi-independent living settings, but not surprisingly, no severely retarded individuals were living independently. Residential placement of subjects is shown in Table 5.

Table 5
Residential Setting by Level of Retardation

Setting	Level of Retardation Mild N (171)	%	Moderate N (137)	%	Severe N (106)	%	Total N (414)	%
Natural parent	20	12	10	8	27	25	57	14
Foster parent	25	15	29	21	15	14	69	17
Group home	71	41	73	53	58	55	202	49
Semi-independent	21	12	14	10	6	6	41	10
Independent	34	20	11	8	—	—	45	10

The severely retarded people in the sample were as likely as other subjects to be living in reasonably clean homelike environments. Also, as might be expected, severely retarded individuals were more often living in more restrictive environments that allowed them less freedom in matters such as going to bed when they wanted, coming and going at will, and deciding what clothes to purchase and to wear. Families of children and of severely retarded individuals tended to perceive the communities as being more friendly than did families of the less seriously retarded individuals. Both the families and the retarded persons themselves generally felt that the subjects were adjusting well in the home. As is shown in Table 6, seriously retarded people were perceived as adjusting well slightly more often than were the less seriously handicapped, but the difference was small. The severely retarded people in the sample were also less likely than other people to have moved while in the community. This is shown in Table 7.

In summary, the severely retarded individuals in the sample had been placed in all major categories of residential settings except independent living. The neighborhoods in which they lived were perceived as friendly. Their placements were somewhat more stable than were those of the less seriously handicapped subjects, and they were generally perceived as adjusting well to their community residence.

Table 6

Resident's Perceptions of Adjustment to House and Residents by Age

Adjustment Rating	Adjustment to the House				
	Children		Adults		Total
	N (55)	%	N (263)	%	N (378)
Good	47	86	185	70	232
Fair	5	9	56	21	61
Poor	3	5	22	9	25
	Adjustment to Other Residents				
	Children		Adults		Total
	N (51)	%	N (253)	%	N (304)
Good	32	63	160	63	912
Fair	12	23	79	29	85
Poor	7	14	20	8	27

Table 7

Number of Settings Lived in by Level of Retardation

Number of Settings	Level of Retardation							
	Mild		Moderate		Severe		Total	
	N (171)	%	N (137)	%	N (106)	%	N (414)	%
One	103	60	99	72	75	70	277	67
Two	31	18	17	12	22	21	70	17
Three	25	15	8	6	5	5	38	9
Four or more	12	7	13	10	4	4	29	7

School/Work Activities

The pattern that emerges from the data on the subjects' day activities is predictable: severely retarded individuals were less likely to be placed in a job, and more likely to be placed in a day activity program. Furthermore, of the severely retarded individuals who were working, virtually all were placed in a sheltered employment situation. In general, severely retarded individuals were somewhat less likely than their counterparts to be in no day placement at all at the time of the interview. These findings are shown in Tables 8 and 9.

Table 8

Current Day Placements by Level of Retardation

Type of Day Placement	Level of Retardation					
	Mild		Moderate		Severe	
	N	%	N	%	N	%
Job (competitive or sheltered employment)	119	70	77	56	39	37
School (attend classes in day or night)	52	30	50	43	45	42
Special day activity center or program	32	19	37	27	44	44
No school, work, or day activity program	18	11	17	12	9	9

Table 9

Type of Work Placement by Level of Retardation

Type of Work Placement	Level of Retardation					
	Mild		Moderate		Severe	
	N (117)	%	N (76)	%	N (39)	%
Competitive job (regular employment)	36	30	18	24	2	5
Sheltered job (sheltered workshop, rehabilitation center, or job training center)	81	70	58	76	37	95

While the severely retarded people who were working tended to like their jobs less than did the more mildly retarded people in the sample, those severely retarded individuals in school overwhelmingly liked what they were doing and were generally more satisfied than the less retarded subjects. In further analysis, it was noted that severely/profoundly retarded people were substantially less "busy" than less retarded individuals as indicated by a measure of day and leisure time activities. Despite this, as shown in Table 10, families of severely retarded persons were considerably more likely than families of less retarded persons to indicate that the individual was adjusting very well in his or her day placement. The generally higher level of satisfaction with the performance of the severely retarded individuals is a recurring theme and raises the question of the influence of family and community expectations on the perception of adjustment, as well as the possibility that the severely retarded individuals possessed some behavioral tendency which facilitated adjustment.

Table 10

Family Perception of Study Group's Adjustment to Work/School Relationships by Level of Retardation

Adjustment Ratings	Level of Retardation					
	Mild		Moderate		Severe	
	N (153)	%	N (124)	%	N (94)	%
Very well	98	61	83	67	68	72
All right	52	32	30	24	24	26
Not very well	3	7	11	9	2	2

Social/Leisure Activities

In general, the severely retarded persons were considerably less likely than their counterparts to participate in social and leisure time activities, particularly those activities requiring more social skills and independence such as going to the movies, going shopping, or having romantic relationships. Still, if severely retarded people did have romantic relationships, families perceived them as handling these relationships quite well, and were less likely than mildly retarded individuals to be perceived as handling them "not very well," as can be seen in Table 11. Tables 12 and 13 show that families generally perceived severely retarded individuals as having less difficulty with social relationships and loneliness than less retarded individuals. Once again the issue of expectations as opposed to actual adjustment has to be raised.

Table 11

Family Ratings of Competence in Managing Romantic Relationships by Level of Retardation

Managed Relationship	Level of Retardation					
	Mild		Moderate		Severe	
	N	%	N	%	N	%
Very well	51	49	32	55	12	46
All right	28	27	16	28	11	42
Not very well	25	24	10	17	3	12

Table 12

Family Perceptions of Problems with Social Relationships by Level of Retardation

Extent of Problem	Level of Retardation					
	Mild		Moderate		Severe	
	N	%	N	%	N	%
Big problem	27	16	22	16	9	9
Somewhat of a problem	44	27	36	27	20	20
Not a problem	95	57	77	57	73	71

Table 13

Family Perceptions of Problems with Loneliness by Level of Retardation

Extent of Problem	Level of Retardation					
	Mild		Moderate		Severe	
	N	%	N	%	N	%
Big problem	26	16	15	11	5	5
Somewhat of a problem	50	30	38	28	17	17
Not a problem	91	54	84	61	79	78

Services and Training

Retarded people receive a wide variety of services and training in the community. Information was gathered on the extent to which people in the sample received and needed certain services and training (see Tables 14, 15 and 16). In general, families of the severely retarded people perceived them as needing less training in various aspects of independent living and utilization of community services than did the families of the less seriously retarded subjects. But the reason for this difference was not that the severely retarded persons already possessed these abilities, but rather that they were not perceived as being able to profit from training of independent community living and service utilization.

Severely retarded individuals were more likely than other people to need and use both physical therapy and speech therapy services. This is consistent with the fact that they are more likely to be multiply handicapped, with speech impairments and mobility limitations as common additional disabilities. Also not surprisingly, severely retarded people used and needed employment services considerably less than their less retarded counterparts. Once again, the issue of family expectation arises. On a score that attempted to measure overall unmet need for services and training, severely/profoundly retarded people were significantly less likely than their counterparts to be perceived as having *unmet* needs.

Table 14

Utilization of and Need for Services by Level of Retardation

Type of Service	Level of Retardation	Used N	Used %	Needed, Not Used N	Needed, Not Used %	Not Needed, Not Used N	Not Needed, Not Used %	Total N	Total %
Medical & Health Care									
Medical services	Mild	160	94	2	1	9	5	171	100
	Moderate	124	93	1	1	9	6	134	100
	Severe	98	94	2	2	4	4	104	100
Dental services	Mild	125	72	18	10	30	18	173	100
	Moderate	112	85	5	3	17	13	134	100
	Severe	74	71	13	12	18	17	105	100
Physical therapy	Mild	14	8	8	5	148	87	170	100
	Moderate	9	7	4	3	123	90	136	100
	Severe	19	18	14	13	72	69	105	100
Speech therapy	Mild	34	20	14	8	122	72	170	100
	Moderate	36	28	23	18	71	54	130	100
	Severe	48	46	31	30	26	24	105	100
Social & Recreational Services									
Recreational therapy	Mild	128	75	18	11	24	14	170	100
	Moderate	113	83	9	7	14	10	136	100
	Severe	92	88	9	9	4	3	105	100
Social & psychological therapy	Mild	103	61	21	13	44	26	168	100
	Moderate	83	61	7	5	46	34	136	100
	Severe	52	50	3	3	49	47	104	100
Camp programs	Mild	51	34	24	10	76	50	151	100
	Moderate	48	45	11	10	48	45	107	100
	Severe	50	53	12	13	32	34	94	100
Occupational therapy	Mild	54	31	15	9	105	60	174	100
	Moderate	38	28	14	10	84	62	136	100
	Severe	40	38	10	10	54	52	104	100
Employment Services									
Employment placement & support services	Mild	112	66	12	7	45	27	169	100
	Moderate	65	49	8	6	81	45	134	100
	Severe	32	31	4	4	67	65	103	100
Housing & Legal Services									
Housing assistance	Mild	51	30	6	4	113	66	170	100
	Moderate	29	22	3	2	102	76	134	100
	Severe	16	15	1	1	88	84	105	100
Legal assistance	Mild	17	10	4	2	148	88	169	100
	Moderate	12	9	2	1	121	90	135	100
	Severe	10	10	2	2	92	88	104	100

Table 15

Utilization of and Need for Training by Level of Retardation

Type of Training	Level of Retardation	Received N	Received %	Needed, Not received N	Needed, Not received %	Not Needed, Not Received: Already had skill N	Already had skill %	Not ready for skill N	Not ready for skill %	Total N	Total %
Personal Maintenance											
Eating	Mild	57	48	1	1	65	53	—	0	123	100
	Moderate	56	50	—	0	56	50	—	0	112	100
	Severe	78	76	3	2	19	10	2	2	102	100
Using the toilet	Mild	12	10	—	0	111	90	—	0	123	100
	Moderate	11	10	2	2	95	88	—	0	108	100
	Severe	32	33	1	1	59	61	5	5	97	100
Dressing	Mild	14	11	—	0	110	89	—	0	124	100
	Moderate	29	26	—	0	82	74	—	0	111	100
	Severe	45	46	4	4	46	45	4	4	99	100
Cleanliness	Mild	65	51	1	1	61	46	—	0	127	100
	Moderate	81	70	—	0	35	30	—	0	116	100
	Severe	76	75	1	1	21	21	3	3	101	100
Grooming	Mild	68	53	1	1	58	45	—	0	128	100
	Moderate	86	74	1	1	29	25	—	0	117	100
	Severe	73	72	1	1	20	20	7	7	101	100
Sensory Development											
Motor	Mild	29	18	4	3	125	78	1	1	160	100
	Moderate	37	29	4	3	87	68	—	0	128	100
	Severe	48	47	8	8	46	44	1	1	103	100
Hearing & vision	Mild	17	11	—	0	139	88	1	1	157	100
	Moderate	19	15	5	4	104	81	—	0	128	100
	Severe	31	31	2	2	67	66	1	1	101	100
Speech & language	Mild	65	41	9	5	83	53	1	1	158	100
	Moderate	58	46	12	10	53	42	2	2	125	100
	Severe	75	75	15	15	8	8	2	2	100	100
Education & Employment											
Preacademic	Mild	42	27	2	1	112	71	1	1	157	100
	Moderate	52	42	5	4	64	52	2	2	123	100
	Severe	75	77	4	4	14	14	5	5	98	100
Numbers & telling time	Mild	79	50	10	6	69	43	1	1	159	100
	Moderate	88	70	12	10	17	13	9	7	126	100
	Severe	62	64	5	5	4	4	26	27	97	100
Reading & writing	Mild	90	55	19	12	47	29	8	4	164	100
	Moderate	56	68	12	10	10	8	17	14	125	100
	Severe	55	55	6	6	4	4	36	36	100	100
Prevocational	Mild	105	65	6	4	45	27	6	4	162	100
	Moderate	83	64	3	2	25	19	20	15	131	100
	Severe	67	68	3	3	1	1	28	28	99	199
Vocational	Mild	100	62	16	10	21	13	24	15	181	100
	Moderate	56	44	11	9	21	16	40	31	128	100
	Severe	41	41	6	6	1	1	53	52	101	100

Table 16

Utilization of and Need for Support Services for Families of the Retarded by Level of Retardation

Type of Service	Level of Retardation	Used N	Used %	Needed, Not Received N	Needed, Not Received %	Not Needed, Not Received N	Not Needed, Not Received %	Total N	Total %
Support and/or training prior to individual's release	Mild	51	38	27	20	57	42	135	100
	Moderate	46	38	28	23	48	39	122	100
	Severe	24	23	28	27	53	50	105	100
General counseling	Mild	77	58	11	8	46	34	134	100
	Moderate	75	61	11	9	37	30	123	100
	Severe	57	54	9	9	39	37	105	100
Consultation for handling specific problems	Mild	105	78	8	6	22	16	135	100
	Moderate	95	77	6	5	23	18	124	100
	Severe	81	76	9	9	16	15	106	100
Temporary relief from responsibilities	Mild	73	63	7	6	36	31	116	100
	Moderate	74	67	10	9	27	24	111	100
	Severe	52	53	14	14	33	33	99	100
Parent or professional associations	Mild	44	33	18	13	73	54	135	100
	Moderate	64	53	17	14	40	33	121	100
	Severe	42	40	21	20	43	40	106	100

Return to the Institution

Finally, as shown in Table 17, severely retarded individuals were somewhat less likely than their less retarded counterparts to return to the institution. In general, they were perceived as having fewer behavior problems and were perceived as adjusting at least as well as less retarded individuals.

Table 17

Level of Retardation Among Those Who Returned and Those Who Remained

Study Group	Mild N	Mild %	Moderate N	Moderate %	Severe N	Severe %	Total N	Total %
Returned	22	42	23	43	8	15	53	100
Remained	155	41	118	31	81	26	374	100

What conclusions, then, can be drawn from the information presented above? Because of the various conceptual and methodological problems to be discussed subsequently, it is difficult indeed to generalize. However, on the basis of the findings it appears reasonable to state the following:

1) It is, in fact, possible to measure at least certain aspects of the community experiences or adjustment of severely and profoundly retarded individuals in much the same manner as it is measured for less retarded individuals;
2) Severely and profoundly retarded individuals appear to be capable of making a reasonable adjustment to the community, at least as perceived by their families;

3) Severely and profoundly retarded people seem to be able to remain in the community despite the fact that they are generally less integrated in terms of day activities, leisure time activities, social relationships, and service utilization than are less seriously retarded subjects;
4) Severely and profoundly retarded people may be judged to adjust better because people, including both the family and community, may have somewhat lower expectations of their performance, and more readily tolerate deviations from "normal" behavior;
5) Severely and profoundly retarded individuals, to a limited degree, express a certain amount of satisfaction with their current community status; and
6) Despite their greater needs, it appears that severely and profoundly retarded persons receive less training and support prior to release from the institution.

Conceptual Issues and Framework

In collecting the data which were summarized above, the project confronted a number of extremely complex conceptual issues, most of which were addressed but not fully resolved. The conceptualizations took place in 1974 before many of the other studies reported on in this volume had been conducted and without the benefit of a clear communication network among the projects that were either completed or were being conducted simultaneously. Although a thorough review of the literature was conducted, there was, in reality, little to draw upon. Most of the previous studies had used relatively narrow approaches, and this project was intended to be comprehensive.

There were a host of broad and complex conceptual difficulties faced in researching the adjustment of deinstitutionalized persons living in a community setting. Three major ones are discussed in this section of the paper:

1) How should community adjustment be conceptualized and operationalized;
2) How should the factors potentially influencing adjustment be identified and measured;
3) How should specific characteristics or experiences be classified: as measures of adjustment (and should they be interpreted positively or negatively); or as factors influencing adjustment?

In addition to these (and other) conceptual difficulties, there were a number of methodological issues and problems that this particular project faced. Four major methodological problems acted as particular constraints on the project's design and adequacy:

1) The information on retarded people was gathered at only one point in time;
2) The sample was selected through voluntary participation, making it virtually impossible to make statistically valid generalizations;
3) Data were generally obtained from only one source (the family) and were not validated from other sources; and
4) Methods for collecting and interpreting data from retarded persons themselves had to be developed.

The conceptual difficulties and methodological constraints will be discussed in detail in the following sections.

How Should Community Adjustment Be Defined?

The fundamental conceptual problem confronting all research in this area has been developing an operational definition of community adjustment. A thorough review of literature reveals that most previous research has relied either on retention in the community as the primary criterion of success or focused on a single aspect of functioning while in the community, such as adjustment on the job. Further, prior to the research summarized in the first part of this paper, virtually no one had attempted to measure the adjustment of severely/profoundly retarded individuals or had included children.

The Abt Associates project, therefore, was required to develop independently a definition of adjustment that met the following criteria:

1) It had to be equally appropriate for individuals of *all ages* and *all levels of retardation*;
2) It had to be measurable *within the resource constraints* of the project. (It was not possible to spend more than an average of approximately 4 hours gathering data on any one individual; to measure at more than one point in time; or to gather data through direct observation or testing);
3) It had to take into account the *actual functioning* of an individual while in the community;
4) It had to take into account the multi-dimensional aspect of an individual's functioning and allow for different patterns of adjustment in different aspects of community living;
5) It could *not hold retarded individuals to standards* of performance that non-retarded individuals would not be held to as well.

Every effort was made to meet these criteria, but it was, of course, extremely difficult and the result was far from perfect. Eventually the following model of community adjustment was used:

1) *Returning to the institution was retained as a "bottom line failure,"* but emphasis was placed on the notion that it was a system failure rather than an individual failure and factors outside the individual were sought as possible explanations for the return of the individual.
2) The community experiences of an individual were divided into *three arenas* in which a person would be expected either to adjust or have difficulties:
   a) *the living environment*;
   b) *the work or school environment* (day environment); and
   c) *social and leisure time activities.*
3) Within each of these aspects of living, the adjustment or experiences were described in terms of:
   a) the family's and the retarded individual's own *perception of how well he or she was getting along* (i.e., of adjustment);
   b) the retarded person's *satisfaction with life in the community*;
   c) the family's and the retarded person's view of the extent to which the retarded person was having specific *problems*; and
   d) the retarded person's overall activity level.

It was assumed participation in a day activity or leisure time activity was better than no participation, and the more participation the better.

The chart which follows illustrates how the arenas and the aspects of adjustment were matched and actually explored in the study.

Specific Criteria of Adjustment for Each Arena

General Criterion	Living Environment	Day Environment	Social/Leisure Activities
Family perception of adjustment	Perception of how well the individual gets along in the home and with the family	Perception of how well the individual gets along at work or school	Perception of how well the individual handles relationships with people of the opposite sex
Retarded individual's perception of his or her own adjustment	Perception of how well the individual gets along at home and with the family	Perception of how well the individual gets along at school or work	
Retarded person's satisfaction	Does the individual like/dislike where he/she lives? What does he/she like/dislike about it? Would he/she rather live elsewhere, either in the community or in an institution?	Does the individual like/dislike school or work? What does he/she like/dislike about it?	
Family and retarded person's perception of problems. Does person have problem with:	Getting along with family	Getting a job; keeping a job	Inappropriate behavior; being lonely. Problems with social relationships
Activity level		In some day placement; number of hours participated per week	Participation in various leisure time activities; presence of friends, romantic relationships

What Factors Might "Predict" or Influence Community Adjustment

The second major conceptual problem addressed by the project was the framework for identifying and measuring the potential predictors of adjustment. Here too there were few precedents in the literature, with the bulk of the literature either being descriptive or, if predictive, relying primarily on characteristics of the individual retarded person (e.g., IQ). As with the concept of adjustment, there were definite criteria that the project attempted to apply to its selection of potential predictor variables. These were:

1) The variables should reflect the fact that many *factors in the environment* could affect the adjustment of the individual and every effort should be made to identify these factors, thus reducing the likelihood that poor adjustment would be seen primarily as an individual rather than a system failure;
2) The variables should be *measurable,* within the same time and resource constraints imposed on the measures of adjustment;

3) The variables should clearly be identifiable as potential *predictors of adjustment* rather than as indicators of adjustment (as discussed below); and

4) To maximum extent possible the variables should measure *policy manipulable* conditions so that if identified as influencing adjustment there could be a specific recommendation made with respect to altering the condition.

As with the measures of adjustment, it was not totally possible to meet these criteria. However, the effort was made, and the following general framework was developed to identify possible factors influencing an individual's adjustment:

1) Characteristics or factors that the individual, in effect, *brought* with him or her *into the community,* including:
   a) inherent characteristics of the individual, such as level of retardation (mild, moderate, severe or profound), age, and sex;
   b) characteristics of the individual's *institutional experience* such as length of institutionalization, and the types and amounts of institutional training received prior to release;
   c) characteristics of the *releasing institution,* such as size, per capita expenditures, on-going relationship with the community, and types and amounts of services offered to residents;

2) Characteristics or factors that could impact on the individual *after release* into the community, such as,
   a) characteristics of the *living environment,* including type of setting (group home, foster home, natural home, semi-independent living setting, independent living), number of people living together, staffing pattern, and rules or housing policies;
   b) characteristics of the *day environment,* including availability of various types of services and training, availability of alternative living environments, and types of providers offering training and service (community or institutional); and
   c) characteristics of the overall *community,* particularly in terms of the extent to which community supports existed. These supports included training and services for the retarded person, alternative living environments, and service for the families. However, the project did not adequately address the issue of the community service network. No information was gathered directly about the overall operations of the non-institutional service system in the communities where the subjects were living. Information about the availability of services was taken only from the perspective of the family and could as well have reflected a lack of awareness as a lack of actual services although it could be argued that, if many people are unaware of services, there is a real problem in making them available to people. The project was designed to trace individuals from the institution into the community, without explicitly acknowledging the presence of a link between the institution and the individual. This is an important aspect of the environment into which an individual is released that should be taken more explicitly into account in future studies.

In general, the interaction between the individual and the community environment was not adequately addressed. There remains a need to identify the ways in which the individual adjusts to the community. This is particularly the case with mentally retarded individuals where the individual represents a burden or responsibility that the community has to incorporate into its social structure. The project attempted to ascertain the extent to which the neighborhood and community at large had responded to the retarded person, but no real effort was made to measure the adaptation that the community (including the home) had to make to the individual. Measuring the interaction between the demands of the community environment and the characteristics of the individual placed in that environment would appear to be essential for a true understanding of adjustment since the same behavior or characteristics of an individual in two environments can result in two very different patterns of adjustment.

The third major problem with which the project wrestled was the interpretation of specific variables. Certain variables seemed to function potentially as either indicators or predictors of adjustment. Other variables had a number of interpretations. An investigation of some of these variables which could be interpreted in multiple ways sheds light on the complexity of the events being studied. As will be seen, decisions about how to interpret the variables were based on a number of factors, including the fact that some variables could only be taken as indicators of success if they had been measured over time (e.g., Adaptive Behavior Scale score and remaining in the community); some variables were difficult to interpret without additional information (e.g., utilization of the institution as a community provider, and perceptions of unmet needs), and others could be seen as positive or negative measures (e.g., movement among day or residential programs and degree of service utilization).

Predictor or Indicator of Adjustment

Score on the Adaptive Behavior Scale (ABS). A one-point-in-time score was obtained on all the retarded individuals in the sample by having a key family member fill out the ABS. The score was ultimately used primarily as predictor variable that was treated as a measure of an individual characteristic much like level of retardation. However, in doing so it had to be acknowledged that ABS score is potentially a function of considerably more than ''inherent'' ability on the part of the individual although it is highly correlated with both age and IQ. The ABS also reflects directly the training that an individual has received in the functional areas measured. With a one-point-in-time measure, however, the ABS would have to be controlled for age and level of retardation or it would consistently indicate that younger and more retarded individuals are less well adjusted or adapted. This analytic process was not feasible within the scope of the Abt Associates' project. Had change scores been available, they could potentially have been used as an indicator of an individual's improved functional level and hence, adjustment (at least in terms of skills).

The utilization of service and training. The extent to which a person used specific types of training and services was reported by families. This information could be interpreted in a variety of ways. High utilization could be seen as an indicator that an individual required a good deal of support and hence was not well adjusted. On the other hand, high utilization could reflect the degree to which the community offered support and the extent to which the family took advantage of it and hence could be interpreted as an indicator of good adjustment and good ability to access community resources. Furthermore, the extent to which an individual receives training and services in the community can be expected to have an impact on that person's adjustment, and hence might be seen as an important predictor of success rather than a measure of it.

Length of time in the community. The length of time a person has been in the community could be interpreted as an indicator of success (the longer the better), or as a predictor of success (the longer a person is in the community, the more adjusted he/she is likely to be). All the people in the sample who were in the community at the time the interviews were conducted had been there between six months and two and one-half years. From other research it appears that most failures or returns occur prior to six months. Since the people who had been in the community only six months had not had an opportunity to remain longer, it was not possible to use duration as an indicator of success. (This would only be approximate in a longitudinal study.) Therefore, length of time in the community was used as a factor potentially influencing adjustment but was not found to be important for the group studied.

Type of community placement. It is clear that the type of community residential setting is a strong determinant of the specific experiences of the individual and, therefore, ought to be considered as an important predictor of adjustment. On the other hand, many of the characteristics of the living setting reflect the abilities and perhaps even the adjustment level of their residents. Thus, a person with more skills and fewer behavior problems is more likely to live in a less structured environment than the individual with fewer skills and more behavior problems. In this way the environment becomes an important indicator or reflection of the adjustment of the individual. Ultimately, in this study the community setting was considered in both ways. It was treated as an important independent variable by examining the differential experiences of individuals in different settings; and an attempt was made to measure the degree of independence that the individual had attained in the living environment.

Positive or Negative Indicator

Movement among day or residential placements. An important aspect of a person's community experiences is his or her movement from one day or residential setting to another. Simple movement is difficult to interpret since it could equally well be an indicator of progress and growth or an indicator of difficulties. Therefore, the project attempted to ascertain the reasons why an individual moved before judging this a positive or negative indicator.

Interpretation

Need for services and training. Families also reported on the extent to which retarded people needed the various services or training that they were not receiving. It appears that the extent to which a family perceived an unmet need was influenced by its expectations of the level of functioning that the individual could attain and of the supports with which they were familiar. Their expectations may or may not have been realistic and appropriate. For example, in the study it emerged that many families with a severely or profoundly retarded individual felt that fewer training supports were needed than did families with less retarded individuals. Thus, low unmet need might reflect low expectations not poor community support. However, reports of high unmet need were considered to reflect poor community support.

Utilization of the institution as a provider after release into the community. One of the most important differences that emerged between the individuals who remained in the community and those who returned to the institution was that the people who returned tended to be more dependent upon the institution after their release into the community. This finding is hard to interpret. Does continued dependency on the institution maintain a link that makes eventual return to the institution more likely, or is it that individuals who have more problems or who live in a community that is less capable of providing support, and thus are already at higher risk of reinstitutionalization, are more dependent on the institution for support services? If the latter is the case, then there is not necessarily a causal link between the institution as provider of support services and eventual reinstitutionalization.

Methodological Issues

There were a number of methodological difficulties and limitations with the Abt Associates' study. Of particular relevance here are those that either point to some key future directions for research or that are likely to continue to plague similar studies. Four of these issues are described here.

The first and most fundamental methodological difficulty was actually a constraint within which the study had to be conducted: information was gathered at only *one point in time*. There was no capacity within the study to gather data on individuals prior to their release, or at specified intervals after release, or immediately prior to or upon return to the institution. The need for prospective and longitudinal studies has been well documented and does not need to be elaborated upon here. It is, however, important to bear in mind that this is a continuing constraint and directly influences both the type and validity of the data collected.

A second basic methodological constraint was that participation of the retarded people was *voluntary*. It was based upon informed consent, with privacy protected not only of those who chose to participate but those who chose not to participate. As a result, the individuals who agreed to participate were not necessarily representative of all persons released. In particular, they tended to be more likely to live in group homes than either natural homes or independently and were likely not to have moved frequently.

The voluntary nature of the participation by the retarded individuals followed the voluntary participation by the institution. The institutions had voluntarily responded both to an initial mail questionnaire and to the opportunity to participate in the follow-up of its released clients. The institutions that were finally included did represent a range in terms of size, age, geographic location, and policies. However, they could not be considered a randomly selected sample, representative of the universe of all institutions releasing retarded people. The institutions were unrepresentative in that they had to have released a sufficient number of people into the community so that a follow-up study would be feasible; they had to be willing and able to work hard to assist in conducting the study; and they had to have procedures for contacting the former residents that were reasonably efficient and minimally time consuming. In addition, no institution was selected that was under court order at the time of the study. In sum, both the institutions releasing the subjects and the deinstitutionalized people who were studied represented somewhat biased samples. This greatly reduced the extent to which generalizations can be made to all individuals released from all institutions.

A third major methodological constraint was imposed by the fact that most information was *obtained from only one source*: the "family." There was no effort to validate information by interviewing other potential sources such as day provider, a community case manager or administrator. In addition, no effort was made to validate information from direct observations of the individual retarded person or the activities taking place within the home setting. This constraint was particularly important for the sample of people who had returned to the institution because it was frequently impossible to interview the family with whom the retarded person had been living in the community, so information was obtained instead from a staff person at the institution (such as a social worker) who was identified as having been informed about the activities of the returnees while in the community. This lack of validation was further confounded for the various historical data by the fact that the study was not longitudinal. Historical data were frequently obtained from a family respondent such as a group home manager who was not familiar with the retarded person during the person's entire stay in the community. Therefore, information about the pre-release experiences and prior day and residential histories were particularly prone to uncertainties.

The fourth methodological difficulty was that information was also obtained *directly from retarded people*. While this effort to obtain information from retarded persons added to the richness of the data in many ways, there had been until recently very little basis for making judgments regarding the adequacy of the data obtained from interviews with retarded individuals (cf. Wyngaarden and Sigelman et al. in this volume).

Recommendations for Future Research

The "wish list" and recommendations for future studies is almost infinite. There are, however, a few key recommendations that can be made as a result of this study that are worth reiterating here.

1) There need to be more in-depth studies that are prospective and longitudinal rather than broad, one-shot pictures of deinstitutionalized mentally retarded people's experiences.
2) More effort needs to be made to understand the relationship between the adjustment of the individual and the adjustment of the environment—between individual behavior and environmental expectations.
3) The community environment clearly emerged as an important aspect of the experiences of the retarded people studied. Stronger efforts need to be made to understand this broader environment, including both the immediate residential and day environments, and the broader community context.
4) The specific role of the institution both in preparing individuals prior to release and retaining a service role after release needs to be understood further to determine how it can be more beneficial to the individual.
5) Increased efforts should be made to determine how best to interview mentally retarded persons about their own experiences.
6) Most information obtained about deinstitutionalized mentally retarded people is obtained from the residence; more effort should be made to focus on other sources as well, such as the day environment.
7) More intensive efforts need to be made to determine the circumstances that appear to make it easier for severely and profoundly retarded individuals to gain acceptance in the community than is the case with certain mildly retarded individuals (particularly those with behavior problems).

References

Gollay, E., Freedman, R., Wyngaarden, M., & Kurtz, N. R. *Coming back: The community experiences of deinstitutionalized mentally retarded people*. Cambridge, MA: Abt Books, 1978.

Nihira, K., Foster, R., Shellhaas, M., & Leland, H. *AAMD Adaptive Behavior Scale*. Washington, DC: American Association on Mental Deficiency, 1975.

Interviewing Mentally Retarded Persons: Issues and Strategies

Marty Wyngaarden

Abt Associates
Cambridge, Massachusetts

In July, 1974, Abt Associates Inc. was awarded a contract by the Bureau of Education for the Handicapped of the United States Office of Education to conduct an assessment of the adjustment of deinstitutionalized, mentally retarded people to community life. As part of the study, 440 deinstitutionalized persons residing in a variety of community settings were interviewed to obtain their perspectives on how effective the institutions were in preparing them for their new lives, how they were adjusting to the community and how satisfied they were with their current residential and day program placements.[1] In addition, extensive demographic, historical and current information was collected about each released person from a variety of other sources: institutional staff and records, community based "families" (natural or foster parent, group home manager) and/or social workers, teachers, employers, friends.

The inclusion of the deinstitutionalized, mentally retarded person as a respondent was one of the unique aspects of the study. The decision to interview these persons and the strategy by which to do so was guided by two assumptions. First, mentally retarded persons are *valid* sources of information with a singular perspective on their experiences that is only obtainable through direct questioning. Second, for some of the information sought, they are the only *appropriate* sources of information. For example, they are the best informants regarding how satisfied they are with their day programs.

This paper reports on the process and outcome of interviewing mentally retarded persons. A description of the process is critical because few studies have attempted to interview retarded persons directly, and thus, few reports on the strategies used in contacting, interviewing and processing the obtained information have appeared. The outcome of this effort is important for it indicates that it is possible and, indeed, critical to seek the personal insights of those most directly affected by shifts in social policy. Mentally retarded persons proved to be one of the valued and valid sources of information in the project.

The following sections of the paper discuss such issues as contacting the respondents and maintaining confidentiality, design of questionnaires and phrasing of questions, training interviewers to conduct the interviews, the dynamics of the interview session, and the general findings on the interviewing process which resulted from this effort.

Contacting the Respondents and Confidentiality

In order to ensure that the privacy of all study group members was protected, participating institutions were asked to make initial contact with the individuals.

[1]For a more detailed description of the project and the characteristics of the respondents, see E. Gollay, R. Freedman, M. Wyngaarden, and N. Kurtz, *Coming back: The community experiences of deinstitutionalized mentally retarded people* (Cambridge, MA: Abt Books, 1978).

Abt Associates developed a standard letter to be sent by the institution to eligible, released individuals describing the study, detailing what participation by the individual and his or her family would entail, and requesting that they sign and return an enclosed consent form.

The consent form, developed by a legal consultant experienced in the field, was written in a style which could be understood by mentally retarded persons and/or their families. Individuals signing the form gave consent both to participate in the study and to allow the releasing institutions to provide basic information about them (e.g., level of retardation, number of years institutionalized). Legal consent was furnished by the parent or guardian if the individual was a minor or was judged legally incompetent. If neither a minor nor judged incompetent, the mentally retarded person was required to sign the consent agreement.

Mentally retarded persons and their families were instructed to return the signed consent forms directly to Abt Associates if they were interested in participating in the study. In this way, Abt Associates did not make any direct contact with the study group members and their families until after they had agreed to participate, and researchers never learned the names of those who declined to participate. Thus, the privacy of both respondents and non-respondents was ensured.

Design of Questionnaires

Two sets of questions were asked of the mentally retarded respondents: those which were asked *only* of the mentally retarded person and those which were asked of *both* the retarded person and also of his/her family respondent in a separate interview.

Questions which were asked only of the retarded person included: likes and dislikes about home, school, and/or work; what he or she would like to have learned in the institution and what he or she wants to learn now in the community; and, what sorts of worries the person faces in the community. These questions were included for two reasons. First, there are no right or wrong answers to these questions, and it was important to avoid a "testing" atmosphere during the interview. Second, since these questions ask for opinions, the mentally retarded person was the only appropriate respondent; and, as noted above, it was a fundamental premise of the study that mentally retarded persons are capable and accurate sources of information concerning what they like and dislike about their lives.

Questions which were asked of retarded persons and family respondents included: factual information on day placements in the community, institutional training received and other skills developed in the community, problems experienced by the person since release, perceptions of the person's adjustment to the community, and perceptions on the degree of friendliness of the neighbors and the community at large to the mentally retarded person. These questions were asked of both types of respondents because it was not clear who would be the most accurate source of information for some of these questions. Many group home managers or foster parents may not have known their retarded family member prior to release from the institution; some social workers may have known the client for only several months. They would, therefore, be unlikely to be thoroughly knowledgeable about institutional training and skill development. Some of the retarded respondents, on the other hand, may not have been capable of addressing those questions which required more detailed and retrospective information. Thus, both types of respondents were asked a duplicate set of questions. As a consequence, it was later possible to compare the agreement between respondents on information supplied by both.

Of the 440 persons contacted for the study, 46 were living independently at the time of the interviews, i.e., in their own apartment or dwelling without supervision. In addition to the questions asked of mentally retarded persons described above, these persons were also asked all the questions for which the family respondent would otherwise have been the source. Such additional areas included were: historical and contemporary information on the services and training received, institutional experiences, community placements and activities, social relationships, and problems.

Phrasing of Questions

Project staff found no other study which had sought to gather all the types of information described from retarded respondents. There were, therefore, few guidelines or rules to shape the way in which questions were asked. One major concern, however, was to avoid questions which might encourage the respondent to please the interviewer by trying to give the "right" or expected answer. Further, the investigators wanted to diffuse any fear that voicing a negative opinion might jeopardize the person's placement in the community. This concern led to the decision to use simply phrased open-ended questions as much as possible. Interviewers were instructed not to supply suggestive answers to questions and to encourage the respondent to answer in his/her own words.

However, interviewers were allowed to rephrase the question, maintaining the original intent, if necessary, to spark a response. For example, "What do you like about living here?" could also be asked, "Is there anything you like about living here?" Thus, the primary concern was to obtain answers to a general set of questions rather than identify specific phrasing of questions most likely to achieve an appropriate response.

Indeed, it was often found necessary to rephrase a question in order to obtain the fullest response. For example, 90% of the respondents said they liked where they live. However, when later asked, "Is there any place else you would rather live?" about one-third indicated that they would rather live elsewhere. It was, therefore, important to ask questions in a number of different ways to elicit the most complete response.

The most difficult aspects of designing a questionnaire for mentally retarded persons revolved around question phrasing, location of potentially sensitive questions, and avoidance of concepts which are not intuitively meaningful to retarded respondents. For example, drafts of the questionnaire asked pre-test respondents to indicate whether a specific problem had been "a big problem," "somewhat of a problem," or "not a problem" for them since release. Rarely was a respondent able to differentiate the severity of a problem; rather, responses simply indicated its presence or absence. For this reason, questions were phrased in the final draft to require a straightforward "yes/no" response or were left open-ended instead of a multiple choice format.

The timing or location of questions during the interview also proved to be extremely important. It was helpful to begin the interview with easy questions such as "Do you go to school?" Respondents could accurately respond to this question and were, therefore, less anxious about their ability to answer appropriately. Questions which were potentially upsetting were placed toward the middle or end of the interview to capitalize on the rapport gradually developed. For example, questions asking what worries the person had about living in the community were asked at the end of the interview when the respondent was more relaxed.

One of the most poignant findings was the inability of some respondents to understand concepts such as "to wish" or "to prefer." One question asked respondents what they wished the institution had taught them to prepare them for living in the community. Another asked where they would prefer to live. These questions often proved exceedingly difficult and needed careful rephrasing in order to elaborate the notion of wish or prefer. Such futuristic or speculative thinking had rarely been asked of many respondents.

Selection and Training of Interviewers

A total of 14 field staff was hired by Abt Associates to conduct the interviews. The field staff, recruited from universities, school systems, and programs and facilities serving mentally retarded persons, included special education teachers, rehabilitation counselors, group home staff, psychologists and staff from state institutions for the mentally retarded. While some staff had previous experience in conducting interviews, they were selected on the basis of their sensitivity toward and familiarity with mentally retarded persons on the premise that it is easier to train sensitive people to be interviewers than interviewers to be sensitive.

All field staff underwent four days of intensive training. The bulk of the training was devoted to developing a thorough understanding of the intent of each question and standard interview techniques and strategies. Each field staff was given a manual which specified the purpose of each question and instructions concerning possible problems which might arise. While staff received adequate documentation and written instruction for conducting the interviews, the primary goal of the training session was to prepare the interviewers for the challenge of interviewing mentally retarded persons. This was accomplished through several strategies. First, each interviewer participated in role-playing sessions in which the questions were asked of a housemanager of a group residence for retarded persons and a mentally retarded person living independently in the community who had agreed to participate in the training sessions. Potential problems were simulated and appropriate responses were discussed.

Second, a locally-based group of mentally retarded adults who present training and sensitivity sessions to professionals were employed to further orient field staff to the process of interviewing mentally retarded respondents. This group was extremely effective in simulating the interview process and alerting interviewers to potential problems. They provided many keen insights which served as guides for interviewers: questions must be asked slowly and without subtle pressure for a hurried response; a sense of trust and privacy must be developed prior to questioning; anxieties and fears which the respondent has must be respected and dealt with.

Dynamics of the Interview Situation

Prior to conducting the interviews, field staff contacted each respondent to arrange the time and location of the interview, to describe the general scope of the questions, the amount of time anticipated for the interview, and to reiterate that answers would be completely confidential. Providing these general guidelines prior to the interview is an obviously advisable procedure; however, it led to several negative consequences. Many of the respondents nervously anticipated the interview and needed careful explanations regarding privacy and confidentiality at the scheduled time. It was also important to stress that there were no right or wrong answers and that respondents were not being evaluated or judged. Others maintained the belief that the field staff were employees from the state institutions and, thus, exhibited mistrust which required dispelling. Some were concerned that their answers not be overheard by anyone and were initially uncomfortable with the interviewer recording verbatim responses.

These reactions were not unexpected as they were among those which had been simulated during training sessions. Anticipating such situations, each interviewer was prepared to spend the necessary time establishing rapport with each respondent and a conversational atmosphere in which a discussion rather than a structured interview might occur. Several strategies were suggested by the interviewers to help establish rapport. First, some found it helpful to ask personal questions of the respondent, such as, "Did you paint that picture on the wall?" or "What sorts of flowers do you grow in the garden?" The point was to draw out something personal and reassuring to elicit friendly conversation.

Second, some noted that by showing the respondent the questionnaire and indicating that whatever was written would be kept very private, the respondent's fears abated. One interviewer remarked that, in response to a particularly suspicious respondent, he drew a map of the United States and indicated that the answers to questions were going back to Massachusetts, not to the institution.

One of the most common interview issues was privacy. Many respondents were most comfortable when the interview was conducted as far away as possible from the rest of the household occupants. Others, however, were less worried about privacy and wanted a friend to sit with them; some wanted the housemanager or parent to remain. While interviewers were instructed to discourage visitors, if the respondent was too uncomfortable without a supportive friend, such persons were allowed to remain.

A potential problem in interviewing concerned questions which sparked unanticipated disturbing or upsetting reactions which interviewers must be prepared to handle. For example, the final question in a set of questions concerning residential satisfaction asked, "Do you prefer living here or at the institution?" Many respondents calmly responded to the question. Some, however, were agitated by the question and were then convinced that the interviewer was from the instititution. The situation was usually handled by stopping the interview for a brief period and reiterating the confidentiality of the interview and the absence of a relationship between the interviewer and the institution. An even less obviously upsetting question was, "Do you like where you live?" For some, the question ignited a host of ambivalences, unmet expectations and perceived injustices. The important point is that it is impossible to predict how a respondent is going to react to a particular question and that the best insurance against a disastrous experience is to properly forewarn and prepare the interviewers to be alert to negative reactions, deal with them immediately and then proceed.

The most important quality an interviewer must possess is patience. The questions need to be phrased slowly, clearly and with a minimum of words. The respondent should not feel that a quick answer is expected. Many prefer to ponder the question and carefully select an answer. Others may provide an immediate one-word response and need prodding for a fuller reply. Others may misunderstand the question and launch into an answer totally unrelated to the question. If an interviewer reacts with impatience or annoyance to these situations, the respondent is aware of the displeasure and will commonly react by becoming fearful and less responsive.

One final aspect of the dynamics of interviewing mentally retarded persons needs to be mentioned. Many of the respondents tended to view interviewers as potential helpers in their problems at work, school, or home. Because employers, teachers, and housemanagers or parents were also being interviewed, there was a tendency to perceive the interviewer as a mediator of difficulties. Some parents also saw the interviewer as a facilitator in obtaining needed services or training for their retarded family member. These perceptions reinforced the researchers' belief that there is a serious lack of outreach by professionals in the community, leaving many retarded residents and their families unaware of the availability of services or training. It also reinforced a belief that retarded persons and their families are effective communicators of their needs and problems. One rather frequent comment made by respondents was that no one had ever asked them before about their satisfaction with their day and residential placements. For them, being interviewed represented a unique opportunity to voice their feelings. However, the expression of difficulties often led to the hope that something would change despite initial explanations that the interviewer would tell no one of what they said and would not be able to change their placements.

Given the above recommendations and precautions regarding interviewing mentally retarded persons about their experiences and opinions, what was the outcome of these interviews? In the following section the retarded persons' comprehension, responsiveness and agreement with the family respondents will be discussed.

General Findings

Of the 440 mentally retarded persons who participated in the study, 19% (84) were 18 years or younger while 81% (356) were 19 years or older. Of the group, 41% were mildly retarded (IQ=68–52), 31% were moderately retarded (IQ=51–36), 24% were severely retarded (IQ=35–20) and 4% were profoundly retarded (IQ=19 or less). A little over half (54%) were males.

Only 57, or 13%, of the 440 retarded persons were not interviewed, most commonly because they were non-verbal or had a level of comprehension which precluded interviewing. Only two persons of the entire study group refused to be interviewed.

At the end of each interview, interviewers provided additional information about the respondents along several dimensions: demeanor and verbal ability of the retarded respondent; level of comprehension; attitude toward the study; and length of time of the interview. About half the respondents were completely verbal or able to respond to questions while about one-fifth had mild speech impediments. While the vast majority of respondents understood most of the questions, less than half understood all the questions asked of them. About a third seemed mildly confused about some of the items, and about 15% reportedly had a great deal of trouble responding to some questions. The overwhelming majority (80%) of the respondents were described as eager and willing to participate in the interview session. For many, this represented the first time that an outside person had asked them about their lives since release to the community, and the response to such an opportunity was typically a mixture of excitement and anxiety. Finally, the average time necessary for completion of the interview was forty minutes.

As noted earlier, there were some questions asked of mentally retarded respondents which were duplicates of those asked of their families. A comparison of the answers received revealed striking agreement between the retarded person and the family respondent on the retarded person's degree of adjustment to other family or house members, school and work relationships and community activities. Both groups cited similar problems in community living and gave similar ratings on the individual's management of personal relationships and overall adjustment to the community.

The ultimate use made of information supplied by mentally retarded respondents was determined after data collection. Prior to the data collection effort, it was not known if the information obtained from retarded respondents could be used analytically. In the end, because of the extensive use of open-ended questions and the frequency of missing data, the information was used qualitatively. In this regard, the verbatim quotations proved enriching to the study by vividly and poignantly illustrating what tables of statistics indicated quantitatively.

Summary

One of the most important findings of the study was that mentally retarded people can and are eager to provide complex and moving accounts of their experiences in returning to community life. Interviewers can be trained, through instruction, experience and role-playing, to elicit this information in a casual atmosphere which removes the risk of failure to answer properly and avoids the pressure to please the interviewer. The most important ingredients are patience and well constructed questions, without forced categories and without ambiguous or complex phrasing. The information collected provides in-depth and highly provocative insights into the experience of retarded persons returning to community life.

Issues in Interviewing Mentally Retarded Persons: An Empirical Study

Carol K. Sigelman
Carol J. Schoenrock
Jane L. Winer
Cynthia L. Spanhel
Sherrilyn G. Hromas
Paulette W. Martin
Edward C. Budd
Gerard J. Bensberg

Research and Training Center in Mental Retardation
Texas Tech University
Lubbock, Texas

Studies of deinstitutionalization and related issues in the developmental disabilities field have relied heavily on survey research methods. Moreover, there is increasing advocacy for allowing retarded persons to speak for themselves rather than relying exclusively on interviews and questionnaires obtained from parents, houseparents, and other presumably knowledgeable persons (e.g., Gollay, Freedman, Wyngaarden, & Kurtz, 1978). At this point, however, virtually nothing is known about the reliability and validity of information gained through survey research with mentally retarded persons. To be sure, methodological critiques of the deinstitutionalization and community adjustment literature abound (e.g., Heal, Sigelman, & Switzky, 1978; McCarver & Craig, 1974; Windle, 1962), but they have tended to emphasize design issues over measurement issues. And data collected from retarded persons (along with those collected from nonretarded informants) have generally been accepted at face value. To cite one example, O'Donnell (1976) concluded on the basis of interview data that multiply handicapped, severely retarded residents of an institution were sensitive to and concerned about issues involving their rights as residents and capable of stating their opinions. However, judging from data to be presented in this chapter, there is serious reason to believe that responses to the "yes-no" questions O'Donnell asked may have been biased by acquiescence, the tendency to answer a question affirmatively regardless of its content (Cronbach, 1946).

Fortunately, there is an extensive literature on systematic biases, or response effects, associated with task, interviewer, and respondent variables in survey research with the general population (cf. Sudman & Bradburn, 1974, for a synthetic review). This literature can and should be applied in the developmental disabilities field to minimize bias in survey research with non-retarded informants. Moreover, while no available literature specifically addresses problems in interviewing mentally retarded persons, there is certainly no reason to think that mentally retarded people are immune from response effects found in the general population. On the contrary, the literature suggests that several response effects are more pronounced among less educated respondents than among more educated ones (Schuman & Presser, 1977; Sudman & Bradburn, 1974). Due to deficient cognitive, verbal, and social skills, mentally retarded persons might be especially susceptible to response effects.

In short, the question of response reliability and validity is by no means trivial. Threats to reliability and validity seriously jeopardize the substantive conclusions reached by researchers as well as by service providers who, in this age of consumerism, are attempting to involve clients in the decision-making process. Assuming that mentally retarded persons should be given opportunities to communicate about their own lives and needs, it is incumbent on researchers to explore the methodological issues involved in doing so.

The present research on the feasibility of interviewing mentally retarded consumers was inspired by the President's Committee on Mental Retardation (PCMR) and funded by the Rehabilitation Services Administration. PCMR suggested a periodic poll of a representative national sample of the mentally retarded about their circumstances, needs, and attitudes which could be used in national policy-making. Before any such national poll was even contemplated, however, it was essential to explore the feasibility and potential productivity of verbal interviews with mentally retarded informants.

In this chapter are reported four separate studies which address several questions about interviewing the retarded:

1. To what extent can retarded persons respond to questions in an appropriate fashion, regardless of the truth value of their answers?;
2. How reliable are such responses, in the sense of being consistent over time?;
3. How valid are such responses, in the sense of agreeing with information in records or provided by parents or attendants and in being free of systematic biases?; and
4. What types of questions appear to optimize responsiveness, reliability, and validity?

Methods

Study 1 focused on 52 children, 12-16 years, who were residents of a state institution for the retarded: 20 severely retarded (IQ 25-39), 16 moderately retarded (IQ 40-54), and 16 mildly retarded (IQ 55-69). Two interview forms were used with some questions repeated and others phrased differently on the two forms and with the forms administered approximately a week apart. Through counterbalancing, half of the children received one form first and half received the other. Half were interviewed by one interviewer first and half by the second, and each child was then administered the other form by the other interviewer. A cottage parent familiar with each subject was also interviewed using an interview schedule which included most of the same questions asked of residents (with "you" changed to "he" or "she").

Study 2 was identical in design, but involved adult residents of the institution, including profoundly retarded persons. A total of 58 adult subjects were included: 16 profoundly retarded, 16 severely retarded, 16 moderately retarded, and 10 mildly retarded.

Study 3 focused on children in the 12-16 year range—57 males and females, 18 severely retarded, 19 moderately retarded, and 20 mildly retarded—none of whom was institutionalized. Students at the lower IQ levels were drawn from a school for the trainable mentally retarded while mildly retarded children were drawn from other special education programs in the same city. This study did not deal with the interview-reinterview reliability issue but instead tested several new questions appropriate to community residents and several alternative question formats on the same topic. Each subject's parent or guardian was also interviewed.

Study 4 centered on techniques for eliciting information from low verbal individuals. It involved new interviews with institutionalized children and adults who had been largely, but not totally, unresponsive in Studies 1 and 2. The 29 participants ranged in IQ from 20 to 48.

Certain methods applied in all four studies. The content areas of interest were always major activities, living circumstances, service and program use, and involvement in decision-making. Moreover, responsiveness to the communication demands of questions was measured in each study through a slight modification of a coding system originally developed by Sigelman and Werder (1975), which includes nine categories: (1) no response; (2) unintelligible response; (3) irrelevant response; (4) don't know, don't remember, not sure; (5) inadequate response (vague or uncodable); (6) request for clarification of the question; (7) refusal to answer; (8) minimally appropriate response (response which meets the formal demands of the question); and (9) expanded response (response which provides qualifying or additional information beyond the formal demands of the question).

Interrater reliability for this coding system has been established at .85 or higher. In all studies, the interviewee's first response to the question was coded in this manner. In the adult institutional sample, responses to a second asking of the question when the first response was inappropriate were also coded. In the children's institutional sample, questions were asked only once while in all other samples questions were asked a second time, if necessary, in exactly the same form. While responsiveness to the first asking formed the measure of responsiveness, codings of the content of responses were based on whichever response, first or second, was at least minimally appropriate. The primary measures of responsiveness used were number of responses coded 8 or 9 divided by the number of questions asked (to form individual responsiveness scores) or by the number of subjects asked a question (to form difficulty scores for each question).

In all four studies a simple screening procedure was used when a person's ability to engage in an interview was suspect. The procedure consisted of three simple questions ("What is your name?" "Is your name [subject's name] ?" "Can you understand me?"). Each of these was asked a second time if no initial response was obtained. If any response (word, sound, or gesture) to one of these questions was given, the person was administered the full interview. Those who could not respond at all were defined as totally unresponsive to all questions in the full interview even though it was not actually administered.

Finally, all four studies utilized contingency tables to examine issues of reliability and validity. In comparisons of participants' responses to a first and second asking of the same question or to alternatively phrased questions on the same topic, contingency tables indicate the percentage of the responding sample providing the same answers on both occasions. Similarly, interviewees' responses can be cross-tabulated with significant others' responses to the same questions. At the same time, cells representing inconsistency between paired answers can be examined to identify particular patterns of response error.

Results

Responsiveness

The first challenge in interviewing mentally retarded persons is to elicit a response of some sort. In Study 1, four interviewees (all males in the severe range) did not respond to the screening questions while the remaining 48 subjects responded at least to some extent. Differences among children were large, with the percentage of the 82 questions on the first form answered appropriately ranging from 0 to 100%. Responsiveness was found to be stable over time, as indicated by a correlation of .96 between percentages of appropriate responses to the two forms. The percentage of questions answered appropriately was also related to IQ ($r = +.62$). The mean percentages of questions answered appropriately for the severely, moderately, and mildly retarded groups were 46.1%, 84.8%, and 90.9%, respectively, pointing to lower responsiveness among the severely retarded, $F(2,49) = 22.51$, $p = .0001$. However, variability was also greater in the severely retarded group (SD = 31.6%) than in the moderately retarded (SD = 17.2%) and mildly retarded (SD = 6.0%) groups, which means that the responsiveness of individuals in the severe retardation range was relatively unpredictable.

Among institutionalized children, neither age nor sex was correlated with responsiveness. In all three IQ groups, responsiveness improved somewhat from first to second administration (71.8% vs. 74.6%, nonsignificant), and the two interviewers did not differ in the responsiveness they elicited from subjects.

Similar analyses in Study 2 confirmed these findings. In this institutionalized adult sample, the only one in which interviews with profoundly retarded persons were attempted, 13 of 16 profoundly retarded subjects failed the initial screening, along with one severely retarded person. The three profoundly retarded persons who passed the screening generally responded to very few of the interview questions, leading to the obvious conclusion that verbal interviews are not feasible for the profoundly retarded. Excluding all profoundly retarded persons, average percentages of appropriate responses for severely, moderately, and mildly retarded groups were 58.5%, 78.0%, and 73.5%, respectively, with variability again high in the severe retardation range but in this case also high in the mild retardation range.[1] In this sample, the correlation between IQ and appropriateness of response was +.51, and age and sex were not predictors of responsiveness. Again, an individual's responsiveness score was stable, with the correlation between individual responsiveness scores on the two forms (+.96) identical to that obtained in the children's institution sample. Finally, while there was some improvement in responsiveness—from 64.6% on first administration to 68.0% on second administration for items repeated across both forms—it was not significant. Again, which person conducted the interview did not affect responsiveness.

Study 2 also focused on whether asking a question a second time if the interviewee had not been able to respond appropriately increased responsiveness. This analysis employed 131 questions drawn from both forms, broken down by question type (yes-no, picture choice, either-or, verbal multiple choice, and open-ended). For all five types of questions, t-tests for dependent means indicated that the mean percent of the sample responsive after two askings of a question was significantly higher than the mean percent of the sample responsive after one asking. While this may seem intuitively obvious, it does suggest the wisdom of giving mentally retarded persons additional opportunities to comprehend a question if they cannot respond appropriately the first time.

---

[1]These figures are based on the 142 items of the first form. They are also somewhat misleading since the mean for the mild MR group (N = 10) was substantially lowered by one subject who was too emotionally disturbed to participate in the interview. Excluding that one subject, the mean responsiveness score in the group increased from 73.5% to 81.1% and the standard deviation decreased from 25.5% to 10.1%.

The relationship between IQ and overall responsiveness also emerged in responses to the very different questionnaire used in Study 3 ($r = +.41$). In this sample, possibly because the design of the questions was guided by knowledge gained from previous studies, severely retarded persons did relatively well, averaging 78.7% responsiveness, compared to 82.1% in the moderately retarded group and 92.7% in the mildly retarded group, $F(2,54) = 5.93$, $p = .005$. In this case, the severely retarded group, instead of being less responsive than either of the other groups, resembled the moderately retarded group, and both groups were less responsive than the mildly retarded.

Overall, then, it may be concluded that responsiveness to interview questions is stable, in the sense that an individual's responsiveness score one week accurately predicts his or her score a week later. Moreover, responsiveness appears to have a cognitive basis, as indicated by its positive association with IQ, and can be expected to diminish significantly as one moves toward the profound retardation range. Responsiveness does not appear to have been affected by factors such as age, sex, or interviewer although it did increase slightly with practice.

Perhaps the finding of most practical importance is that responsiveness was clearly a function of the type of question asked—some types of questions being answerable by vast majorities of subjects and others representing major challenges. Table 1 presents the mean responsiveness scores in Studies 1, 2, and 3 for each type of question. As the table indicates, the relative difficulty of the various types of questions was quite stable across samples. Consistently, questions which could be answered by pointing to a picture or by answering "yes" or "no" (with the occasional exception of yes-no questions asking for subjective perceptions) were easiest to answer appropriately. This is not surprising in view of the fact that both of these types of questions could be answered nonverbally (by pointing in the first case, by nodding or shaking the head in the second). Either-or questions typically elicited the next highest rates of responsiveness and were easier (for all but community children) than both verbal multiple choice and open-ended questions. The multiple choice questions typically required choice among four, or sometimes three, alternatives (e.g., "never," "not much," "sometimes," or "a lot"). Apparently, either because a quantitative concept was involved or because subjects were unable to process so many options, these questions proved difficult, as difficult as open-ended questions that required respondents to generate responses independently, without benefit of structure.

Table 1
Mean Percentages of Appropriate Response to Various Types of Questions in Three Samples

	Sample		
Question Format	Institution Children (N=50)	Institution Adults (N=42)*	Community Children (N=57)
Pictorial Choice	83.3	(Not used)	96.1
Verbal Yes-No (Activities)	82.2	84.8	94.0
Verbal Yes-No (Subjective)	76.5	81.7	81.7
Verbal Either-Or	68.7	65.7	72.5
Verbal Multiple Choice	49.7	51.9	72.9
Open-ended	51.0	50.6	69.9

*Excludes profoundly retarded group

Thus the responsiveness data suggest that yes-no and pictorial choice questions are the methods of preference if the goal is to obtain information from as many mentally retarded persons as possible. However, obtaining an appropriate answer is only part of the battle; one must ask whether answers are reliable and valid.

Reliability

Drawing on data from the Studies 1 and 2, the extent to which answers to questions one week were consistent with answers to the same questions a week later was examined.

In the children's institution study, 30 questions repeated on both forms were examined for reliability. Twelve yes-no questions pertaining to activities, quality of life, and rules and decision-making were repeated on both forms. On the average, 85.2% of those able to respond "yes" or "no" to both askings of these 12 questions gave the same answer both times. Consistency was particularly high on questions about activities (93.5%) and lowest on questions about rules and decision-making (77.3%), with the lowest consistency figure (56.1%) obtained on the question, "Are you allowed to hit people?" The fact that a "no" answer to this question is socially desirable is not coincidental. On many of the questions (8 of 12), the predominant type of consistency was saying "yes" both times in cases where "yes" represented the socially desirable answer. As will be noted later, acquiescent responses were common in these samples; thus one might suspect that the reliability figures for yes-no questions are generally inflated. In any case, the relatively high reliability figures for yes-no questions are not necessarily evidence of validity.

An additional four questions of the yes-no variety, this time asking about chores and presenting pictures of each chore, also yielded high reliability (89.8% on the average). Again, however, since "yes" responses to both askings accounted for almost all of the consistency, one cannot rule out the operation of acquiescent response sets.

Six multiple choice questions repeated across forms also posed interpretive problems. Three of these questions—asking interviewees to identify the extent of their activity as "a lot," "sometimes," "not much," or "never" (or in one case "a lot," "some," "not many," and "none" in reference to number of friends)—yielded 71.9% consistency on the average. This figure is relatively high considering the fact that the probability of matching responses by chance is lower for a four-choice question than for a two-choice, yes-no question. However, three other questions, asking respondents to point to one of four faces (degrees of frowning or smiling) to indicate how they felt about aspects of institutional life, yielded extremely low consistency (46.2%). It is impossible to determine whether this was the case because of the subjective and mood-dependent nature of the questions or because a greater proportion of the sample was able to respond to these pictorial choice questions than to the verbal multiple choice questions. In any case, this format was not successful.

The remaining eight questions repeated on both forms were open-ended. Four were factual in nature, calling for name, spelling of name, birthday, and characterization of the state school. Roughly two-thirds of those asked these questions were responsive to the first and second administrations of each. Of these, 63.3% were consistently able to give their full name correctly; 42.9% were consistently able to spell their names; 63.6% consistently identified their birthdays; and 61.9% consistently described the place in which they lived. This finding is rather discouraging, not only because many persons could not answer these basic questions, but also because those who did often gave incorrect or incomplete information both times.

The remaining four open-ended questions were each analyzed by response categories, which were based on responses given by both residents and attendants. In these cases, both the total percentage consistent (i.e., either mentioning an item in a category on both askings or failing to mention it both times) and the percentage mentioning something both times were examined. There were marked differences between the two measures. On a question asking for an enumeration of activities with friends, for example, the average total consistency figure across all eight categories was 70.7%, but the average percentage of respondents consistently mentioning something both times was only 18.1%. Virtually the same thing occurred for the other questions asked. For example, asked about what they were being taught in school, 69.6% of those who could answer both times referred to academics of some kind, but for each other category of response, high total consistency was achieved by failing to refer to a category both times. There seems to be no satisfactory way of analyzing such questions, for consistency depends on the verbosity of the respondents and the number of categories developed by the coders. Perhaps the major conclusion to be drawn is that open-ended questions calling for enumerations yield very little information, partially because many mentally retarded persons cannot respond appropriately to them in the first place, and partially because when they do respond, they say very little. However, since the total consistency figures for all 35 response categories of four questions averaged 83.9%, one can at least conclude that it was relatively rare that a respondent mentioned something one time but failed to mention it the other time.

Judging from this sample, reliability of response from one week to the next can generally be considered marginally adequate, except for the subjective questions mentioned previously about rules and decision making and the picture-choice questions about the quality of institutional life. Reliability did vary as a function of both question format and question content, but for the most part answers to questions repeated a week apart were largely similar.

Similarly, reliability over a one-week interval appeared to be relatively adequate in the adult institution sample. For 29 yes-no questions, the average percentage of cases in which responses to the two askings agreed was 81.2%. Consistency did not vary as a function of whether these questions were factual or subjective. The average consistency figure for four, either-or questions was similar (82.2%), as was the figure for categories of response to eight, open-ended questions (86.8%). Again, the potential for acquiescence on yes-no questions and the predominance of "no mention-no mention" consistency on open-ended questions suggest that reliability figures may be artificially inflated. As measurement specialists well know, reliability does not necessarily imply validity.

Validity

The validity of answers was examined both by comparing subjects' responses to alternative questions on the same topics and by comparing their responses with information provided by significant others (attendants or parents). Technically, neither of these approaches fully addresses the validity question. A respondent can be consistent in his or her responses to alternative questions without necessarily revealing the truth; similarly, lack of agreement with a significant other cannot necessarily be construed to mean that the retarded respondent is wrong. However, these two sources of information do provide suggestive evidence about response validity. What follows will highlight some of the findings, starting with a type of response bias that has major implications for interviewing the mentally retarded.

Acquiescence. This research clearly indicates that acquiescence—the tendency to answer yes-no questions affirmatively regardless of their content—is more common among mentally retarded respondents than in the general population (cf. Rosen, Floor, & Zisfein, 1974, for related data) and is a serious enough problem to invalidate yes-no questions, despite the fact that they are associated with high rates of responsiveness. In part this issue was approached by asking, within the same interviews, oppositely worded questions where "yes" answers to both questions are contradictory. Table 2 presents rates of acquiescence (yes-yes combinations of response) in three of our samples for two such sets of questions: "Are you usually happy?" vs. "Are you usually sad?"; and "Are you usually by yourself?" vs. "Are you usually with other people?" As can be seen, rates of acquiescence on these subjective questions were alarmingly high in all three samples. Moreover, in most cases persons with lower IQs were more likely to acquiesce as indicated by correlations between IQ and acquiescence versus nonacquiescence.

Table 2
Percent Saying "Yes" to Both Questions in Pair and Correlations of Acquiescence and IQ in Three Samples

	Percent Acquiescing	r with IQ
Are you usually happy?		
Are you usually sad?		
Community Children (N=55)	50.9	–.30*
Institution Children (N=32)	43.8	–.40*
Institution Adults (N=38)	44.7	–.41*
Are you usually by yourself?		
Are you usually with other people?		
Community Children (N=50)	50.0	–.24*
Institution Children (N=33)	39.4	.03
Institution Adults (N=36)	41.7	–.04

*p<.05

A second approach was used to "smoke out" acquiescence in the sample of more severely retarded residents of the institution. They were asked questions that should have elicited "no" answers, e.g., "Are you Chinese?" and "Are you a school bus driver?" In response to a set of these questions, 44% would have the investigators believe that they are Chinese, 41.7% that they are school bus drivers, 52.0% that they know how to fly an airplane, and 73.1% that it snows (in Arkansas) in the summer! The only question in the set which yielded a low rate of acquiescence (28.0%) was more immediately verifiable and was phrased, "Right now, is it raining outside?" (or sunny outside, whichever question should have been answered "no" at the time).

To further illustrate the implications of acquiescence, Table 3 presents four sets of alternatively worded yes-no and either-or questions, along with the percentages of the institutional children's sample responding in various ways. In each case, positively worded yes-no questions yield a very rosy picture of the group, perhaps because "yes" responses in these cases also represent socially desirable responses while negatively worded yes-no questions give a relatively bleak picture. As Table 4 indicates, inconsistency of response was higher for paired yes-no questions than for paired either-or questions, with acquiescence rather than nay-saying accounting for the vast proportion of inconsistency. By comparison, although there was some tendency to choose the last choice on either-or questions, consistency of response was relatively good.

Table 3
Mean Rates of Inconsistency and Response Content for Four Question Sets (Institutional Children)

	Mean % Inconsistent	*% Happy*
Are you usually happy?		91
Are you usually sad?		47
Are you usually happy or sad?	29.2	67
Are you usually sad or happy?		85
		% Nice
Do people here treat you nice?		88
Do people here treat you mean?		57
Do people here treat you mean or nice?	24.2	68
Do people here treat you nice or mean?		69
		% Big Enough
Is this place where you live big enough?		86
Is this place where you live too little?		64
Is this place where you live big enough or too little?	26.1	71
Is this place where you live too little or big enough?		88
		% Other People
Are you usually with other people?		82
Are you usually by yourself?		42
Are you usually by yourself or with other people?	32.9	70
Are you usually with other people or by yourself?		67

Moderate negative correlations were repeatedly found between acquiescence and IQ, indicating that while moderately and mildly retarded respondents are by no means free of a tendency to acquiesce, the more severely retarded the respondent, the greater the likelihood of acquiescence. For example, in the children's institution sample, the relationship between IQ and an acquiescence index based on the four pairs of yes-no questions in Table 3 was –.35. Moreover, it was found that acquiescence on oppositely worded questions predicts "yes" answers to some other sets of yes-no questions. For example, in the children's institution sample the

Table 4
Specific Response Biases Underlying Inconsistency of Responses to Alternative Questions (Institution Children)

	Mean % of Paired Answers
Yes/No Questions	
Acquiescence	36.9
Naysaying	3.5
Total	40.4
Either/or Questions	
First Thing Mentioned	9.2
Last Thing Mentioned	18.6
Total	27.8

acquiescence index predicted endorsement of items about negative treatment by others even with IQ controlled (partial $r = .35$). In the community children's sample, those high on acquiescence and low in IQ were likely to claim they were being taught a greater number of subjects in school (partial correlations of .38 and –.33 for acquiescence and IQ, respectively, controlling the other variable). While this is not the case for all sets of items examined, many mentally retarded persons do have a strong acquiescent response set which invalidates their answers to some yes-no questions. At the very least, these findings suggest that yes-no questions should not be employed without checks for the operation of acquiescence; beyond that, it is also arguable that they should be avoided whenever possible.

Agreement with significant others. To what extent do the answers of retarded persons and those of nonretarded informants match? Findings from the children's institution sample are instructive. Across 56 questions, the average percentage of agreement between residents and attendants familiar with each resident was 62.8%, which suggests a rather mixed pattern of agreement and disagreement.

As was the case with reliability, child-attendant agreement varied from question type to question type. For yes-no questions, the average was 73.2%, but agreement was greater on questions about activities and relationships than on questions about rules and decision-making and knowledge of various topics relevant to independent living. Even within topical categories, agreement was mixed. For example, subjects and attendants readily agreed (95.7%) that subjects watched television. However, for less commonly performed activities, agreement was lower, typically because clients said "yes" while attendants said "no." This was especially true of a series of questions asking if subjects knew how to read and write, cook, keep house, and count money. On all but the housekeeping question, the most frequent response combination (from 45% to 58% of the paired responses) was "yes" from the client and "no" from the attendant. This pattern is very likely a function of acquiescence on the part of retarded persons.

Resident-attendant agreement was lowest on multiple choice questions (29.9% on the average) and higher on open-ended questions (74.8% across categories). However, as was the case with reliability, this relatively high agreement was typically a product of both parties' failing to mention a category. Positive agreement was very rare, and, of course, relatively few paired responses could be compared in the first place because of the difficulty participants had in responding to open-ended questions. At the same time, there were several instances in which an attendant mentioned something which was not mentioned by the client, suggesting that just as yes-no questions may lead to overreporting by mentally retarded persons, open-ended questions, which demand verbal skill, may lead to underreporting.

In the adult institution sample, client-attendant agreement for 126 questions averaged 59.3%. In the community children's sample, child-parent agreement across 61 questions averaged 64.5%. Further comparisons of these three samples using only questions asked in all three studies have confirmed the conclusion that child-parent agreement is not significantly greater than resident-attendant agreement (Sigelman, Schoenrock, Spanhel, Hromas, Winer, Budd, & Martin, 1980). Instead, whether it is a community sample or an institutionalized one, and whether the respondents are adults or children, retarded persons and informants speaking for them agree about two-thirds of the time on the average. Percentages agreeing do vary greatly from question type to question type, with, for example, multiple choice questions with quantitative options consistently faring miserably but either-or questions and some open-ended questions consistently yielding high agreement. Thus, while retarded persons can be expected to give the same answer on two occasions about 80% of the time, that answer is not as likely to be confirmed by an informant. Certainly these agreement figures are low enough to suggest that versions of reality obtained from retarded persons and nonretarded persons who know them may differ substantially.

What can be done to circumvent this problem and others identified above? It is to this question that attention next is turned.

Comparison of Alternative Questions

A major purpose of this study has been to compare alternative questions in hopes of identifying techniques that optimize responsiveness, reliability, and validity. To illustrate the approach used and the types of insights which emerge, consider one comparison made in the adult institution sample, summarized in Table 5.

Table 5
Comparison of Alternative Formats
Yes-no versus Open-ended
("Do you decide what chores you do?" versus "Who decides what chores you do?" —Adult Institution Sample)

1. *Which Question Yields Higher Responsiveness?*
   Percent Responding Appropriately: Yes-no 54.4%
   Open-ended 34.5%
2. *To What Extent Are Answers Consistent*?
   With answers coded client decides versus someone else decides, percent consistent =56.3%. All of rest (43.7%) are instances of "Yes, I decide" on yes-no and mention of someone else on open-ended—i.e., acquiescence.
3. *To What Extent Do Client and Significant Other Agree*?
   For yes-no; 34.6% agree. Remaining 65.4% are cases in which client says, "Yes, I decide," while attendant mentions someone else in response to open-ended question.
   For open-ended question, 88.2% agree, both saying "someone else."

Conclusion: While more subjects can answer the yes-no question, acquiescence invalidates response. Open-ended question is preferred on grounds of validity.

In comparing two questions—in this case a yes-no and an open-ended question— the responsiveness test was first applied and it was concluded that the yes-no question yielded responses from a higher proportion of the sample. Turning to the issue of reliability, however, consistency of response to the two questions was relatively low, and error was systematic—specifically, consisting of "yes, I decide" responses to the yes-no question paired with mention of someone else in response to the open-ended question. As a result of acquiescence, answers to the yes-no question were also not as valid (in the sense that they agreed with the attendants' answers) as responses to the open-ended question. As was found on numerous occasions, there are trade-offs to be made. While the yes-no question is to be preferred on grounds of responsiveness, it is clearly deficient on grounds of validity because of the strong influence of acquiescence. The open-ended question should therefore be the method of choice, but neither is very attractive.

To illustrate that validity does not always have to come at the expense of responsiveness, consider the picture choice, open-ended, and multiple choice questions on the same topic presented in Table 6 and based on the children's community sample. Here, as expected, the picture choice question optimized responsiveness, but interestingly, the verbal multiple choice question on this topic was easier to answer than most multiple choice questions which were examined. Comparison of children's responses to the alternative formats provides little

Table 6
Comparison of Alternative Formats

Picture Choice vs. Open-ended vs. Multiple Choice
(Child Community Sample)

A. (Pictures of bus, car, walking, and bicycle) "Which way do you get to school most days? Point to the picture."

B. "Most days, how do you get to school?"

C. "Most days, do you get to school on the bus, in a car, by walking, or by riding a bicycle?"

1. *Responsiveness*: Picture Choice: 100%; Open-ended: 73.6%; Multiple Choice: 94.5%

2. *Consistency*: 95.2% between picture choice and open-ended, 86.9% between picture choice and multiple choice, 95.1% between open-ended and multiple choice.

3. *Agreement with significant other*: Picture Choice: 85.8%; Open-ended: 85.4%; Multiple Choice: 77.4% (tendency to choose last option where no parent chose it)

Conclusion: The major disadvantage of the open-ended question is that it yields low responsiveness. Picture choice appears to optimize responsiveness with no sacrifice in validity. Verbal multiple choice was associated with a slight tendency to choose the last option.

guidance, for responses are generally reliable and free of bias. However, child-parent agreement figures suggest that, on the verbal multiple choice question, children tended to select the last of the four options (bicycle), whereas such bias was not evident on the picture choice question. Although the open-ended question also yielded valid answers, the picture choice question is ultimately preferable because it optimized responsiveness without sacrificing validity.

Based on many such analyses, one is reasonably confident in several conclusions about alternative questions. First, as noted previously, acquiescence is a serious threat to the validity of yes-no questions. Acquiescence does not appear to be reduced through the use of pictures or drawings accompanying yes-no questions. Moreover, the impacts of acquiescence are evident in numerous comparisons between yes-no questions and other formats, especially open-ended ones. When yes-no lists and open-ended questions on the same topic (e.g., activities with friends) are compared, there is a clear trend toward overreporting on the yes-no questions and underreporting on the open-ended questions. This finding is consistent with the literature for the general population (Belson & Duncan, 1952; Schuman & Presser, 1977), but is highly exaggerated in retarded samples. Therefore, just as yes-no questions create validity problems, open-ended questions appear to reduce responsiveness and create validity problems of their own.

Another conclusion reached is that multiple choice questions involving quantitative concepts (e.g., a lot, sometimes, not much, never) appear to create numerous reliability and validity problems. Comparisons of such four-choice questions with two-stage counterparts (e.g., Does your family come to visit you? (if yes) Do they visit you a lot, some, or not much?) have revealed that both formats are unsatisfactory. Such multiple choice questions are also subject to a response bias—a tendency to choose the last option in the series. Pictorial multiple choice questions requiring a selection among happy and sad faces have also proved unsatisfactory. At best, reliability figures for them suggest that satisfaction as measured by such questions is highly mood-dependent and changeable from week to week, in which case questions can be raised about the utility of such information. At worst, mentally retarded informants appear to choose responses randomly. In any case, neither these picture formats nor verbal multiple choice counterparts are adequate.

Having detected serious problems with yes-no questions, quantitative multiple choice questions, and many open-ended questions, these researchers are most optimistic about the potential of either-or questions, which appear to be associated with relatively high reliability and validity without sacrificing a great deal in responsiveness. Multiple choice questions with discrete rather than quantitative options (e.g., the one in Table 6) and open-ended questions calling for a single answer rather than an enumeration of activities also show promise as methods of obtaining meaningful answers from retarded persons.

Finally, not only does question format affect answers, but there is evidence about the influence of question wording. Several comparisons have been made of questions like, "Do you play any sports?" and "Do you play any sports, like baseball or football?" both followed by an open-ended question, "Which ones?" The use of examples, which might appeal as a means of making an abstract concept concrete, creates problems. It generally produces slightly higher responsiveness to the follow-up open-ended question, but this gain in responsiveness is associated with a higher-than-normal tendency to echo back the items used as examples. To cite another example, comparisons have indicated that, in asking about rules and decision-making, choice of words influences findings. For one set, for example,

77.6% on the average answered "no" to a series of questions about rules using the phrase "are you allowed," while only 57.3% responded "yes" to parallel questions with the phrase "it is against the rules," a finding which replicates one in the general literature comparing the terms "allow" and "forbid" (Schuman & Presser, 1977).

Summary and Conclusions

This paper has provided an overview of several findings from studies of the feasibility of interviewing the mentally retarded. To summarize briefly, it has been found that:

(1) The ability to respond to questions is a stable individual behavior, partially a function of intelligence, and is optimized by certain types of questions, especially those that allow nonverbal responses. Verbal interviewing techniques appear to be infeasible in the profound retardation range, applicable with some severely retarded persons, and generally applicable in the moderately and mildly retarded ranges.

(2) Reliability of response to questions asked a week apart generally averages around 80% but varies quite substantially for different formats and content areas.

(3) Agreement between mentally retarded clients and parents or attendants appears to be lower than the reliability of client responses and is low enough to suggest that substantially different information may sometimes be obtained from the two sources.

(4) Response effects found in the general population appear to be pronounced in mentally retarded populations. In particular, acquiescence is a significant enough problem to make the use of yes-no questions suspect, despite the fact that they optimize responsiveness. To a lesser extent, a tendency to select the last option on multiple choice questions and to say little in response to open-ended questions are also problems.

(5) Comparisons of alternative questions on the same topics, while not always pointing to the superiority of one question or another, have revealed recurring biases associated with certain types of questions and indicate that the extent to which clients' answers are congruent with information provided by significant others depends on how the question is asked.

These findings are highly relevant to both past and future studies of deinstitutionalization. Unfortunately, they are rather discouraging. They suggest that obtaining answers, especially reliable and valid answers, from mentally retarded persons is a challenging task; moreover, they imply that the validity of some data obtained in previous studies is suspect. For instance, yes-no checklists have been a common technique of obtaining information about activities, services received, and so on; yet these findings suggest that such checklists are likely to produce overreporting. More important, since acquiescence is generally more common among the more severely retarded than among the less severely retarded, the acquiescence phenomenon may well obscure relationships between IQ and extent of involvement in activities. At the same time, it is important to recognize that parents, attendants, houseparents, and other informants are by no means immune from response effects themselves, judging from the survey research literature.

In short, the findings reported here underscore the need for further attention to reliability and validity issues in mental retardation research. The present study has emphasized the effects of question format and wording, leaving many other issues (for example, order of questions, familiarity of interviewer and interviewee, site of interview) unexamined. Indeed, some unanticipated threats to validity were encountered, such as the dampening effect of Elvis Presley's death during one of data-gathering trips and the tendency of some respondents to stop talking when they saw that the interviewer had run out of space for writing. To put things in perspective, however, it must be noted that emphasis has been given to reliability and validity of information provided by *individual* respondents. If response error is largely random, the picture of a *sample* which emerges from a study may not be greatly affected by variations in question format and wording (although one cannot be heartened when respondents appear to be answering as if they were flipping coins). Systematic bias (e.g., acquiescence) is the primary validity threat, for pictures of the aggregate may then be distorted. It should also be noted that many problems encountered in our research are not as pronounced in the mild range of retardation, suggesting that previous studies, by restricting interviewing to more verbal clients, may have fewer reliability and validity problems than the present investigators uncovered.

This research group strongly believes that clients' perspectives should be considered in evaluating policy and program alternatives. In many instances, the group's interviews have yielded a great deal of insight into the lives of mentally retarded persons. This implies that it is the researcher's responsibility to improve rather than shut off the communication process by designing questions (and perhaps creative nonverbal or behavioral observation techniques) that optimize responsiveness, reliability, and validity. It also implies that researchers should concern themselves with reliability and validity issues, for example by using multiple approaches in inquiring about a given topic and incorporating systematic checks for response bias. Researchers should be impressed and confident when findings from different studies concur despite method variation, as witnessed in the present volume, but they should devote more attention to identifying implications of method variation.

While the present research has not identified sure solutions, a great deal has been learned about what to expect from mentally retarded persons in interviews, about what approaches are clearly faulty, and about what approaches appear to have potential. At the very least, it is hoped that these findings will make researchers more sensitive to methodological issues as they seek information directly from mentally retarded persons.

References

Belson, W., & Duncan, J. A. A comparison of the checklist and the open response questioning systems. *Applied Statistics,* 1962, *11,* 120-132.

Cronbach, L. J. Response sets and test validity. *Educational and Psychological Measurement,* 1946, *6,* 475-494.

Gollay, E., Freedman, R., Wyngaarden, M., & Kurtz, N. R. *Coming back: The community experiences of deinstitutionalized mentally retarded people.* Cambridge, MA: Abt Books, 1978.

Heal, L. W., Sigelman, C. K., & Switzky, H. N. Research on community residential alternatives for the mentally retarded. In N. R. Ellis (Ed.), *International review of research in mental retardation* (Vol. 9). New York: Academic Press, 1978.

McCarver, R. B., & Craig, E. M. Placement of the retarded in the community: Prognosis and outcome. In N. R. Ellis (Ed.), *International review of research in mental retardation* (Vol. 7). New York: Academic Press, 1974.

O'Donnell, B. Resident rights interview. *Mental Retardation,* 1976, *14*(6), 13-17.

Rosen, M., Floor, L., & Zisfein, L. Investigating the phenomenon of acquiescence in the mentally handicapped. I. Theoretical model, test development and normative data. *British Journal of Mental Subnormality,* 1974, *20,* 58-68.

Schuman, H. & Presser, S. Question wording as an independent variable in survey analysis. *Sociological Methods and Research,* 1977, *6,* 151-170.

Sigelman, C. K., & Werder, P. R. The communication skills of the mentally retarded: A new analysis. *Journal of Developmental Disabilities,* 1975, *1,* 9-16.

Sigelman, C. K., Schoenrock, C. J., Spanhel, C. L., Hromas, S. G., Winer, J. L., Budd, E. C., & Martin, P. W. Surveying mentally retarded persons: Responsiveness and response validity in three samples. *American Journal of Mental Deficiency,* 1980, *84,* 479-486.

Sudman, S., & Bradburn, N. M. *Response effects in surveys: A review and synthesis.* Chicago: Aldine, 1974.

Windle, C. Prognosis of mental subnormals. *American Journal of Mental Deficiency,* 1962, *66*(5) (Monograph Supplement).

III. Recent Research on Community Placements

Qualitative Methods and Cultural Perspectives In the Study of Deinstitutionalization

Sylvia Bercovici

The Neuropsychiatric Institute
University of California
at Los Angeles

The classical model of qualitative methodology[1] is the traditional anthropological ethnography of non-Western cultures. The ethnographer's principal task is to produce a faithful description of the phenomena under study employing a holistic perspective and naturalistic data collection procedures such as participant observation.[2] A qualitative approach may be defined as a way of viewing and understanding human beings and cultural phenomena which takes into account: 1) the system or environments of which the subject is a part, and 2) the perspective(s) of the individual(s) under study.

While the need for direct observation and holistic description is obvious in cross cultural research where there may be little or no prior knowledge of the society, it is less so when studying people and institutions in one's own society. There is a feeling, in the latter case, that researchers already know the essential natures of these phenomena and that they can proceed to "zero in" on specific targets of inquiry. This seems to be the case in the current study of deinstitutionalization, particularly the community placement phenomenon.

In speaking of the "community" and in employing terms like "community adaptation," a very general construal seems to satisfy most discussions and premises for research. This construal is based on a taken-for-granted familiarity with the subject matter in question. Quantitative research methods, then, "take off" from this point, requiring reduction of data, the precise measurement of variables, and the testing of hypotheses. This kind of approach does not question its assumption of familiarity and rarely considers a holistic description of the subject under study to be of value. In the case of the above-mentioned subject, although there have been many studies as to what degree deinstitutionalized individuals are "successful" in adapting to the "community," it is still not known specifically and in detail, what might be the nature of such persons' actual daily contacts with this "community." Neither is it known what this phenomenon of "community" might mean to a developmentally disabled person who is living in a

---

The research on which this paper was based was supported in part by the Neuropsychiatric Institute, UCLA Center for the Health Sciences, and by DHEW/Office of Human Development, Grant #50-P45564/9-01.

[1]*Introduction to qualitative research methods: A phenomenological approach to the social sciences* by Robert Bogdan and Steven J. Taylor (New York: John Wiley & Sons, 1975) is a basic text on qualitative methodology that has particular relevance to research in developmental disabilities. An account of anthropological field methods as employed in mental retardation research is found in R. B. Edgerton and L. L. Langness, Observing mentally retarded persons in community settings: An anthropological perspective. In G. P. Sackett (Ed.), *Observing behavior Vol. I: Theory and applications in mental retardation*. Baltimore: University Park Press, 1978, 335-348.

[2]Participant observation generally refers to "...a period of intense social interaction between the researcher and the subject, in the milieu of the latter. During this period, data are unobstrusively and systematically collected" (Bogdan & Taylor, 1975, p. 5).

residential facility or what might be this person's concerns, reflections, and attitudes about the particulars of his or her daily life.

Similarly, in referring to community-based alternatives to state institutions, we proceed as if these have some kind of familiar counterpart or model in the larger society. Experience in these settings, however, would suggest that they comprise a social entity (or entities) with no real precedent in the society. "Group homes," for example, may not only bear little resemblance to each other (Baker, Seltzer & Seltzer, 1977), but additionally, they may not bear any resemblance to, or duplicate the functions of, other human habitats or social settings known to the society. It is possible that this is an emergent form, a response to a particular and unprecedented set of social conditions. However, among all the finely honed research that has been done in the area of community placement, the writer has yet to see a complete description of even one residential facility and the daily life of its residents—one that, following the ethnographic model, assumes nothing and records everything, including, and especially, the "natives'" concerns as expressed in their own words. While this is not a critique of quantitative methodologies, it is a suggestion that researchers might be using their techniques too exclusively in attempting to understand and direct what is a complex situation of social change.

The basis for this argument is a body of exploratory, descriptive research done on community placement viewed as a cultural phenomenon. An initial descriptive survey was made of 40 residential settings for developmentally disabled persons in the Los Angeles area. This included extensive observations of, and personal contact with the residents of these facilities. This preliminary investigation generated a number of questions, among which were: 1) What is the nature of daily life in the particular social system(s) of community based residential settings? 2) What is the nature of the contact that developmentally disabled individuals from these systems have with the larger community? 3) What is the nature of programmed efforts to normalize these persons?

To approach these questions, a sub-sample of 10 group homes was chosen for more detailed ethnographic investigation.[3] As a second stage of the research, this study was carried out under the auspices of a research/service program. The researcher worked in collaboration with a team of occupational therapists who provided habilitation services to residents in the facilities. In this way it was possible to gain greater access to the facilities than otherwise might be the case, and the researcher was able to observe changes in resident behavior when different conditions and experiences were made available to them.

The following is a presentation of some of the features and conditions of the community placement situations that were observed. The descriptive data relating

---

[3]In choosing this sample of 10 facilities, an attempt was made to include variation in size (small, medium, large), location (urban-suburban), and resident level of functioning (severe, moderate, mild retardation). The length and intensity of contact varied from setting to setting due to the varying requirements of the ethnographic task; for example, some facilities were very large with over 100 residents and required many hours of observation just to obtain a basic description. Facilities varied also in their receptivity to the presence of the researcher and the occupational therapy team; the amount of time spent in a facility was greatly affected by this factor. Finally, practical considerations such as distance unavoidably affected the degree and frequency of contact—two facilities were an hour away. The length of contact ranged from 8 months to 3 years. Descriptive data were collected principally through participant observation at the residential facility, by accompanying subjects to settings outside the facility that were part of their natural routines, by observing subjects in activities with the university occupational therapists, and by visiting other habilitation programs, they were ordinarily involved with. Audio and videotaping of informal interviews and naturally occurring interactional events augmented daily fieldnotes as data-recording methods.

to the first question regarding daily life in the residential facility setting are only touched upon here due to the limitations of space. The material presented here is more involved with questions of community contact and selected normalization efforts.

Contact with community. Most of the individuals who were observed had spent a portion of their lives in state institutions; however, many had been living in the community for five years or longer. Observations of these persons revealed a general lack of familiarity with the most commonplace aspects of community life. Investigation revealed various factors and circumstances which served to isolate these persons from the community and thus limit possibilities for acquiring and improving adaptive skills and behavior.

One isolating factor was the demographic location of many of the facilities and the sociological conditions of the immediate neighborhoods. Because of zoning restrictions, many group homes for developmentally disabled persons, especially the large ones, are found in low-rent, commercial areas or in economically depressed residential neighborhoods. In 7 of 10 facilities developmentally disabled residents were justifiably fearful of their physical safety should they venture too far from the facility. For example, one facility was surrounded by liquor stores, bars, and adult motels. The women residents repeatedly warned the researcher to be careful—that rape and robbery were common events in the area and occurred even during the day. Careful mapping of this neighborhood and excursions with the residents revealed that the nearest shopping area was several miles away—a long walk for these persons, many of whom have physical disabilities, are in poor health and physical condition, or perhaps labor under the effects of tranquilizing medications. Few of the residents of this facility, as was the case for the sample in general, knew how to use the bus or had a special reduced fare bus pass.

In half the cases, the facility residents were a racial minority in the immediate neighborhood. Congregates of these developmentally disabled persons in such areas then tend not only to be stigmatized by physical and behavioral handicaps and by the label "retarded," but also by their minority status. Contrary to some expectations, observations in this study suggest that while developmentally disabled persons may be tolerated by inhabitants of lower income or economically depressed neighborhoods, they are not necessarily any more accepted than they are in more affluent neighborhoods, and they are certainly not exempt from victimization.

In addition to certain features of the surrounding community that might make developmentally disabled persons reluctant to venture out of the facility, there are discouragements that stem from the management concerns of the facility operator.

While the residential facilities in the study varied in size, type, and location, within the greater Los Angeles area, with only two exceptions, they had one important feature in common—the residents were not permitted to, were discouraged from, or were not shown how to go out into the community to make use of resources available to "normal" persons, or to establish relationships with persons other than those in the facility, workshop, or activity center. Rigidity of routine due to cost-efficiency concerns and caretaker avoidance of risk are just two among several factors which promote a general conservatism among home operators regarding the issue of community experience for their developmentally disabled residents. This situation held particularly true for the smaller group homes with 10 or fewer residents.

Another generalization that may be made from the observational evidence is that in addition to not preparing their charges for, or encouraging them to experience the world outside the facility, caretakers tend to discourage, even prohibit residents from maintaining contacts with friends or acquaintances or inviting them to visit at the facility. This seemed especially true of the smaller facilities and was the case in 6 of the 10 group homes in the study. In homes that are not large enough to warrant a pay phone, residents' use of the facility's phone is frequently limited. Residents may be prohibited from using the phone at all to make calls and are frequently told that they may not give the telephone number to anyone outside their families. Incoming calls are answered or may be intercepted by the caretaker or staff. Many otherwise competent individuals in the study did not know how to use a telephone and had not developed social communicational patterns that would require this skill—the lack of which, in turn, prevented increased social communication. Similarly, it was the experience of the researcher, and that of other service personnel in the field who were interviewed, that most facility operators do not like visitors of any kind to come to their facility. "Resident privacy" is the reason frequently offered, but it also seems to be the case that operators are apprehensive that licensing violations will be witnessed and reported. The overall impression this "closed-door" policy makes is that caretakers are trying to maintain as much autonomy as possible in a situation where they feel overburdened by bureaucratic surveillance. It is clear from any brief conversation with residential facility operators that they feel they have proprietary rights in their enterprises and that these rights are being increasingly violated. As one caretaker commented, "Everyone talks about *client* rights, but nobody talks about *caretaker* rights."

Confirmation of the picture of isolation from the larger community just presented comes from developmentally disabled persons themselves. Some of the men and women in the study who were former state hospital patients still seemed to perceive themselves as being on the "inside" while others (that is, "normal" persons) are on the "outside." The following quotations typify the kind of statements that are made by informants from various facilities:

Roger, the resident who made the following statement, is a man in his thirties who has been "in the community" for over five years and lives in a small group home.

> I'm not really a mentally retarded patient. I figure I can do things on my own more than anybody else can do. I can go *out in the public* right now if I wanted to. . . . Because, I figure it this way. Every person's gotta have their own life to live and go *out in the public* and show the public what they can do *out there* more than people *out there* can do when they could be *in here* helping us, helping the mentally retarded, you know what I mean? . . . Like if we were *out there*—they're sicker more than we are . . . than *we are in here*. . .They need to be *in here* more than we should. And we could be *out there*. Because I figure this way, it's not right to call a person mentally retarded.

The next quotation is from an interview with Arline, a woman in her middle forties, who has been in the community for over 20 years. Fourteen years were spent on a work placement program. For the past seven years Arline has lived in a large board and care facility.

> I just want to *get out* and live a good normal life. . . . Live like other people—normal. Talk normal, work, have a nice place to live. *Get out* and meet other people . . . I get forty dollars a month. It's be less than that if I'm living on the *outside*. That what the social worker said.

Contact with "normal" others. In the absence of significant contact with the larger community for these developmentally disabled persons, the preponderance of interaction with "normal" others is with the facility staff. In the facilities studied, the bulk of personal contact with residents fell primarily to custodial personnel. In only one facility of the 10 in the sample was the owner/operator the person with whom the residents had most contact. The other facilities were characterized by absentee owner/operators who only visited their facilities—sometimes on a daily, sometimes on a weekly, basis. All but one of the caretakers owned and operated one or more facilities *in addition* to the one in the study. Only three of the facilities (the larger ones with resident capacities ranging from 35 to 140 persons) had hired administrators; the other facilities, in the absence of the owner/operator, were run by custodial personnel.

It is not any news that custodial personnel in such settings generally receive very low wages and are commonly unskilled, under-educated, and untrained for working with developmentally disabled persons. In a number of facilities, custodial staff also tended to be ethnic minorities or recent immigrants, adding language and cultural barriers to an already problematic situation. In some of the larger facilities, custodial personnel such as kitchen help and janitorial staff, were sometimes hired from local "skid row" boarding houses. Not only could these persons be classified as "deviants" themselves, but they greatly increase the already high staff transiency rate in these facilities.

One might hope that persons from the lower socioeconomic levels of society would be more likely than, say, "middle-class" citizens, to befriend or feel sympathy for developmentally disabled persons and "take them under their wings," as it were. The observations made in this research, however, revealed otherwise. In setting after setting it was observed that the quality of the interaction between these "normal" custodial persons and developmentally disabled residents was characterized primarily by what King, Raynes and Tizard (1971) termed "social distance." Social distance in institutional settings is characterized by the physical segregation of staff and residents during meals and recreation; and, more important, by interaction which is limited to commands and admonishments. This was true of all but two of the facilities in the sample. In cases where one observed more "friendly" interaction or relationships between a staff member and a developmentally disabled resident, it was characterized by a strong degree of inequality. In some of the "friendlier" relationships between facility personnel and residents, the resident was treated like a small child or even a pet by the staff member. For example, one of the cooks at a large facility had befriended a resident with Down's syndrome. His "pet name" for this 50-year-old man was "Baby Billy—Bow Wow—Porky Pig." A common interaction between them consisted of the cook's getting Bill to "bark" to the song, "How Much Is That Doggy in the Window?" At first, this pattern of social distance and superordination on the parts of custodial persons was difficult to understand, until one realized that such persons are themselves on the bottom of the social ladder, so to speak. A reason for this situation may be that it is critical for the social self-esteem of these low-status persons to maintain a distance from, and not be associated with the next rung down—the retarded. Persons with higher social status such as professionals do not have this kind of fear (although this does not mean there is no social distance between professionals and developmentally disabled persons—it is merely a different kind).

From observing relationships such as these within the residential facility setting, a sense of the social structure of this system began to emerge. It became clear that there were some important basic differences between the daily life experiences of developmentally disabled persons in residential placement and "normal" persons in the larger community that deserved further attention.

Subcultural Features of Community Placement

The observations made during the course of this study revealed that many dehospitalized mentally retarded persons are not, and do not perceive themselves to be, living in the normal community, contrary to the assumptions that are generally held. The data indicate that these persons may be seen, instead, as inhabitants of a physically segregated and perhaps culturally distinct social system.

The culture concept has been used by social scientists in an effort to understand more traditional institutional settings and the human beings within them (Caudill, 1958; Edgerton, 1963; Edgerton et al., 1961; Goffman, 1961; Henry, 1973; Salisbury, 1961). In a similar fashion, a cultural analysis may further a more complete understanding of some of the fundamental dynamics of community placement for the mentally retarded, a phenomenon which, thus far, has been apprehended only in some of its more superficial aspects. There are four major points that support an argument for a cultural view:

1. Although only touched upon in this paper due to the demands of brevity, the ethnographic study revealed that community-based residential facilities because of their custodial practices manifested a number of features of institutional culture.
2. With respect to the resident population, the fact of separation, segregation and isolation from the larger community or culture is, in itself, conducive to the development of "subculture."
3. The kind of social system observed in these settings has no counterpart in the larger culture and hence can be seen as "subcultural."
4. The individuals concerned, in addition to being inhabitants of a segregated social system, differ from "normal" persons in the mainstream culture not so much for reasons of physical or mental disability but because their life histories and their socialization experiences (which amount to their acculturation) have resulted in a view of both self and the social world that may differ significantly from the "Weltanschauung" of the dominant culture.

This last point perhaps needs some further explanation. Most, if not all, individuals who have been institutionalized or who are in any kind of residential placement have been drastically diverted from culturally prescribed life-patterns. Their "normal" fellows in mainstream society (those who have not been removed or isolated), by and large, engage in all or many of the important institutions of the society that mark the progression of an individual along the path from birth to death. Experiences, accomplishments, and rites of passage (such as family life, early schooling, high school graduation, courtship, work/career, marriage and parenthood, are not only chronological events, they are indicators of cultural membership. These "human career" (Kielhofner, 1979) experiences that are taken for granted by "normals" are not generally shared by this population of physically and mentally handicapped persons, many of whom were removed early in life from the mainstream of society to total institutions for the duration of their formative years and beyond. These individuals, having been inhabitants of a separate sub-system, have acquired over long years (sometimes a life-time) not just different "behaviors," compared to mainstream persons, but a *different set of assumptions* about the world and *different strategies* for physical survival and for the maintenance of self-esteem. The sum total of these orientations is what anthropologists call a "cognitive map."

As was discussed earlier, there are aspects of the community placement situation itself which add to the argument that deinstitutionalized persons are not of the dominant culture, but, instead, participate in a lifestyle that has certain subcultural features. Some are echoes of the custodial practices of the larger institutions; others are unique to the community placement situations, which include not only the residential facility but other agents and organs of the service system.

One example might serve to illustrate the peculiar structure of this postulated subcultural social system and how it gives rise to a set of assumptions and consequent action on the parts of its members. One significant and visible feature of the lives of developmentally disabled persons in residential placement is that they are subject to the surveillance and control of what can be seen as a "collaborative network" of "normal" others. Information about the "client" freely circulates through communications among caretaker, social worker, workshop director, family, physician, and researcher, at the same time that this person's contact with others outside this system may be severely limited. A person in community residential placement, very much like a patient in a large institution, leads a "goldfish bowl" existence. As members, or "natives," of this system, mentally retarded and other developmentally disabled persons know very well how it works.

During the initial stages of the research contact with persons in community placement, it was almost always assumed by them (particularly those in small facilities) that the researcher would be in communication with the other "normal" persons in their lives to whom they were answerable, especially the caretaker, and would report on their behavior. At first, clients were understandably circumspect about what, and how much, they told the researcher about themselves and were cautious about talking about their thoughts and feelings. It would also happen that when out of the facility clients would implore the researcher not to tell the caretaker when they felt they had done something wrong—even something as trivial as spilling food on their clothing. In some cases, it took many months to convince "natives" of this system that the researcher was not part of the collaborative network they saw as an immutable fact of life. It is not that these individuals are any more "reactive" or unrealistic than anyone else. They used their own background knowledge to make sense of the identity of a person who suddenly came into their lives. They had had no social type in their cultural classification system that corresponded to the identity the researcher wanted them to perceive and understand.

This feature of the subculture of community placement, like many others, has important implications for research, service, and facility monitoring. It would seem to be the case that one cannot simply "walk in off the street," interview a few residents of a facility and expect them to reveal critical information either about themselves or others. One group of residents of a large facility who complained regularly and bitterly to the researcher about conditions in the facility gave a positive report to a visiting committee from the licensing bureau because, as one of them put it: "We didn't want to get anybody in trouble."

Another example of a subcultural "cognitive map" has to do with *time*. Initially, one encounters in these inhabitants of the board and care world what appears to be constitutional apathy or cognitive disability in the form of their responses to the mainstream culture's conceptions about, and management of, time. Efforts to introduce activity programs in these settings invariably encounter this "obstacle." It was not until a considerable number of observations had been made on the daily patterns of the residents in these facilities that it was understood that the temporal framework in residential placement situations is different from that of mainstream culture. This has been described elsewhere for both the community-based setting (Kielhofner, 1979) and for the large institution (Biklen, 1977).

An institutional temporal pattern can best be characterized by saying that the inhabitants of the system are passive respondents to a time framework established by the institution. Major daily events such as rising, meals and bedtime, are not scheduled by the resident of such a system, nor can he or she ordinarily vary or change them. Other significant regular occurrences such as outings, the doling out of spending money, visits from the social worker or family members and trips home are most always initiated by, and under the control of, "normal" others. Thus, "waiting time" is a significant feature of daily life and even an activity in itself in both large institutions and smaller, community-based facilities. Autonomy is the key issue here. An individual whose daily life pattern is so preordained and so dominated by an imposed and immutable schedule has no opportunity to develop a more active role vis-a-vis the management of time. A frequently reported problem in community adaptation is the failure of a client to be on time or to keep appointments. This and other traits such as "dependency" can be seen as the manifestation of mental disability. A *cultural interpretation*, however, enables one to see them as *rational and adaptive behavioral patterns* in the setting(s) that constitute the cultural universe of these persons. A strictly clinical view, therefore, can be seen as ethnocentric insofar as it is restricted to the perspective of an "outsider" or "non-member" of this system.

Culture-bound features of assessment and habilitation. Most assessment instruments are designed to measure discrete behaviors. However, the measurement of physical functioning, cognitive capacity, or cosmetic appearance can result in a reductionistic approach to a person if the environment, way of life, and viewpoint of the individual are not taken into account. The demand for, and requirements of, measurability may create a Procrustean bed in the sense that the totality of the individual is reduced to that which will conform to the configuration of the particular instrument at hand. One of the natural outcomes of reductionistic assessment is that the items assessed also appear to be logical intervention targets. A common assessment made of retarded adults is their inability to read, count, and handle money; an equally common recommendation is formal instruction in these skills areas.

Ethnocentrism enters the picture here in that other areas of adaptive functioning are seen to hinge on these accomplishments. This recommendation followed an assessment of one of the individuals in the study cohort: "Due to his inability to read or handle money, it is not recommended that he take a bus or live independently. Considering his age he would benefit from instruction in simple money management and possibly simple reading. Thus he could be able to read street signs, etc., and handle himself independently in a store." The individual who received this evaluation subsequently demonstrated his ability, with some initial assistance, to travel around the city on the public bus system without problems or mishap, without first having acquired further reading or money handling skills. Unaided, he now regularly uses public transportation to avail himself of various resources in the community outside the residential facility and to visit his family.

It is probably fairly safe to say that either because of age, cognitive inability, or the absence of an appropriate pedagogy, very few adult retarded persons will be taught to read effectively, write, or count money. This does not mean, however, that they cannot acquire considerable mobility. Observations of nonliterate "retarded" persons who are not able to do simple arithmetic reveal that some of them have developed strategies other than the supposedly "normal" ones for getting around on buses, making purchases and ordering in restaurants. It also seems to be the case that when some of these persons have acquired some skill, say, in word recognition, it is a *result* of their exposure to the community. The culturally biased insistence that formal instruction and the achievement of cognitive skills *precede* practical experience may be quite mistaken. Not only might this insistence be in error with respect to logic and efficacy but it may be guilty of abetting a discriminatory process. These signs of "normality" which the retarded are required to produce before they are considered able to live in anything but a totally protective environment may be more a matter of "ideal" culture than "real" culture. Menu planning, budgeting, and banking are fairly high-level operations that many "normal" individuals in the larger culture do not, or cannot, perform, and yet they are not asked to relinquish their personal freedom.

Formal skills as passport to the dominant culture. It has been observed that in a society like ours which values and stresses the acquisition of formal techniques of symbolization (reading, writing, arithmetic), these techniques can become ends in themselves and are not necessarily related to the requirements of physical survival or cultural adaptation (Dexter, 1958).

Assessment approaches often reflect this cultural predisposition, and recommendations are frequently along the lines of this one: "If a tutorial program was available, he could benefit from instruction in reading, writing, and handling money." Many persons, like the adults in this study who are considered to be mentally retarded and who cannot perform these cognitive operations, not only lament their inability, but have a very clear understanding of the "passport" value of such skills. Being able to read and write as a symbol of being "normal" may be valued more than its potential practical benefits. The following comments by retarded individuals were made in the context of a general dialogue on their lives:

> Roger (a 37-year-old man who has spent most of his life in state hospitals and who now lives in a small group home): I figure it this way, it's not right to call a person a mentally retarded patient—mentally retarded. 'Cause I'm not. I can take care of a house and I can remember names pretty good. But I can't write no phone numbers down. If I could have help writing—writing numbers down and remembering them, that way I could prove to people that I could be on my own.
>
> Arline (a 44-year-old woman who has lived at a large board and care facility for 5 years): I was retarded but I snapped out of it when I was 13....I feel I can act just like the rest of you people in here....Do you feel I can talk just like all of you?...It's very mild, Dr. A said, very mild....A lot of people didn't want to have anything to do with us (referring to her twin sister) when we were that way. The other kids, they used to throw rocks at us, just because I didn't know what two and two was. But I know what it is now. Two and two is four. Ten and ten is five—I mean ten and ten is twenty. And five and five is ten.
>
> Marie (a 23-year-old woman who has lived for the past 5 years in a group home with 16 other developmentally disabled women):
>
> Researcher: Have you spoken to your parents about wanting to get married?
>
> Marie: I did talk to my mother about it once, but it didn't work out the way I wanted it to because she doesn't think I'm quite ready for the big step yet... She said she thinks I'd better wait.
>
> Researcher: Until when?
>
> Marie: Until the time comes—until it's time, when I'm good and ready.
>
> Researcher: What do you have to be able to do to get married?
>
> Marie: Cook, sew, read, count money, tell time, add, subtract, stuff like that....When I first came out of the hospital the doctor asked me if I could have three wishes what would I wish for. My first wish was that I could see Bobby Sherman (a popular singing star) in person—and I wanted to learn how to read and write—and I wanted (there) to be peace in the world....I was supposed to get a tutor to teach me how to read and write, but I haven't heard anything.

Given the emphasis in the society on the acquisition of formal skills and the general view that retarded persons suffer primarily from cognitive deficits, it is natural that the classroom and its teaching methods be recruited in the cause of normalization. For those mentally retarded persons in residential placements who do receive regular outside habilitative services (and many do not) these are likely to take the form of an instructional program in a classroom setting (with the exception of workshop programs). Formal skills such as reading, writing, and math are a major content area of such programs along with instruction in daily living skills. Four such programs were observed in the course of the study.

Behind the widespread reliance on the classroom for the habilitation of the developmentally disabled is the premise that skills needed for adaptive functioning in the community are effectively learned in a formal educational setting and can be generalized to the daily life situations of the students. Instruction in such practical skills as preparing meals, using money, ordering in a restaurant, looking for a job, improving one's appearance, acquiring culturally appropriate behaviors, getting along with others, budgeting and banking in a classroom context often employs many of the teaching methods and devices that are used in the traditional teaching of formal skills. In addition to personal instruction from the teacher, such methods include manuals, guides, and workbooks. Such a formal approach may or may not be augmented by actual experiences in naturally occurring situations.

Regarding the population in this study, it was consistently the case that individuals were not provided with natural opportunities to learn and practice many daily living skills that were included in one form or another in the educational program, e.g., the restrictions imposed by the residential facility prevented many of these individuals from acquiring practical experience in the community. Other barriers between developmentally disabled persons and community learning experiences were posed by the educational program itself. The refusal or inability of such programs to deviate from the classroom model and to extend the teaching to the natural contexts outside the classroom was seen as having non-normalizing results. There was frequently a "let's pretend" quality to these preparations for real contact with the community when no such contact was being allowed or even planned for.

Normalization and normal appearances. The rationale for including formal academic components in special programs for adults is the normalization principle. However, observations made of educational settings for mentally retarded adults show that what is frequently achieved in the place of, and at the expense of, normalization is the production of "normal appearances." At first glance, there is something gratifying and reassuring about a classroom of substantially handicapped persons busily working with pencil and paper at their desks or tables. Closer inspection and repeated observations may, however, reveal the "normal appearances" or cosmetic value of such activities. Some of the mentally retarded adults observed in classroom settings have spent years daily tracing and copying letters and numbers without having acquired any ability to understand or use these symbols. One 38-year-old man in the study cohort, Joe, was able to copy entire articles from magazines without making any errors at all. He was, however, unable to read or write anything on his own. Joe would carry around a sheaf of papers, a pencil and a magazine or two, and could be seen when not otherwise occupied, busily "writing away." In many respects, Joe is much more competent and potentially independent than his fellow residents at the group home and his peers at the activity center. He is very aware of this and is particularly sensitive about being associated with people who appear retarded or who are obviously handicapped. Any chance he gets, Joe separates himself from his house or classmates and does his "writing." He explains, "It gives me something to do." An unlit pipe that Joe constantly has with him greatly enhances his production of normal appearances.

This kind of thing is similar to the "Cloak of Competence" described by Edgerton (1967) in his study of dehospitalized individuals attempting to make an adjustment to life in the community. In both cases there is a recognition of status differential and relative deprivation on the part of this subdominant group vis-a-vis the dominant culture. The point here is that these individuals, who have been diagnosed as mentally retarded, demonstrate an awareness of the dominant culture's template. In the classroom situation, and in other normalization efforts, this template is frequently employed by "normals" on behalf of their "retarded" students, who may or may not themselves manufacture "normal appearances" as a strategy for eliciting more favorable responses from others. The teacher-imposed production of normal appearances may subtly become a goal in itself in such educational programs. Classroom and administrative personnel have to comply in one way or another with how the culture defines "education" and "teacher" and often lack an alternative educational approach.

Another feature shared by educational programs observed is the unintended socialization experience they provide for these marginal members of the culture. The classroom model dictates that there be a teacher and that there be students. It also contains an inherent element of conflict. It has been noted that in every teaching situation the teacher, because he or she is knowledgeable, is superior, and that the pupil, because he or she does not have that knowledge, is inferior (Geer, 1968). Even in "normal" classroom teaching situations the teacher must control the interaction; in effect, the student role is one of submission. In mainstream society, however, this subordinate/superordinate relationship has certain restrictions imposed upon it. It usually occurs during a particular period in a person's life and is further limited by the fact that the role of submissive pupil takes place, at most, on a six hour a day basis and that outside the framework of school, a child has the chance to meet others on a equal footing. In the case of this population of marginal adults, the classroom, because of its organizational needs, can only perpetuate and reinforce subordination. It thus unwittingly joins other social forces in the lives of these individuals in socializing them to be inferiors, or like children.

There is an additional element that combines with those already outlined to make "closed systems" of such habilitation environments. This is an underlying operating principle that does not allow normal risks to be taken in these settings, with this population. For example, while even the youngest "normal" school children are allowed to exit the school alone and even cross the street by themselves without the school necessarily assuming responsibility for their welfare, organized services for the "handicapped" generally assume a much more protective, even custodial position. At one educational foundation in the study, at no time could a client, regardless of his or her physical or intellectual competence, be sent on an errand to the corner shopping center, cross the street alone to get to the park, or even leave the school building to wait in the foundation's parking lot without being accompanied by a "normal" adult.

The classroom model produces a very limited perspective of the client and has the effect on the teacher and other classroom personnel of underestimating a client's overall competence. This perception, in turn, reinforces the fear of risk and results in the constant monitoring and controlling of these individuals. An environment which consists extensively of these attitudes and practices is, in some ways, *institutional* as opposed to *normalizing*.

Summary and Conclusion

This ethnographic research examined several key issues in deinstitutionalization. It focused on the interface between developmentally disabled individuals in residential placement and the communities in which they live. Observations of this sample of dehospitalized persons revealed that they are isolated in many ways from the larger society and that the community placement way of life contains several elements of a subculture. In addition to the residential facility itself, certain habilitation settings and programs were observed and analyzed within a cultural framework. These settings were seen to exhibit features and mechanisms that further isolate developmentally disabled persons from the larger society and help to perpetuate a subcultural system.

Qualitative methodology is uniquely suitable for an examination of the complex phenomenon of deinstitutionalization. The holistic framework that underlies a qualitative approach, in requiring researchers to view the individual as an integral part of its system, allows them to discover elements in the lives of developmentally disabled persons that might otherwise go unnoticed.

Participant observation, an essential feature of a qualitative methodology, provides the means to obtain a detailed and in-depth understanding of the everyday lives of these human beings. This methodology recognizes the need to understand the problems and issues involved in deinstitutionalization from the perspectives of the persons involved; it also provides the techniques for doing so. Without such an understanding, can one really be sure that services to these individuals are relevant?

References

Baker, B. L., Seltzer, G. B., & Seltzer, M. M. *As close as possible: Community residences for retarded adults*. Boston: Little, Brown & Company, 1977.

Biklen, D. The politics of institutions. In B. Blatt, D. Biklen, & R. Bogdan (Eds.), *An alternative textbook in special education*. Denver: Love Publishing Co., 1977.

Bogdan, R. & Taylor, S. J. *Introduction to qualitative research methods: A phenomenological approach to the social sciences*. New York: John Wiley & Sons, 1975.

Caudill, W. *The psychiatric hospital as a small society*. Cambridge: Harvard University Press, 1958.

Dexter, L. A. A social theory of mental deficiency. *American Journal of Mental Deficiency*, 1958, *62*(5), 920-928.

Edgerton, R. B. A patient elite: Ethnography in a hospital for the mentally retarded. *American Journal of Mental Deficiency*, 1963, *68*, 372-385.

Edgerton, R. B. *The cloak of competence*. Berkeley: University of California Press, 1967.

Edgerton, R. B., Tarjan, G., & Dingman, H. F. Free enterprise in a captive society. *American Journal of Mental Deficiency*, 1961, *66*, 35-41.

Geer, B. Teaching. In *International Encylopedia of the social sciences* (Vol. 15). New York: Macmillan & Free Press, 1968.

Goffman, E. *Asylums*. Garden City, NY: Doubleday, Anchor Books, 1961.

Henry, J. *On sham, vulnerability and other forms of self-destruction*. New York: Vintage Press, 1973.

Kielhofner, G. The temporal dimension in the lives of retarded adults: A general problem of interaction and intervention. *American Journal of Occupational Therapy, 1979, 33*(3), 161-168.

King, R. D., Raynes, N. V., & Tizard, J. *Patterns of residential care: Sociological studies in institutions for handicapped children. London: Routledge & Kegan Paul, 1971.*

Salisbury, R. F. *Structures of custodial care: An anthropological study of a state mental hospital*. Berkeley: University of California Press, 1962.

Wolfensberger, W. *Normalization: The principle of normalization in human services*. Toronto: National Institute on Mental Retardation, 1972.

Crime, Deviance and Normalization: Reconsidered

Robert B. Edgerton

Mental Retardation Research Center
University of California, Los Angeles

When beliefs about social realities change over the course of time, the basis for this change can only sometimes be shown to be the emergence of new factual information. So it is with the history of beliefs concerning the criminality of mentally retarded persons; new "facts" are sometimes presented, and revised, but as far as policy change is concerned, these facts will be interpreted in a variety of ways if they are not ignored altogether. Over the past 70 years or so there has been an impressive change in public and scientific beliefs concerning the likelihood that mentally retarded persons will commit crimes. For example, in a review of the scientific literature, the distinguished criminologist, E. H. Sutherland (1931), found that the average percentage of delinquents reported to be mentally retarded fell from 55% for the period 1910-1914 to 20% for the period 1925-28. As early as 1930 some investigators found no evidence for a relationship between mental retardation and crime while others, even in subsequent decades, continued to raise alarms about the menace posed by "defective delinquents" (Brown & Courtless, 1971; Davies, 1930; Goldstein, 1964).

By the 1960's the presumed criminality of mentally retarded persons had lessened so much that it was common to find reports that asserted mentally retarded persons to be no more criminal than normal persons, and perhaps even less so (Beier, 1964). Indeed, by the late 1960's when deinstitutionalization was well underway, the pendulum had swung so far from the days when Fernald and Goddard fulminated about the inherent and inevitable criminality of the retarded that Richard Allen (1968) was able to summarize the historical record as follows:

> "About half a century ago it was pretty widely believed that every mentally impaired person was a likely delinquent, and that most criminal offenders were such because of impaired intellect. The polemicists have now come full circle and it is today just as stoutly maintained by some members of the scientific, legal and correctional communities that mental retardation bears no causal relationship to crime" (1968, p. 22).

This viewpoint was exemplified by the influential "Task Force on Law" of the president's Panel on Mental Retardation, chaired by Judge Bazelon (1963), when it focused its report not on the criminality of retarded persons, which was assumed to be inconsequential, but instead on the responsibility of society and the law to provide mentally retarded offenders with therapy and justice.

This research was supported by NICHD Grant No. HD 09474-02, The Community Context of Normalization, and by NICHD Grant No. HD 04612, The Mental Retardation Research Center, UCLA. I am most grateful to my associates on this research project: Lorel Cornman, Candy Fox-Henning, Laurel Haas, Patti Hartmann, Keith Kernan, Cheryl Killion, Paul Koegel, L. L. Langness, Don Sutherland, Jim Turner and Rob Wittemore. I also appreciate the suggestions and assistance of Ronald Gallimore, Barbara Herr, Harold Levine, Nancy Miller, Lupe Montano, Kazuo Nihira, Lenda Walker and Douglass Price-Williams.

This report by the President's Panel did not itself review the empirical data regarding the criminality of retarded persons, but it did lead others to re-examine the evidence concerning mental retardation and antisocial conduct, especially violence. Thus, after concluding that there was "little or no" systematic information on the subject, Brown and Courtless (1967) examined one aspect of the phenomenon, the extent to which incarcerated offenders were mentally retarded. Although they found substantial geographic variation, they concluded that about 10 percent of the prison population in the U.S. was mentally retarded, a finding supported by Allen (1968) and presaged by numerous earlier studies (Goldstein, 1964). But in addition, Brown and Courtless found that 57 percent of prisoners with IQs below 55 had been convicted of crimes against persons. Indeed, when a sample of prisoners in five states was retested to determine the accuracy of their IQ designation, 40 percent of all those found to be mentally retarded had committed some form of homicide and 21 percent had been convicted of first degree murder. On the other hand, sexual offenses were uncommon (Allen, 1970). It was certainly not the intent of these investigators to resurrect the spector of the violent mentally retarded person, but their findings nevertheless contrasted starkly with the calm assurances of previous writers.

As various authors have noted, there are compelling reasons why inferences drawn from incarcerated populations of mentally retarded offenders must be treated cautiously. For example, such data are often confounded with the class and ethnicity of the offenders; 80 percent of the retarded inmates identified by Brown and Courtless were either Black or Hispanic. There are also obvious biases in IQ testing with such populations, just as there are manifest inequities in society and the criminal justice system that could lead to a higher probability of criminality and arrest for ethnic minority persons whether retarded or not (Biklen, 1977; Marsh, Friel, & Eissler, 1975; Santamour & West, 1979). Moreover, mentally retarded prisoners are less likely to be paroled than non-retarded offenders who commit the same crimes (Lomastro, 1976). Therefore, they are more likely than non-retarded offenders to remain in prison and to be enumerated when an assay of incarcerated offenders is made.

Building on the report of the Task Force on Law, research of the kind carried out by Brown and Courtless (1967), Allen (1968) and others contributed to the recognition that retarded offenders face special problems, a realization that has led to the development of programs intended to reduce hazards and inequities for mentally retarded persons in the criminal justice system (Browning, 1976). However, in the decade that has passed since Brown and Courtless wrote, there has been no concerted effort to determine the extent to which mentally retarded persons do in fact pose problems for society by their criminal or deviant acts, even though it was during this same decade that the national policies of deinstitutionalization and normalization were implemented. These policies have been based on the assumption that relatively few mentally retarded persons commit crimes, particularly serious crimes of violence. Wolfensberger (1975, p. 55) reflected the prevailing view when he wrote: "Today, of course, we know that most retarded adults make an adequate adjustment in the community, and that they are more likely to be the victims rather than the perpetrators of social injustice." Edgerton (1967) expressed a similar view some years earlier.

This paper will reconsider the empirical literature concerning the criminality of mentally retarded persons in community settings. It will also present relevant findings from a 30-month study of the community adaptation of a sample of mildly retarded adults.

Antisocial Behavior in Community Settings

As virtually every review of the literature on the behavior of mentally retarded persons in community settings has noted, this research is flawed by poor research design, lack of adequate comparison populations, and heavy sample attrition, as well as superficial and reactive methods of data collection (Butler & Browning, 1970; Cobb, 1972; Edgerton, 1967; McCarver & Craig, 1974). In addition to these problems, the study of antisocial behavior among retarded persons has been limited by inexact criterion measures and reliance on official records. Despite these limitations, some of which beset criminological research in general (Farrington, 1979), there is a large body of literature which should not simply be dismissed.

There are numerous studies in print that report the frequency with which retarded individuals come into conflict with the law (Goldstein, 1964; McCarver & Craig, 1974). Some, like that by Andron and Sturm (1973), report rather frequent conflict (nine of 24 persons studied had such problems), while others, like Stabler (1974), report far less trouble (only seven of 103 persons studied had legal problems). Still others, (e.g., Edgerton, 1967; Hamlett & Engle, 1950; Henschel, 1972; McDevitt, 1978; Rosen, Clark, & Kivitz 1977) report that the antisocial behavior (usually defined as violation of the law) of the retarded persons they studied was neither frequent nor serious.

However, other investigators have reported that the "antisocial" behavior of the retarded persons they studied was neither infrequent nor inconsequential. Indeed, several reports have identified antisocial behavior as a major reason for failure in community placement. For example, Craft (1958) reported that 21% of his sample which had been deinstitutionalized in the western counties of England had to be returned to the hospital due to antisocial behavior. Similarly, Windle, Stewart, and Brown (1961) found that many of the mildly retarded patients who were returned to community settings from Pacific State Hospital in California in the early 1950's had to be reinstitutionalized as a result of antisocial behaviors. Specifically, of the 48 patients on vocational leave (usually residing in or near their place of employment), 14% were returned to the hospital for antisocial behavior; of the 84 patients placed in their parents' homes, 63% were returned for these reasons, but only four percent of the 164 patients placed in family care homes (small residences in which a family provided room, board and supervision for four or fewer clients) were returned for similar reasons. Whether these dramatic differences in return rates were due to selective factors in the placement settings themselves, to differential closeness of supervision or the varying tolerance levels of persons in the settings, or to other factors was not determined. Neither of these two studies reported the extent to which the so-called antisocial behavior was violent in nature, and the definitions of "antisocial" were not always clear.

More recently, Pagel and Whitling (1978) examined the reasons why 117 mentally retarded persons were returned to Pacific State Hospital as community placement "failures" in the period 1974-1976. They found that 50% of the moderately retarded persons and 62% of the mildly retarded persons were rehospitalized for "maladaptive behavior," the most common forms of which were acts or threats of physical violence. Moen, Bogen and Aanes (1975) reported that 13 of 85 retarded adults placed in group homes in Minnesota from 1970 to 1974 had to be rehospitalized; the principal reason for rehospitalization was aggressive behavior. Other investigators have noted that aggressive behavior can be a significant problem in group homes in California (Mink, 1978; Nihira & Nihira, 1975). On the other hand, there are studies of group home placement that have not reported either antisocial behavior in general or violent behavior in particular to be frequent or serious (Baker, Seltzer & Seltzer, 1977; Birenbaum & Seiffer 1976).

The studies mentioned are but a few of many that reflect the same inconsistency—some report that crime and violence are common and seriously affect community adaptation while others report quite the opposite. Not only is the evidence conflicting, it is usually so lacking in details about the context of the reported "antisocial" or criminal behavior that interpretation of these various studies is hazardous at best. For example, Saenger's (1957) well-known study of 520 moderately retarded adults who had formerly been pupils in special classes in New York City reported that 7% of the sample had been in some difficulty with the law in the community, and only a handful had been involved in a violent offense. Yet given the very limited access that these persons had to community settings, is 7% remarkably low as Saenger contended, or might it be surprisingly high?

Another example of interpretive difficulty is provided by the research of Deno (1965). There have been many studies of the community adjustment of special class graduates (e.g., Jackson, 1970; MacMillan, 1977), but Deno's research is of particular interest because of her effort to compare the criminality of special class graduates with that of the general population in Minneapolis where the research was conducted. Examining 423 students who graduated from special classes in 1957-1960, Deno found that by the age of 18, 57% of former special class boys had police records compared with 37% of all boys in Minneapolis; the rate of special class girls was 24% compared with 11% for girls in the general population. These figures seem to point to a higher rate of criminality among the special class graduates, but Deno points out that the worst delinquency among the special class graduates was found among non-white students of lower socio-economic status. Her comparison with crime percentages for all of Minneapolis, then, is misleading. Had the comparison been confined to juveniles from similar ethnic and socio-economic backgrounds the results would have been more meaningful. It should be noted that other investigators (e.g., Lee, Hegge, & Voelker 1959; Peterson & Smith 1960) who have compared special class graduates with normal controls have also reported that the delinquency of the retarded persons was substantially greater than that of the controls.

Another interpretive problem is exemplified by the research of Muehlenberger (1972). Using a participant-observation research procedure, Muehlenberger carefully documented various aspects of the community adjustment of ten mildly retarded adults randomly selected from a universe of 59 persons discharged in 1969-1970 from Empire State School in New York. Muehlenberger noted incidents of victimization (e.g., one retarded woman was raped by three men), but he also recorded criminal offenses, some of them rather serious. One retarded man was awaiting trial on a charge of first degree sodomy with a child. Another man was serving a jail term for first degree forgery, a crime which he admitted practicing repeatedly. Others were occasionally in lesser kinds of trouble. Setting aside questions about the size of his sample, Muehlenberger's data raise another point. To find two persons out of ten facing serious criminal charges would be alarming indeed if this percentage were found to extend to larger samples of deinstitutionalized retarded persons. However, it may be useful to keep in mind that this sample, like many that were once institutionalized, had a previous history of frequent law violation. The literature on the pre-institutional delinquency of mentally retarded persons is difficult to assess (Robinson & Robinson 1976), but it is clear that a very large percentage of those persons had records of pre-institutional delinquency. It also seems to be true that these persons have had many fewer brushes with the law after release than they had before they were institutionalized (a pattern which holds for many non-retarded delinquents as well). From this perspective, then, it is possible to conclude that the community adaptation of most of Muehlenberger's sample was improved. Needless to say, however, from a community perspective, a 20% rate of serious crime would still be alarming.

In an effort to reduce interpretive difficulties such as these, some investigators have utilized comparison populations. First, an early study (Fairbanks, 1933) in a suburb of Baltimore compared 122 mildly retarded persons with 90 persons of normal intelligence. The mentally retarded persons were first identified in 1914 when they were in school. Consistent with the climate of those times, the explicit expectation for the post-school lives of these children was an adulthood of poor social adaptation, including crime and serious social deviance. However, when Fairbanks located these retarded adults in 1930, she was surprised to discover that most had married, held jobs, had children, and had generally done well in life. She noted that promiscuity, prostitution, and illegitimacy were somewhat more frequent in the retarded sample, as were alcoholism and criminality, but she emphasized that the differences were not great. This was especially noteworthy given the fact that 25% of the retarded sample had records of delinquency as juveniles. Although this study, like others, was flawed by sample attrition, imperfect matching of controls, and somewhat superficial data collection, it presents a positive portrait of the community adaptation of mildly retarded adults, and its flaws are no greater than those of the often-cited studies of the community adaptation of mildly retarded adults that also attempted to use non-retarded comparison populations.

The well-known and influential comparison study is the work of Baller, Charles, and Miller (1966) concerning the community adaptation of mildly retarded adults in Nebraska. In 1935 Baller compared the frequency of criminality in his mentally retarded sample with matched controls of normal intelligence and reported that there were three to seven times as many violations of the law charged to the retarded sample. When Charles restudied the two samples in 1950, he reported that about 50% of the retarded persons had been in trouble with the law for civil charges (mostly misdemeanors), a rate well above that of the controls. When Miller re-examined the adaptation of these populations in 1960, he reported that the retarded group had become more law-abiding, with their offenses being largely minor. The picture drawn is one of a retarded population which becomes less and less likely to violate the law as years pass; it adds that most of these retarded persons in all periods were consistently law-abiding. Nevertheless, in all periods the mentally retarded persons were more likely to violate the law than were the controls. Moreover, there was substantial sample attrition that, as the authors themselves noted, probably involved the loss of the less successful and perhaps more antisocial members of the retarded sample (Jackson, 1977). As a result, the findings are inconclusive and may not be as positive as they are commonly taken to be.

In another well-known study, Kennedy (1966) compared persons identified in school as mentally retarded with matched, non-retarded controls in the same Connecticut community in 1948, then again in 1960. When Kennedy compared the two populations in 1948, the retarded group had a higher frequency of court records, a higher rate of recidivism, more frequent jail sentences, more commitments to correctional facilities, and a greater variety of offenses. Indeed, 21% of the retarded sample had been arrested, although 85% of their offenses were misdemeanors. When the two groups were restudied in 1960, the retarded population (especially the men) still had a substantially higher incidence of criminality than the controls although the incidence was only about half as great as it had been in 1948. However, there was a 30% sample attrition in the retarded sample and 21% in the controls. Whether those who could not be relocated were more or less law-abiding, or more so in one population than the other, could not be determined. Once again, the results are inconclusive.

Much of the available research implicates an association between delinquency, low socio-economic status, and ethnicity—a relationship which is also well-documented in the general criminological literature. For this reason, a study from the Federal Republic of Germany is of interest, especially so since West Germany is more homogeneous ethnically than the United States. Utilizating files from the Federal and State police, public prosecutors and courts, as well as mental hospital records, Häfner and Böker (1973) were able to determine that detected crimes of violence committed by mentally retarded persons are proportional to the number of such crimes committed by the general population. For example, the authors found that the risk for homicide by retarded persons as well as the general population, was six per 100,000. While socio-economic status was *not* a factor in predicting violence among mentally retarded offenders, it was found that most of the violent retarded offenders were single males from broken homes or ''antisocial'' milieus. These offenders also showed ''behavioral disturbances'' (usually threats of violence) before committing their violent crimes. These findings may or may not be generalizable to the United States.

In summary, while the bulk of the literature from the United States and the United Kingdom seems to show that mildly retarded adults are more likely to be involved in antisocial behavior than their non-retarded counterparts, this differentially high rate of antisocial behavior has not been shown to be independent of ethnicity, low socio-economic status, or a less than normative early family environment (e.g., absent father or alcoholic parent). What is more, the literature is limited by its reliance on police or court records of crime, rather than more direct measures, including unreported crime. In what follows the writer shall attempt to provide a record of the unreported as well as reported criminality or serious deviance of a sample of mildly retarded, ''middle-class'' Caucasian adults who were living in various community settings.

The Sample

Beginning in May 1976 and continuing through 1978, 48 mildly retarded persons have been studied by intensive, naturalistic methods. The goal of this research was to understand the community adaptation of mentally retarded adults who were considered to have the potential for normalization, particularly independent living and competitive employment. More specifically, it was sought to identify phenomena that facilitated or thwarted their normalization. The sample was selected by soliciting the names of persons who were classified as being mentally retarded by some component of the mental retardation system (special education, regional centers, sheltered workshops) within the catchment areas of three regional centers for developmental disabilities in Los Angeles. Individuals in the delivery system were then asked to identify persons on the lists whom they thought capable of independent living. Some 120 individuals were nominated, each of whom was interviewed to ascertain how well he/she met the criteria for inclusion in the final sample: (1) Caucasian, (2) ''middle-class'' family background, (3) no major physical handicaps that would preclude independence, and (4) willingness to participate in the study. Estimation of socio-economic status was not precise, but it was adequate to eliminate persons whose family background included low-income, or low-education parents. Although persons with disabling physical handicaps were eliminated, it is likely that most members of this white, middle-class sample suffer some degree of central nervous system dysfunction. Similar dysfunctions may also be common in other mildy retarded populations.

In all, 50 persons were selected for intensive study. Early in the course of the research, four members of the sample dropped out; two others were added, yielding a final sample of 48 persons who were studied for a period of 30 months. These 48 persons were chosen by means of a quota sample intended to represent a range of individuals in the various categories thought to be theoretically relevant for a longitudinal study of community adaptation. Thus at the inception of the research there were 22 males and 26 females, 30 of whom were single, the remainder married or separated; 22 were unemployed, 13 were in sheltered workshops and 13 in competitive jobs, while 23 lived independently, 14 with their parents and another 11 in group homes. The age range was 18 to 52 with a biomodal distribution of young adults (aged 23-27) and older persons (aged 33-37); the mean age was 27. Current IQs for all members of the sample are not available, but it would appear that all members of the sample had recorded IQs between 65 and 70 when the research began.

Data Collection

The principal means of data collection was a form of participant-observation. Use of this procedure has been discussed in detail elsewhere (Edgerton & Langness, 1978; Taylor & Bogdan, in this volume), but in brief its essence is the prolonged and unobtrusive presence of a sensitive, disciplined observer with the person or persons being studied. When the procedure is used well, the persons being studied will in time learn to take the observer for granted, behaving almost as if he or she were not there, and the observer will come to see the world almost as these persons do.

Each member of the sample was visited on the average of every ten to 14 days. These visits sometimes consisted of only an hour or two of conversation but as often they involved many hours spent in varied forms of interaction: in a restaurant, on a shopping trip, on an excursion to visit friends, family, or Disneyland, or simply talking to one another. Over the period of this research, sample members were seen repeatedly in the various settings of their everyday world (home, work, transportation, leisure). In between visits, there was regular telephone contact, sometimes on a daily basis. Fieldworkers also had frequent contact with significant persons in the lives of sample members (spouse, parents, siblings, friends, caretakers, employers, social workers).

To assure comparable coverage of topics, fieldworkers were provided with a field guide of topics and questions that allowed them, when appropriate and natural, to collect the same kinds of information on each member of the sample. These topics included various aspects of work, self-maintenance in everyday activities, family relationships, leisure, behavior in public places, communicative competence, involvement with the service delivery system, and even fantasy. One of these domains focused on deviance, crime, and any involvements with the legal system either civil or criminal. The resulting corpus of data provides a detailed record of the lives of these 48 persons as they, the researchers, and others observed and interpret them.

Although one cannot be certain, it is unlikely that more than a few crimes were committed—whether detected or not—that the researchers did not learn about either from the retarded person, or from someone else intimately involved in his or her life. Also learned about were the most conspicuous forms of deviance, such as sexual promiscuity or wife beating, and for most of the sample members various minor forms of impropriety or inappropriate behavior were also discovered. Even learned about were many of these peoples' deviant fantasies. The concern here is only with serious deviance—i.e., rule violation that is seen as being sufficiently bizarre, offensive, dangerous, or the like by persons in the community or the delivery system (Edgerton, 1976) that it could lead to a variety of negative consequences including the imposition of limits on the retarded person's access to a more normal life. While the data record undoubtedly contains omissions and is therefore an underestimate, it is probably the most complete record available of the deviance and criminality of a sample of mildly retarded persons in community settings.

The methods employed are subject to certain limitations. For one thing, because of the time these procedures require, as well as the expense of training and maintaining a staff of fieldworkers, the sample was small. A second issue involves the subjectivity inherent in the process of participant observation. Employed were a variety of procedures to minimize such bias (Edgerton & Langness, 1978), but participant observation requires rapport, and rapport requires a give-and-take of human concern and emotion. Fieldworkers have an effect on sample members who in turn affect fieldworkers. However, no direct effects were discerned that relate to crime or deviance beyond the undemonstrated possibility that the presence and concern of the fieldworkers may have reduced either the occurrence of some forms of crime or deviance or, perhaps, the willingness of some sample members to discuss such behaviors.

Findings

The most compelling finding concerning criminality and deviance among the 48 persons in this sample is variety—these people represent everything from model citizens who engage in no wrongdoing whatsoever to persons who commit repeated and sometimes dangerous criminal acts. The extent of this variation is significant and it will be considered later, but in spite of the variation found, it is possible, and useful, to place sample members in various categories determined by the frequency and seriousness of their criminality or deviance. When this is done, it is seen that approximately one-third (18) of the sample has engaged in no criminality or serious deviance, another group of 20 persons has committed various kinds of minor or victimless deviant acts or offenses, while a final group (10) has committed more serious offenses, often against other persons.

"Model Citizens"

Eighteen members of the sample lived such trouble-free lives during the period of this research that there is nothing hyperbolic about the designation of them as model citizens. Nothing antisocial could be discovered about their behavior, nor was there any noteworthy deviance. Instead, most were consciously concerned (but only a few were obsessed) with following the "rules" and not breaking the law. The trouble-free adaptation to community living by these 18 persons was not a result of being sheltered against the opportunity to violate social rules. They had as varied a set of experiences as the rest of the sample. For example, ten of the 18 were living independently, and only six were living with their parents; ten were married. As one would predict from a knowledge of previous research, more women (12) than men (six) belonged to this model citizen category. The only one of these 18 persons to receive a "ticket" during the period of this research was a woman who was walking with her upper-middle class mother when the mother chose to save time by jaywalking. When this sample member objected, pointing to the fact that jaywalking was illegal, she was told not to be so "rigid" and was led across the street where a waiting police officer ticketed them both. The ability of these 18 people to avoid trouble of any kind is more remarkable when it is realized that three of these people had records of delinquency in the years (usually during high school) before this research began and two were married to men who were rather frequent and sometimes serious troublemakers with police records.

Minor or Victimless Offenders

Another 20 of the 48 persons studied sometimes committed minor acts of deviance or victimless crimes. Like the model citizens, most (12) of these persons were women, and the settings in which they lived were similarly diverse. Eleven lived independently and only three lived with parents. Six of these people were married. Since their deviant acts were so varied, the best characterization possible is a brief summary of each person's deviance or crime during the 30-month period of research. Beginning with the eight men, their deviance was as follows: (1) a major but injury-free auto accident while driving without a license; a fistfight with a co-worker at the workshop; (2) Three psychotic episodes leading to a diagnosis of schizophrenia; two bad checks; several visits to prostitutes; occasional use of marijuana; frequently expressed threats of violence against a former girlfriend (none of these was reported to the police); (3) hiring two prostitutes to visit his apartment at the same time; (4) one drunk driving arrest (there were other undetected acts of this kind); accepting $500 to marry an immigrant woman from Taiwan in order to permit her to remain in the U.S.; selling farm produce at a roadside stand without a police permit; (5) frequent acts of passive homosexuality; knowingly buying stolen property for his own use; (6) occasionally brushing against or touching women on buses or other public places; instigating fights on buses; (7) regular attendance at pornographic movies; attempting to use an illegal electronic device in an undetected attempt to defraud the telephone company; (8) a psychotic episode leading to hospitalization, during the course of which he committed $150 worth of property damage to parked cars; some homosexuality; two fist fights at a workshop. Some of these eight men (e.g., number 3) engaged in very little that could be construed as serious deviance or violations of the law, but others were involved in deviance or crime which sometimes had the potential for more serious consequences.

The deviant acts of the 12 women in this category are as follows: (1) some homosexuality; threats of violence against co-workers at a workshop; (2) occasional use of marijuana; frequent promiscuity which in one instance involved the death of a boyfriend in her bed (the cause of death was chronic illness and there were no police charges); (3) several fistfights with co-residents in group home; flagrant promiscuity; contracting a venereal disease; (4) several periods of hospitalization for diagnosed schizophrenia; threats of suicide; some promiscuity; (5) repeated adultery; two physical assaults against her ex-husband (a sample member); various threats of violence; eviction from her apartment for maintaining it in such a filthy condition that the Bishop of her church threatened her with excommunication; (6) eviction for the filthy condition of her apartment; speeding ticket (80 mph); refusal to return overpayment on SSI (leading to a threat of litigation); (7) homosexual seduction of a teenager leading to her expulsion from day-camp program; dependence on various medications including Librium and phenobarbital; driving without a license and under the influcence of tranquilizing drugs; (8) adultery resulting in her disfellowship from the Mormon Church; (9) repeated suicide threats and gestures with a knife; (10) occasional use of marijuana; suicide threats; illegal income while receiving Supplemental Security Income (SSI); birth of an illegitimate child which was given up for adoption; (11) outbursts of temper and obscene language while working as a babysitter, leading to the loss of these jobs; (12) frequently riding a motorcycle without a license; attempting to falsify her work records in an effort to increase her earnings (since she did not understand the differences between piece-work and an hourly salary, her falsification was counter-productive).

Obviously, these brief depictions tell us very little about the context of these acts of deviance or the persons involved. They are presented simply to indicate the range of acts involved, their approximate frequency and their potential for serious consequences. With the women, as the men, there was a great range of deviant acts some of which could have led to personal injury or to criminal charges. However, in fact there were no injuries requiring more than first aid, and while church officials twice intervened, there was no police action taken, except for three motor vehicle citations.

For men and women alike in this category, the most general pattern is one of relatively minor deviance, often of a sexual nature, with very little criminality of any kind, especially of a violent sort. Although there were various acts, or threatened acts, that violated the law, these were not reported to authorities, and on the whole, the deviance of these men and women was neither very frequent nor very serious. The deviant behavior of the final ten members of the sample was a good deal more frequent and serious.

More Frequent and Serious Offenders

These ten more serious offenders live in a variety of circumstances; four live with their parents, four live in group homes, and two live independently. Three are married, one is divorced, the rest are single. Unlike the previous categories, nine of these more serious offenders are men; only one is a woman. As before it is impossible to do more than sketch the outlines of their deviance; but, since this deviance is more frequent and more serious, the sketches will necessarily be somewhat longer. First, the woman (married to, then divorced from, a sample member to be next discussed) who has engaged in a great array of troublesome and illegal activities. For example, in addition to almost ceaseless adulterous affairs with men, she has maintained a prolonged homosexual relationship and had two abortions. She has frequently threatened suicide and several times made what appear to be serious attempts. She often drove recklessly and received several speeding tickets. She has become dependent on Valium, has cheated on her SSI payments, and has been evicted for the filthy condition of her apartment. She has stolen small items from coffee shops (an activity she boastfully calls a "five-finger discount"), but has not been detected. She has been arrested for breaking and entering the house of her ex-husband (the charges were later dropped). Finally, she received an 18-month probated sentence for assaulting her second husband.

The first husband of this woman has an equally extensive list of offenses. For example, he often drove recklessly and drunkenly without being detected by the police; nevertheless he amassed five speeding tickets and was arrested and jailed for drunk driving. He also had two major accidents, at least one of which was due to his recklessness. Like his former wife he attempts to defraud SSI by not reporting outside income. He keeps a loaded gun under his pillow and often threatens to use it; once he arranged to have friends physically assault one of his wife's lovers, and later he attacked this same man on a bus. Finally, he and a friend stole a newspaper-dispensing machine for the coins it contained; they were arrested and convicted with a sentence of 12 months probation plus a fine of $150.

A second man who was convicted of manslaughter in an automobile accident some years before this research began has recently had his license returned, and he continues to drive well over the speed limit. He has yet to be ticketed. He has been threatened with eviction due to the unsightly and unhygienic condition of his apartment. He also has an explosive temper that leads him to attack inanimate objects as well as people; he often puts his fist through walls, sometimes beats his wife, and has twice assaulted co-workers, although in no instance has there been serious injury or police involvement.

Another man has also engaged in violence, twice beating his girlfriend, but his principal deviance involves bad checks and credit card debts which he cannot pay. He acquired a credit card by falsifying the application form, and he has only remained out of jail in the face of repeated threats of litigation because his mother has paid his debts. He has attempted to defraud SSI by not reporting extra income. He has also had two major auto accidents, one of which occurred in Mexico where he was jailed for failure to have proper insurance.

A fourth man has a history of violence. He once attacked his mother, with whom he then lived, throwing her across a room. He also pushed a co-worker off a loading dock and threatened his employer with a knife. Although he has been fired from jobs for his violence, no charges have been filed with the police. Another man, who had been institutionalized as a teenager for sexually molesting a child, has also developed a pattern of violent behavior. For example, he has threatened (or attempted) to attack a co-worker with a metal garbage can, he has repeatedly put his fist through the bedroom wall of his group home, and he has threatened a visitor to his home with a gun that belonged to the caretaker. Again, there was no police action in these cases.

A sixth man, formerly married to a sample member, has frequently reported violent dreams and fantasies, and has several times directed verbal aggression at strangers in public places. He has also expressed violence openly as, for example, in three fights with co-workers and various conflicts with his ex-wife, which included once standing over her with a knife pointed at her throat while she slept. His only arrest was for loitering, although he has sexually molested a nine-year-old niece (he kissed her and masturbated toward her). Most of these acts are said to have occurred during his "blackouts" which were variously diagnosed during a voluntary stay at a mental hospital as schizophrenia or epilepsy. He now overtly uses his blackouts to excuse continued sexual misconduct.

A seventh man, who is a heavy user of alcohol, has threatened a co-resident at his group home with a knife (no police charges filed) and has several times engaged in theft or robbery. He is a "street-wise" man who has several times stolen from friends and co-residents. He has also collaborated with an attractive girlfriend who leads on a victim sexually while he steals the man's money. He has never been arrested.

An eighth man was convicted of a felony charge of aggravated assault when he attacked a ten-year-old neighbor boy and kicked him repeatedly with his heavy boots. The boy had apparently taunted him. This was not an isolated act of violence; he often beat his wife, sometimes savagely so, once dislocating her ankle. He also struck a woman at a bowling alley and threatened a member of a social group for retarded persons with a knife. He drove recklessly on many occasions causing his license to be suspended and finally leading to a three-day jail sentence. He has also stolen money, usually to spend at massage parlors, or to hire masseuses to come to his apartment (sometimes while his wife was locked in another room). On more than one occasion he has said, "I never lie except to the police."

The final man in this category has had 12 known arrests, four of which occurred during this study. Most were for theft or breaking and entering homes or cars. In addition to the robberies for which he was arrested, he has admitted to stealing from the manager's office of a movie, from a parked car, and from friends. He has also had several fights including one in which he fought with inmates while he was in jail awaiting trial. He carries a knife which he puts under his pillow at night and he sometimes carries a realistic toy gun. On some occasions he has carried both a switchblade knife in his pocket and a six-inch hunting knife in a scabbard on his belt. He often drinks beer excessively and sometimes smokes marijuana, and he has been accused of masturbating publicly on at least one occasion. His last conviction for robbery led to a sentence of 18 months probation under the supervision of the caretaker of his group home. He freely admits that his thefts are planned in advance and says that he has been stealing since he was eight.

Discussion

Without comparable data from other populations it is impossible to determine whether the offenses sketched here are more or less frequent or serious than would be found in a sample of non-retarded persons. There was no comparison population in this research project, and a search of the literature has revealed no fully comparable corpus of data for a non-retarded population.[1] Despite this limitation, some conclusions about the deviance and criminality of this sample may be possible.

First, and most important, is the intra-sample variation that was discovered. The frequency of deviant or criminal acts ranged from never at all for more than a third of the sample, to being virtually an everyday occurrence in the lives of five or six of these people. The form and seriousness of these offenses were similarly varied. This variation is significant because it emphasizes once again what sometimes seems to be forgotten, namely that antisocial behavior should not be thought of as a problem for *all* mentally retarded persons. It is a problem for *some* mentally retarded persons but not others. In this sample it was a significant occurrence in the lives of ten persons, or approximately 21% of the sample.

Because of the findings by Brown and Courtless (1967, 1968) that a disproportionate number of mentally retarded offenders across the country had been found guilty of crimes of violence, the violent behavior of these sample members is of particular interest. Fifteen members of the sample physically assaulted another person at least once. Most did so on several occasions and two were convicted of violent crimes. Much of this violence was directed against spouses, as is common in the general population. Thus, five members of the sample (three men and two women) struck or kicked their spouse on more than one occasion. Weapons were never used in these attacks and with one exception the resulting injuries were minor. The most common target for physical violence, however, was not a spouse but a co-worker or supervisor; six men and one woman assaulted co-workers, sometimes using a chair or garbage can as a weapon, and two men attacked their

[1]For a discussion of the adequacy of existing methods of eliciting data about crime—official records, self-reports, and reports by the victims of crime—see Hindelang (1978). For a discussion of more general issues of research design in these studies, see Farrington (1979).

supervisors. Three men attacked unrelated persons, and two men and one woman attacked or physically threatened a co-resident of a group home. Six of the men who engaged in violence either used or threatened to use a deadly weapon; in one instance the weapon was a hand gun, in four others it was a knife, and in another it was heavy workboots. Five men possessed and sometimes carried knives, while two of them possessed handguns, although these weapons were never fired to the researchers' knowledge.

Despite the various acts of violence by these 15 people, there were only three complaints made to the police during the period of this research. One of these was dropped, but the other two led to convictions—one for battery against a woman who fought with her husband (he too was convicted), a second for felony aggravated assault when a man kicked and beat a neighbor boy who allegedly taunted him. Both offenders were placed on probation.

In summary, although only two members of the sample were convicted of violent crimes, four others could have been charged with aggravated assault and several others could have been charged with simple battery. Almost all of this violence was impulsive although one man twice planned assaults and once arranged for friends to assault someone for him. Yet, given the fact that six men in the sample had ready access to knives or guns, the consequences could have been more serious than they were. It should be repeated that there were no homicides, no injuries inflicted by a deadly weapon (except for the kicking incident), and no brutal or sadistic acts of violence.[2]

The same prison-generated data that pointed to the frequency of crimes of violence for retarded offenders indicated that sexual offenses were infrequent. In this sample, 19 persons engaged in sexual behavior that could be considered either deviant or criminal. As labeling theorists have demonstrated, whether an action is regarded as offensive, and whether it is labeled as such, varies greatly from time to time and place to place (Edgerton, 1976). Opinions could vary widely regarding the impropriety of these sexual behaviors, but all the behaviors listed here were considered wrong by at least one person who was in an important relationship with the actor. None of this behavior was violent and rarely were "nonconsenting" persons involved (one man occasionally rubbed against women on buses or other public places; another kissed and masturbated toward his nine-year-old niece; another masturbated in semi-public view). In none of those cases was there any police involvement. In the remaining instances of sexual deviance, five women were engaged in flagrant sexual promiscuity. One of these women contracted gonorrhea (which led her to be ostracized by co-residents of her group home), and a second had an illegitimate child which was relinquished for adoption. Three other married women were involved in adultery, but only one of these women was indiscreet about her behavior. Three men employed prostitutes, but never on a regular basis. Three men and three women had homosexual encounters or relationships, but none appeared to have accepted a homosexual self-definition. Only one of these encounters could be considered seductive or aggressive, and here the evidence is equivocal. Thus, while it appears that about one-third of the sample had some sort of difficulty relating to sexual conduct, very few in the sample could be considered "antisocial" in their sexual behavior, and none of these sexual behaviors led to police action.

---

[2]While they are too complex to be considered here, we should note that many of the violent members of our sample had violent fantasy lives, and others sought employment as police officers or security guards. The literature reports no relationships between violent behavior and violent fantasies among institutionalized retarded people (Sternlicht, 1966; Silber & Courtless, 1968), but this research did not consider naturally occurring (versus explicitly elicited) violent fantasies in community settings.

On the other hand, theft was an antisocial behavior for some of these retarded persons. While only five persons in this sample were involved in theft, four of these were repeated offenders. All four of these persons stole in a premeditated fashion, and while their thefts were always petty, their approach was usually rational, with the motive clearly that of profit, and with no remorse for the victim. Three of these four persons were arrested and convicted.

Another area of concern involves the operation of motor vehicles. Previous research on the community adaptation of mentally retarded persons has not emphasized traffic violations as a major form of antisocial behavior, although Baller, Charles, and Miller (1966), and Kennedy (1966) noted in passing a high rate of traffic violations in their retarded samples, and Henschel (1972) reported that 55% of the drivers in her mentally retarded "Chicano" sample and 30% of drivers in her "Anglo" sample had received one or more traffic tickets. Henschel also noted that some of the "Chicano" drivers frequently drove while under the influence of alcohol. A report from Australia (Boyce & Dax, 1976) found that drivers from special schools for the mentally retarded had more traffic offenses than their normal counterparts, but concluded that there were so few retarded drivers that they did not consititute an appreciable danger on the road.

Thirteen members of our sample drove at least occasionally. Three of these did so without any known traffic violations, but the remaining ten drivers committed many violations. For example, three of these drivers accounted for five accidents, one with injury. Four repeatedly drove recklessly; the ten speeding tickets those four persons received represent only a small percentage of the violations known to the researchers. Two persons were arrested for drunk driving; these same two people, plus two others, often drove while intoxicated and were not detected. Finally, three persons drove without licenses; two of these were ticketed.

As before, there are no comparable data for undetected traffic violations, but in terms of officially reported violations it is clear that the driving records of ten of the 13 drivers in this sample are worse than "average." For example, during the year 1977, in the city of Los Angeles (population 2,900,600 plus several million drivers from adjacent communities) there were 594,391 traffic tickets issued for moving violations, or approximately one ticket for every five or six residents in Los Angeles. In this study 13 drivers accumulated seven moving violations in 1977, and 12 over the 30 months of the research. There were 71,510 accidents in Los Angeles in 1977, 31,207 of which involved injuries. Sample drivers were involved in five accidents, one with injury; four of these occurred in 1977. Thus while three of the sample members are exemplary drivers, the remaining ten drivers are more likely to commit traffic offenses than the average citizen, and many of these offenses are dangerous.

Are These Retarded Persons More Deviant Than Non-Retarded Persons?

It is possible to approach this question by comparing the rates of criminality or deviance of a group of mentally retarded persons with non-retarded controls. When this has been done in other studies, the retarded samples are usually more criminal (data on non-criminal forms of deviance are seldom available). As has been seen however, these studies have either failed to match their controls adequately or they have suffered great sample attrition. Comparison can also be made with groups whose rates of official or self-reported deviance are known (e.g., teen-aged gang members), or with overall crime rates (e.g., the estimated crime rate for Los Angeles in 1977 was 5 per 100; the violent crime rate was .05 per

100).[3] When such group comparisons are made it is possible to show that, more often than not, mildly retarded persons commit crimes more frequently than most groups of non-retarded persons do, although there are exceptions, such as young black males of low socio-economic status or mentally ill persons (Farrington, 1979; Mednick & Christiansen, 1977; Rabkin, 1979). In the view of the writer, these group comparisons are of limited value and can be misleading. That is so because in *every* known sample of mentally retarded persons, some commit crimes or otherwise get into trouble, but many others do neither. To repeat, in this sample 18 persons got into no trouble at all, 20 more were occasionally involved in relatively minor deviance or victimless crimes, while ten persons committed serious or frequent offenses. Group comparisons suggest a homogeneity concerning criminality that simply does not exist.

The question that has the greatest practical importance for deinstitutionalization, as well as the greatest theoretical relevance, is this: Can one explain why some retarded individuals become criminal while others do not? Although it is important that this question replace the more global one about the criminality of retarded persons, it must be obvious that the present research was not designed to provide an answer. For one thing the sample was too small for such an explanatory enterprise; for another, it was also too homogeneous with regard to such relevant variables as age, ethnicity, socio-economic status, and IQ. Also, the data available for periods of time prior to the onset of research, especially for early childhood, were imprecise. Despite these serious strictures, a few comments may be warranted. First, the near universal finding that males are more delinquent than females—whether mentally retarded or not—was once again clearly demonstrated. On the other hand, the presence of deviant peer or parental models in this sample was not related to criminality (Shapiro, 1968). For example, conspicuous models for criminality or deviance (e.g., some were thieves, some drove recklessly, others were violent) occurred twice in the model citizen group, five times in the middle group, and only three times in the most deviant group (Butler & Browning, 1970). Since the presence of family disruption and alcoholic fathers has so often been linked with delinquency, it is of interest to note that before the age of eighteen, twenty members of this sample lived in seriously disrupted families due to divorce, parental death, or desertion, and four others had alcoholic fathers. However, neither the criminality nor the deviance of sample members was unrelated to these prior family disruptions (Robins, 1966).

The most suggestive prognostic finding involves teen-aged delinquency. Only two of the 18 of the model citizens was a teen-aged delinquent, but nine of the 20 persons engaged in minor or victimless crimes and nine of the ten most deviant members of the sample had records of teen-aged delinquency. Given the small sample size, this finding must be treated cautiously, not simply because there have been as many putative causes of delinquency as schizophrenia, but also also because there have been as many refutations. The most powerful research designs for discovering possible antecedents of delinquency—as in schizophrenia —are prospective, long-term studies in birth cohorts, not retrospective studies that compare known delinquents with matched controls. Based on his review of the best available research, some of it his own, Wadsworth (1978) has been forced to conclude that one cannot now predict delinquency with any accuracy. What is more, available models predict far too many false positives. Just as one is manifestly unable to predict which mentally retarded persons will succeed in

[3]See *FBI, Uniform Crime Reports*. U.S. Department of Justice, 1977.

community adaptation (Cobb, 1972), one cannot now predict which ones will engage in deviant or criminal behavior.

One can say that it is now quite clear, if not widely accepted, that officially detected as well as self-reported delinquents and criminals in the United States, United Kingdom, and Denmark, for example, have lower IQs than the general population (Mednick & Christiansen, 1977; Wadsworth, 1978). While this differential in IQ is not great enough to put the low-IQ offenders in the mentally retarded range, it is as strongly related to criminality as social class or race, variables that are widely accepted as having an undeniable relationship to criminality (Hirschi & Hindelang, 1977). Lefkowitz, Eron, Walder & Huesmann (1977) have linked low IQ to a propensity for violence. Because of the homogeneity in IQ within this sample one cannot comment on this argument. However, there is nothing in the published literature on mental retardation to demonstrate that IQ differences within the mild range are predictive of criminality in community adaptation.

But the question about mental retardation and crime cannot be confined to IQ, it must also include a complex of experiences having to do with isolation from ordinary social learning opportunities, stigmatization, parental and peer rejection, school failure (through which low IQ may be mediated), and loss of self-esteem. What is more, mildly retarded people in this sample evinced a high rate of emotional traumata, mental illness, convulsive disorders, brain injuries, and other central nervous system related dysfunctions. This is presumably so because mentally-retarded persons from white middle-class backgrounds are likely to be clinically retarded (Tarjan, 1970). These condictions may involve confusion, rage, impulsivity, anxiety and other emotional states that could be related to deviance. Given the common presence of such central nervous system dysfunctions in middle-class, white retarded populations, the problems of matching with "normal" controls are highlighted, as is the need for research that focuses on the possible relationship of these phenomena to deviance and crime.

Are the Mentally Retarded More Often Victims than Victimizers?

That mentally retarded persons are more often victimized than they are victimizers in the process of deinstitutionalization is an underlying assumption in the normalization movement (Wolfensberger, 1975). It is commonly believed that even if the retarded may offend against others in the process of adapting to community settings, they are more often and more seriously offended against. Is this assumption merely a shibboleth? Even if one ignores the subtle forms of humiliation and exploitation which all members of this sample have experienced and limits discussion to overt and reasonably serious occurrences, one finds that 26 members of the sample have suffered some noteworthy kind of victimization. Therefore, even if one disregards the common phenomena of parental control, caretaker dominance, and neglect by caregivers, one finds that victimization is as common a feature of the lives of these persons as is deviance or crime. To provide some sense of these occurrences, the writer once again sketches them, beginning with the persons in the model citizen category.

Seven of the 18 "model citizens" experienced marked victimization: (1) without her consent a woman regularly had most of her SSI income expropriated by her sister; (2) a man was fired from his job when he was accused of theft (evidence demonstrates that he was "framed"); (3) a woman's purse was stolen from her residence and she was accosted on a bus; (4) a man was accused of fondling a young woman and was dismissed from a day camp as a result; the person who dismissed him admitted that he was innocent but that he made a necessary scapegoat; (5) a woman's apartment was burglarized; (6) a woman was sexually exploited by a normal man who took her to a motel where they had intercourse despite her apparent protests; (7) a man was questioned by the police while he stood in front of his group home because he looked suspicious; as he walked home from a sheltered workshop, boys in the same neighborhood several times shouted insults and threw stones at him. While many of these episodes are trivial, they are much more serious than anything done by *any* of these 18 "model citizens."

Thirteen of the 20 persons who committed minor or victimless crimes were also victimized: (1) a woman's money was often misappropriated by her mother; (2) a woman had her purse snatched while walking to the bus; she was also sexually seduced (and threatened if she complained) by her group home caretaker; (3) a woman was struck by a panhandler when she ignored him; without her consent, a boyfriend pawned her furniture and wedding ring after their relationship broke up; (4) a woman's apartment was twice burglarized and she was once mugged; on several occasions friends borrowed sizeable sums of money which were never repaid; (5) a woman who was living in a motel after her husband had died was raped; (6) a man was exploited by an employer who paid him less than was promised and forced him to work excessive hours; (7) a woman was taunted and physically threatened by co-workers who objected to her appearance and retardation; (8) another woman was forced to work for 33½ cents an hour; a member of her church "borrowed" her entire savings and disappeared; her in-laws forced her to turn over her SSI money to them; she was also burglarized and sold an expensive encyclopedia—when she could not keep up the payments, the books were repossessed; (9) a man was similarly exploited when a salesman sold him a useless medical insurance plan; his apartment was burglarized five or six times; (10) a man was robbed in the street and so cruelly teased by children in public that he called the police; his sister several times misappropriated his income; (11) a woman was several times beaten by her father who also regularly misused her money; (12) a woman had many of her possessions stolen (usually by men whom she invited home for sexual relations); on occasion, a man struck her and she may have been raped by one; her family did not administer her trust fund as required by the court; (13) a woman was stopped for questioning (and held for several hours) at the U.S.-Mexican border because her speech impediment made her speech seem suspicious to the American immigration officers on duty. Arguably, these persons have suffered more at the hands of others than others have from their acts.

Seven of the ten persons who have engaged in the most serious and frequent misconduct have also experienced some form of exploitation. As may be seen, however, in this group the exploitation seems to be both less frequent and less severe than in the others: (1) a man who was hired by a firm engaged in illegal activities was not paid when the firm suddenly went out of business; (2) a man's apartment was robbed; (3) a man was cheated by a used car salesman; (4) a woman was struck once by her father and repeatedly by her husband; (5) a man may have been the victim of police harrassment (this is difficult to assess, especially so since he was engaged in various criminal activities); (6) a man often had his SSI checks taken by his step-uncle; and (7) a man's residence was burglarized four times and he was mugged once and perhaps twice.

While it is difficult to make any precise comparison of the seriousness of the offenses these persons committed versus those committed against them, it seems reasonable to conclude that as a group they were as often the victims of offenses as they were the perpetrators of them. But again a "group" comparison is misleading. The least troublesome members of the sample were more often victimized than were the ten serious offenders. With the exception of the ten serious offenders, the offenses committed against members of this sample were at least as serious, and possibly more so, than the ones they committed.

Conclusion

The most compelling finding of this research is the *variation* in crime and deviance among 48 ostensibly similar persons. These white, middle-class, mildly retarded persons were studied in an effort to determine how such a homogeneous population of persons would experience the process of adaptation to community living. Yet this sample of persons thought to be capable of successful normalization was far from homogeneous in deviance and criminality. This intra-sample variation in deviance makes it manifestly unnecessary—and perhaps even mischievous—to continue to ask whether some group of retarded people is more or less criminal or violent than some group of non-retarded people. The reality reflected by this sample is not fundamentally different from that reported elsewhere; that is, while the proportions vary, it seems to be the case that any sample of mildly retarded persons will contain a substantial number of persons—perhaps a majority—who are able to adapt to community living in a relatively troublefree manner, but it will also contain others—usually a substantial minority—whose community behavior is troublesome, sometimes involving criminal conduct. Many of these persons will be the victims of wrongdoing at the hands of non-retarded persons.

Given this reality and present inability to change it by predicting who will become socially troublesome in the course of community living, one must confront the apparent fact that any time mildly retarded people are placed in community settings, some will become victims, some will become victimizers, and many will experience both roles. In this regard, it is difficult to ignore the fact that more and more mentally retarded persons are being reinstitutionalized (Conroy, 1977) and that a principal reason for this retrograde movement is deviant behavior, especially aggressive behavior.

How does it happen, then, that although more than 20% of this sample was quite deviant—and most of these were guilty of crimes—no one was imprisoned or institutionalized for more than a brief period (Edgerton, 1979)? Almost all the offenses of these persons were known to someone within the delivery system (social workers, regional center counselors, group home caretakes, workshop operators), and many were also known to parents, relatives, and friends. Yet the police were rarely informed, and when informed they seldom took action. At other times, or in other places, offenses such as these could have led to incarceration—and to resulting "failure" in community adaptation. Since the most unquestioned criterion of failure in community adaptation is incarceration or reinstitutionalization, and since such action is relative to the conditions that exist in various places and at various times, one is confronted by a possibility that would seem to have been invented by labeling theorists, namely, that wherever one has evidence, some retarded persons (like some non-retarded persons) commit rule violations that could be construed as deviant or criminal. In years past, such acts often led to hospitalization. In some towns or cities today, they still do so, as reinstitutionalization rates attest (Conroy, 1977). But in this sample, nothing of the kind took place. The violations took place, but the societal reaction was benign.

The point of this is that the relationship of crime and deviance to success in community adaptation is anything but simple. It is relative to a complex of social, economic, and political factors that determine how such behaviors will be responded to under various circumstances. In Los Angeles, during the time of this research, the prevailing sentiment with regard to mentally retarded persons seemed to call for a resolution to troublesome behavior within the least restrictive setting possible. Perhaps this was due to the pervasive effect of penal codes[4] that call for mentally retarded offenders to be dealt with in ways other than by incarceration whenever possible, and enable many regional center counselors to "rescue" their clients from the criminal justice system. This mood and practice of "permissiveness" was accurately perceived and manipulated by a few of the serious offenders in this study who said that they did not fear criminal prosecution because no serious punishment would result. If normalization is meant to include normal risk for criminal acts, these individuals are not being normalized.

If it is correct that any population of mildly retarded young adults from white, middle-class backgrounds will contain a majority who adapt without any socially troublesome behavior and a minority who create trouble for themselves and others, then the policy implications are substantial. If there had been a strict meting out of jail terms for retarded persons who committed crimes, then more than 20% of the persons studied could have been incarcerated. The prevailing policy kept all of these people—several of whom were repeated and flagrant offenders—in the community. Since most available research evidence seems to indicate that most retarded persons—even those whose early years of community adaptation were highly troubled—achieve a progressively more stable and troublefree pattern of life as years pass, it is possible to interpret the present policies as encouraging this pattern of growing civility over time, and it may also be possible to commend it for choosing long-term gains despite short-term risks. As a result, many retarded persons who engage in socially troublesome behavior will be given time to develop more acceptable patterns of community conduct. Whether those few members of this sample who repeatedly and flagrantly violated the law will also benefit by such a policy or will simply continue to exploit it, is something that only time, and continued research, will tell.

References

Allen, R. C. The retarded offender: Unrecognized in court and untreated in prison. *Federal Probation*, 1968, *32*, 22-27.

Allen, R. C. The law and the mentally retarded. In F. J. Menolascino (Ed.), *Psychiatric approaches to mental retardation*. New York: Basic Books, 1970.

Andron, L. & Sturm, M. Is "I do" in the repertoire of the retarded? A study of the functioning of married retarded couples. *Mental Retardation*, 1973, *11*, 31-34.

Baker, B., Seltzer, G. B. & Seltzer, M. M. As close as possible: Community residences for retarded adults. Boston: Little, Brown, 1977.

Baller, W. R., Charles, D. C. & Miller, E. L. *Mid-life attainment of the mentally retarded: A longitudinal study*. Lincoln, NE: The University of Nebraska Press, 1966.

Bazelon, D. L., Boggs, E. M., Hilleboe, H. E. & Tudor, W. W. *Report of the Task Force on Law*. Washington, DC: President's Panel on Mental Retardation, United States Department of Health, Education and Welfare, 1963.

Beier, D. C. Behavioral disturbances in the mentally retarded. In H. A. Stevens & R. Heber (Eds.), *Mental Retardation: A review of research*. Chicago: University of Chicago Press, 1964.

---

[4]California Penal Code 1370:1 provides that a criminal defendant who is mentally incompetent because of a developmental disability will be treated differently than a criminal defendant who is not so disabled. Such a defendant will become a client of a regional center, become eligible for their services and programs, and except for extreme offenses, will not receive a jail term.

Biklen, D. Myths, mistreatment and pitfalls: Mental retardation and criminal justice. *Mental Retardation*, 1977, *15*, 51-57.

Birenbaum, A. & Seiffer, S. *Resettling retarded adults in a managed community*. New York: Praeger, 1976.

Boslow, H. M. & Kandel, A. Psychiatric aspects of dangerous behavior: The retarded offender. *American Journal of Psychiatry*, 1965, *122*, 646-652.

Boyce, L. & Dax, E. C. The special school pupil as a motor car user. *Australian Journal of Mental Retardation*, 1976, *4*, 53-61.

Brown, B. S. & Courtless, T. F. *The mentally retarded offender*. Washington, DC: The President's Commission on Law Enforcement and Administration of Justice, 1967.

Brown, B. S. & Courtless, T. F. The mentally retarded in penal and correctional institutions. *American Journal of Psychiatry*, 1968, *124*, 1164-1170.

Brown, B. S. & Courtless, T. F. *The mentally retarded offender* (DHEW Publication No. (HSM) 72-9039) Rockville, MD: National Institute of Mental Health, Center for Studies of Crime and Delinquency, 1971.

Browning, P. L. *Rehabilitation and the retarded offender*. Springfield, IL: Charles C Thomas, 1976.

Butler, A. J. & Browning, P.L. Methodological issues in the prediction of rehabilitation outcome with the mentally retarded. In H. J. Prehm (Ed.), *Rehabilitation research in mental retardation*. Eugene: Rehabilitation Research and Training Center in Mental Retardation, University of Oregon, 1970.

Cobb, H. *The forecast of fulfillment: A review of research on predictive assessment of the adult retarded for social and vocational adjustment*. New York: Teachers College Press, 1972.

Conroy, J. W. Trends in deinstitutionalization of the mentally retarded. *Mental Retardation*, 1977, *15*, 44-46.

Craft, M. Withdrawals from license in mental deficiency. *American Journal of Mental Deficiency*, 1958, *63*, 47-49.

Davies, S. P. *Social control of the mentally deficient*. New York: Crowell, 1930.

Deno, E. *Retarded youth: Their school-rehabilitation needs*. Minneapolis: Minneapolis Public Schools, 1965.

Edgerton, R. B. *The cloak of competence: Stigma in the lives of the mentally retarded*. Berkeley: University of California Press, 1967.

Edgerton, R. B. *Deviance: A cross-cultural perspective*. Menlo Park, CA: Cummings, Publishing Co., 1976.

Edgerton, R. B. Failure in community adaptation: The relativity of assessment. Paper presented at a joint conference sponsored by The National Institutes of Child Health and Human Development and the University of California, Los Angeles, September 25-27, 1979.

Edgerton, R. B. & Langness, L. L. Observing mentally retarded persons in community settings: An anthropological perspective. In G. P. Sackett (Ed.), *Observing behavior* (Vol. 1): *Theory and applications in mental retardation*. Baltimore: University Park Press, 1978.

Fairbanks, R. F. The subnormal child—seventeen years later. *Mental Hygiene*, 1933, *17*, 177-208.

Farrington, D. P. Longitudinal research on crime and delinquency. In N. Morris (Ed.), *Research in criminal justice* (Vol. 1). Chicago: University of Chicago Press, 1979.

Goldstein, H. Social and occupational adjustment. In H. A. Stevens & R. Heber (Eds.), *Mental retardation: A review of research*. Chicago: University of Chicago Press, 1964.

Häfner, H. & Böker, W. Mentally disordered violent offenders. *Social Psychiatry*, 1973, *8*, 220-229.

Hamlett, I. C. & Engle, T. L. Mental health analyses of furlough patients. *American Journal of Mental Deficiency*, 1950, *55*, 257-263.

Henshel, A. *The forgotten ones: A sociological study of Anglo and Chicano retardates.* Austin: University of Texas Press, 1972.

Hindelang, M. J. Race involvement in common law personal crimes. *American Sociological Review*, 1978, *43*, 93-109.

Hirschi, T. & Hindelang, M. J. Intelligence and delinquency: A revisionist review. *American Sociological Review*, 1977, *42*, 571-587.

Jackson, N. Educable mental handicap and delinquency. *Educational Research*, 1970, *12*, 128-134.

Kennedy, R. J. *A Connecticut community revisited: A study of the social adjustment of a group of mentally deficient adults in 1948 and 1960.* Hartford, CT: Connecticut State Department of Health, Office of Mental Retardation, 1966.

Lee, J. L., Hegge, T. G. & Voelker, P. H. *A study of social adequacy and of social failure of mentally retarded youth in Wayne County, Michigan.* Detroit: Wayne State University Press, 1959.

Lefkowitz, M. M., Eron, L. D., Walder, L. O. & Huesmann, L. R. *Growing up to the violent: A longitudinal study of the development of aggression.* New York: Pergamon, 1977.

Lomastro, J. A. *The retarded offender: A new perspective.* Unpublished Ph.D. Dissertation, Brandeis University, 1976.

MacMillan, D. L. *Mental retardation in school and society.* Boston: Little, Brown & Co., 1977.

Marsh, R. L., Friel, C. M. & Eissler, V. The adult MR in the criminal justice system. *Mental Retardation*, 1975, *13*, 21-25.

McCarver, R. B. & Craig, E. M. Placement of the retarded in the community: Prognosis and outcome. In N. R. Ellis (Ed.), *International review of research in mental retardation* (Vol. 7). New York: Academic Press, 1974.

McDevitt, S. C., Smith, P. M., Schmidt, D. W., & Rosen, M. The deinstitutionalized citizen: Adjustment and quality of life. *Mental Retardation*, 1978, *16*, 22-24.

Mednick, S. & Christiansen, K. O. *Biosocial bases of criminal behavior.* New York: Gardner Press, 1977.

Mink, I. T. Disruptive behavior of residents and caretaker response: Community and institution. Paper presented at the Annual Meeting of the American Anthropological Association, Los Angeles, November, 1978.

Moen, M., Bogen, D. & Aanes, D. Follow-up of mentally retarded adults successfully and unsuccessfully placed in community group homes. *Hospital and Community Psychiatry*, 1975, *26*, 754-756.

Muehlenberger, C. E. The social-psychological experiences of adult former residents of a state school for the mentally retarded. Unpublished Ph.D. Dissertation, Syracuse University, 1972.

Nihira, L. & Nihira, K. Jeopardy in community placement. *American Journal of Mental Deficiency*, 1975, *79*, 538-544.

Pagel, S. E. & Whitling, C. A. Readmissions to a state hospital for mentally retarded persons: Reasons for community placement failure. *Mental Retardation*, 1978, 16, 164-166.

Peterson, L., & Smith, L. L. A comparison of the post-school adjustment of educable mentally retarded adults with that of adults or normal intelligence. *Exceptional Children*, 1960, *26*, 404-408.

Rabkin, J. G. Criminal behavior of discharged mental patients: A critical appraisal of the research. *Psychological Bulletin*, 1979, *86*, 1-27.

Robins, L. N. *Deviant children grown up: A sociological and psychiatric study of sociopathic personality*. Baltimore: Williams & Wilkin, 1966.

Robinson, N. M. & Robinson, H. B. *The mentally retarded child: A psychological approach*. (2nd Ed.). New York: McGraw-Hill, 1976.

Rosen, M., Clark, G. R., & Kivitz, M.S. *Habilitation of the handicapped: New directions in programs for the developmentally disabled*. Baltimore: University Park Press, 1977.

Saenger, G. *The adjustment of severely retarded adults in the community*. Albany, NY: Interdepartmental Health Resources Board, 1957.

Santamour, M. B. & West, B. The mentally retarded offender in the social context. *Amicus*, 1979, *4*, 23-28.

Shapiro, A. Delinquent behavior and disturbed behavior within the field of mental deficiency. In A. V. S. de Renck & R. Porter (Eds.), *The mentally abnormal offender*. London: Churchill, 1968.

Silber, D. E. & Courtless, T. F. Measures of fantasy aggression among mentally retarded offenders. *American Journal of Mental Deficiency*, 1968, *72*, 918-923.

Sternlicht, M. Fantasy of aggression in delinquent and nondelinquent retardates. *American Journal of Mental Deficiency*, 1966, *70*, 819-821.

Sutherland, E. H. Mental deficiency and crime. In K. Young (Ed.), *Social attitudes*. New York: Henry Holt, 1931.

Tarjan, G. Some thoughts on socio-cultural retardation. In H. C. Haywood (Ed.), *Social-cultural aspects of mental retardation*. New York: Appleton-Century-Crofts, 1970.

Wadsworth, M. E. J. Delinquency prediction and its uses: The experience of a 21-year follow-up study. *International Journal of Mental Health*, 1978, *7*, 43-62.

Windle, C. D., Stewart, E. & Brown, S. J. Reasons for community failure of released patients. *American Journal of Mental Deficiency*, 1961, *66*, 213-217.

Wolfensberger, W. *The origin and nature of our institutional models*. Syracuse: Human Policy Press, 1975.

Zeleny, L. D. Feble-mindedness and criminal conduct. *American Journal of Sociology*, 1933, *38*, 564-576.

A Letter to a Developmental Disabilities Administrator

Gershon Berkson
Daniel Romer

Institute for the Study of Developmental Disabilities

Arthur Lawrence Christopher
Administrator, Worldsend Region
Department of Developmental
Disabilities
State Office Building
Cornfield, Illinois

Dear Art:

This is a response to your memo of October 1 asking for input regarding the proposed guidelines for new standards for funding of community facilities. We do not ordinarily offer our opinion about such things, but for once, our research seems relevant to the Department's concerns. So we offer our suggestions in hope that they can be helpful.

As is usual with us, we won't come to the point immediately. We think that guidelines come from a philosophy of service, and we will try to make ours explicit at the beginning. We believe that service systems for the mentally retarded spring from three general ideologies: caregiving, training and social ecology. These ideologies sometimes clash, but they are complementary in a first-class service system. It is only when one of them dominates the purposes of the program and excludes others that the lives of the mentally retarded who are being served become more restricted than necessary.

Three Concepts of Service

Caregiving refers to the maintenance of good health. Good nutrition, cleanliness, and freedom from disease are obvious prerequisites to any decent program. On the other hand, services built solely around the need for maintaining good health produce stultifying psychological environments. Instances of such inadequate environments may be seen in state-operated custodial institutions and community-operated sheltered care facilities and nursing homes which provide food in a regimented atmosphere, maintain cleanliness on a rigid schedule and control behavior with drugs.

The second ideology, *training*, has as its central assumption that what prevents mentally retarded people from living normal lives is that they lack the necessary skills for adaptation to society. It is believed that these prerequisite skills can be defined at least in broad terms and that, given adequate behavioral technology, the mentally retarded can be trained and then "placed" into general society.

The research reported in this paper was supported in part by a grant from the National Institute for Child and Health and Human Development (HD-10321) to the Illinois Institute for Developmental Disabilities, Department of Mental Health and Developmental Disabilities. This paper is based on a presentation at the study group meeting of the Society for Research in Child Development entitled Development of Friendship, held at the University of Illinois-Urbana, November, 1978.

The success of special education, vocational rehabilitation, and specifically programs based on so-called behavior modification principles has been spectacular. When skills have been lacking, formal tuition on the basis of coupling of skill structures with reinforcement principles has dramatically changed the lives of many mentally retarded people. Training programs have allowed previously unskilled mildly retarded people to work at normal jobs, learn money systems, and maintain independent households. More severely disabled people have learned self-help skills, language, and other social skills which have helped others to care for them.

On the other hand, it must be said that expectations based on the training perspective have not been completely fulfilled. Sometimes it is not so easy to describe all of the skills necessary for adaptation. Sometimes scheduling of situations and of rewards is difficult. Moreover, when not managed by professionals, there is the danger that the power for good of the principles of programmed learning can degenerate into a system of random rewards and nonfunctional record keeping done without reference to the purposes of the program or even to the progress of the individual for whom training is supposedly being carried out.

Programs which purport to prepare people for normal community life through training also sometimes fail to acheive their aims because they do not adequately take into account the environmental contexts which the aims assume. An example (which is by no means isolated) is the failure of some sheltered workshop programs to arrange for contracts that are appropriate for training—sometimes these workshops have no work at all for extended periods. As a result, not only is training not possible, but clients become demoralized and learn to spend their time in ways which would be inappropriate in regular employment.

An overemphasis on a training ideology that ignores the context in which training is done is therefore inappropriate. General concern for the *social ecology* in which clients live and work would strengthen the success of both caregiving and training approaches. In this approach, programming is focused on the creation of social and environmental settings that enable handicapped persons to lead maximally satisfying and productive lives. We believe, therefore, that the guidelines which you are preparing should include specifications which assure maintenance of health and adequate staff training. They should also deal with ecological factors which will promote full expression of caregiving and training approaches.

Our recommendations are based on our research which, in turn, is based on recent changes in the society, especially the normalization or deinstitutionalization movement. It is not necessary to go into the deinstitutionalization movement in detail here. However, there are certain points which should be expressed briefly. The shift of mildly and moderately retarded adults from state-operated institutions in rural areas to privately run facilities in both urban and rural settings has been going on for about 20 years now.

This shift in population has not reduced the total number of people in state-operated institutions as markedly as it has changed the character of institutional populations. Whereas a generation ago, institutions were typically very large and served all levels of functioning among the mentally retarded, now the typical modern institution tends to be smaller and devoted almost exclusively to severely disabled people.

Mildly and moderately retarded adults, who were once in rural institutions, now live near their homes either with their families or more often in large sheltered care facilities and sometimes in small group homes. In these community living facilities, they have some opportunity to participate in the community in which they live through work and recreational activities. A most important aspect of their life situation, however, is that most of their time is spent with mentally retarded and mentally ill people. In this sense, their "community" consists not so much of normal people who consider them as friends to invite for an evening of beer and cards as it does other mentally disabled people who share with them common histories and life problems.

Thus, mentally retarded adults in the service system to which your guidelines will apply live in supervised communal settings with other mentally disabled people. These organizations have some similarity to the nuclear families we sometimes like to use as a standard of normalized living. However, they are vastly more complex than families, and they deserve study in their own right. There is, in fact, a fair amount of research on staff of such facilities, mainly directed to evaluating their attitudes toward working with retarded people. There is rather less known of what the staff actually do, and what is known does not offer much encouragement to proponents of progressive services.

Social Relations of Mentally Disabled Adults

Our research has attempted to look into the relationships between clients of community facilities for mentally disabled people. Our purpose has been to discover some of the dimensions which determine degree of involvement of mentally retarded adults in the social organizations in which they live and work.

Before we began our studies, we knew that retarded people living and working with each other are capable of social relationships. Edgerton and his associates, for instance, had described a friendship between two severely retarded individuals in an institution and had also described an informal car-washing business initiated and carried on by a group of mildly retarded people. The literature, therefore, confirmed what any worker in a service agency for the retarded knows: peer relationships among the retarded are complex and form an important part of their daily lives.

Although the existence of complex social relationships is well accepted, the characteristics, correlates and determinants of their social interaction have not been intensively investigated. Our approach has been to choose well-established concepts and methods from general social psychology and apply them to the analysis of social relationships among mentally retarded persons. First of all, we wanted to know whether objective methods of studying social behavior are reliable and valid with this population. Second, we studied how sociability is expressed and whether social behavior is related to work productivity. We have also been interested in whether cognitive level is a predictor of the amount and type of social interaction. Employing a similarity choice principle, we have asked whether retarded people tend to associate with individuals of similar cognitive level, age, sex, and diagnosis. Beginning from "mere exposure" theory, we have asked whether past opportunity to interact with another individual predicts probability of associating with him or her. We have also been interested in whether social interaction of retarded adults is particularly sensitive to physical attractiveness.

In addition to using concepts and methods of general social psychology to help analyze the social behavior of retarded persons, we believe that, in the situations we have studied, it has been possible to test some traditional predictors of social choice in ways that have not been previously accomplished. For instance, similarity choice for IQ is a classical finding in the social psychology literature.

However, previous tests of this hypothesis have confounded social class and exposure with IQ. In our studies, this confounding does not occur, and we are therefore able to make a somewhat more adequate test of similarity choice by intelligence than has been possible before. Also, classical tests of exposure effects in humans have confounded exposure in the past with recognition at the time of testing. Again, we have been able to eliminate this confusion of variables by the nature of our population and test situation.

As might be expected, our findings have been complex. We can describe social interactions, but we find that we need a variety of methods to do so adequately. Direct observation procedures are useful, but they are expensive. More traditional questionnaire approaches are relatively easy to use, but they give only a partial picture of what is happening. We find that social relationships of retarded adults are qualitatively similar to that of normal groups. But there are interesting quantitative differences. Some of the variables which we thought would be obviously correlated with social behavior are not related at all.

However, we are getting ahead of our story. Let us tell you, then, about some of the details of procedure of our main study. We have worked with a ''not-for-profit'' service agency which manages four large sheltered workshops for mentally ill and mentally retarded adults. We chose to study these workshops because they provide services that are typical: neither exemplary nor abominable. The many problems that this agency faces are typical of those of many community facilities. These problems include high staff turnover rates, inconsistent management practices, lack of consistent contract work, morale problems, strikes, and so forth. On the other hand, the agency provides a place for the clients to spend their days in productive activity, receive a certain amount of training, and experience acceptance by others. Many of the people we have studied also reside in a single sheltered care home, and we have studied people there also. Table 1 outlines some basic demographic characteristics of our sample.

The data we will present include information on 326 separate individuals among 894 admissions to the agency. As you can see from Table 1, there are generally more males than females, more younger adults than older people, and more mentally retarded than mentally ill people in our sample. The racial distribution is typical of the areas in which the workshops are located. The high ratio of mentally retarded to mentally ill clients reflects certain funding policies of the ''department'' and perhaps also a higher dropout rate among the mentally ill (Heller, Romer and Berkson, 1978; Heller, Berkson & Romer, in press).

The data we will describe come from four sources: client records, interviews with staff, interviews with clients, and direct observations. In all cases, we studied and report data only on clients who have agreed to participate in the study. Data collection and analysis procedures carefully maintain confidentiality of information on individuals.

From client records, we obtained historical and demographic information and information related to diagnosis. When records were inconsistent, we determined the accuracy of the statements through consultation with staff. All IQ scores were corroborated with a Peabody Picture Vocabulary Test administered by an experienced tester.

Interviews with staff were conducted by questionnaire. The first of these questionnaires included items intended to determine whom the staff thought the clients' friends were. The second questionnaire concerned the rated physical attractiveness of each client. Each questionnaire was administered to at least two staff members.

Table 1

Characteristics of the Sample on Which Observations Were Done

Characteristic		Facility					
		WE	WI	WH	WA_1	WA_2	H
	Number	116	66	55	49	47	118
Sex	M	65	44	35	33	32	88
	F	51	22	20	16	15	30
Age	18-20	4	2	0	0	0	1
	21-45	85	33	25	20	19	53
	46-60	22	24	22	23	22	47
	61-99	3	6	8	5	5	15
	Missing	2	1	0	1	1	2
IQ	10-30	0	5	5	11	9	23
	31-50	13	16	17	10	10	42
	51-75	57	18	21	21	15	42
	76-90	26	10	7	3	8	5
	91-110	12	3	4	2	3	3
	<110	6	2	0	0	0	0
	Missing	2	12	1	2	2	3
Diagnosis	MR	84	38	32	33	31	88
	MR-MI	13	8	10	8	8	21
	MI	14	16	10	7	7	6
	Other	4	4	3	1	1	2
	Missing	1	0	0	0	0	1
Race	White	101	39	50	35	33	96
	Black	7	11	5	9	9	19
	Latin	3	1	0	4	4	2
	Oriental	2	0	0	0	0	0
	Missing	3	15	0	1	1	1

Client interviews were done privately and also included an assessment of who their friends were. In addition, a "social self concept" scale was administered to each client. This scale determined the kinds of activities that clients preferred to engage in and provided an index of sociability from the clients' perspective.

The fourth source of information was a series of about 100 behavioral observations done on each client in the workshop. An additional 100 observations were done on 118 clients in the sheltered care residence where they lived. These observations were made only when the clients were free to associate with whom they wished. That is, they were not observed in situations to which they had been assigned by staff (at work stations or in classes). In the workshops they were observed at break periods or lunch. In the residence their behavior was recorded in many free situations in and around the home, including a recreation room, halls, bedrooms (when doors were open), the dining room, in television rooms, and in stores and on the street near the facility.

The basic procedure for each observation was a five-second look at the client followed by a recording of the observation. Observations were carried out on different clients in a predetermined random order and individual observations on the same client were separated by at least five minutes to minimize redundancy. The behaviors and their definitions are listed in Table 2. Agreement between observers was maintained above 85% in all studies.

Table 2
Behavior Category Definitions

COMFORT	(CO)	show genuine effort to ease the sadness, disappointment, failure of another person
HELP	(HE)	aid another to accomplish a given task or to more effectively deal with a given situation, verbal included
APPEASEMENT	(FR)	use friendly restraint on person acting violently
AFFECTION	(AF)	any flirtatious or courting behaviors including affectionate touching such as stroking, pat on back—examples: asking someone for a date; holding hands and talking, smiling and dancing closely with another
SEXUAL ACTIVITY	(SX)	specific sexually-related activities, alone or with others, involving direct physical contact in an intimate manner
SUPERVISION	(SU)	Assume a leader-instructor role related to routine or household tasks, including evaluation and planning of such activities
OFFERING	(OF)	altruistic behaviors related to distributing resources in a generous or equitable manner
VOCALIZATION	(VO)	S utters sound not recognizable as language
VERBALIZATION	(VE)	speak in a recognizable language, or use a formal symbolic substitute such as finger spelling or American sign language
UNCLEAR VERBALIZATION	(UV)	same as verbalize but observer cannot understand or hear. Excludes symbolic substitute
AMBIGUOUS SOUND	(AS)	observer cannot determine whether subject's sound is interactive or not
GESTURE	(GE)	primitive movements of the body, hands, face, etc. to express a meaning (like hand waving, hand out, palm up to receive handout)
TELEPHONE	(OT)	S is talking on telephone
LETTER WRITING	(LW)	S has writing implement and paper and is expressing himself to another on the paper, or S is dictating a thought to a staff member who is writing it down for him or the S is dictating a tape to be sent to an acquaintance
ANNOYANCE	(AN)	pester, irritate, persistently follow, whine; tease in nasty way
AGGRESSION	(AG)	angry disagreement with or without physical violence
APPROVAL	(AP)	social behavior involving bestowing sanction or "positive" reinforcement on others for identified action
TEACHING	(TE)	inform another person about specific facts, usually in an educating manner either verbally or physically—examples: showing how to make change, teaching about moral issues, explaining how to fix something broken, or how to say a new word
DISAPPROVAL	(DA)	indicate clearly that actions of another are not acceptable, liked, etc. by reprimanding, scolding, depriving privileges, etc.,—clearly educational reprimands should be scored under teaching

Table 2 (Continued)
Behavior Category Definitions

ROUGH PLAY	(RP)	push or shove another person in a playful manner
INFORMAL PLAY	(IP)	joke or tease in a cheerful pleasant way; casual play in which no rules are used, such as ball tossing
INTERACTIVE GAME PLAY	(IG)	S plays game with other people
ISOLATED OBSERVATION	(IO)	attends to the activity of a group but is not a particpant in it; or S watches another person with great interest
OTHER SOCIAL	(OS)	a specific social behavior for which we have no code
OTHER NON-SOCIAL	(ON)	a specific non-social behavior for which we have no code; will be recorded if nothing else can be recorded
DISRUPTIVE BEHAVIOR	(DB)	S acts out alone (cries, speaks in loud violent tone to no one, bangs or throws, etc.)
STEREOTYPY	(ST)	S engages in repetitive behavior which has no apparent function (eye-poking, rocking, hand and finger movements)
ABNORMALITY	(AB)	very atypical, unacceptable or asocial, maladaptive behaviors (pica, exposure)
ODDITY	(OD)	less deviant abnormal behavior
MUSIC LISTENING	(ML	S is actively involved with equipment or singing along or tapping foot
TV VIEWING	(TV)	S's attention is focused directly on the monitor and appears to be watching the action on the screen
BODY CARE	(BC)	bathing, grooming, dressing, toileting, health-related activities
SLEEP	(SL)	eyes are shut, breathing regular and subject does not respond to the others around him
EAT AND DRINK	(ED)	ingesting or preparing to ingest food and/or beverages
WORK	(WO)	staff-assigned task which produces income
SELF MANIPULATION	(SM)	S manipulates part of his body (picks nose, rubs genitals, scratches)
PURCHASE	(PU)	buy goods either from the machines or from an attendant who is dispensing merchandise
INDEFINITE SOCIAL	(IS)	S is judged to be a member of a group and is not doing anything else interactive
UNABLE TO OBSERVE	(UO)	the S was not observed during an observation period —this designation is only given after observers have consulted following an observation period
ABSENCE	(AT)	the S has been determined not to be in attendance at the facility being studied—this designation is given only once during a day's observations
SIGN LANGUAGE	(VS)	S uses a nonverbal language substitute, e.g., ASL

The information we will present to you is the result of a first look at the data set. We will present it in three sections. In the first section, we describe some general features of the behavior we saw in the various facilities. The main principle we will emphasize is that while there are important quantitative behavioral differences between facilities, the character of the behaviors our sample engaged in is similar from workshop to workshop and that the behaviors are reasonably normal.

The second section of the data is an analysis of the various observation behavior measures and of the client self-concept scales. In the analysis, we looked at the correlations among the various behavioral measures in an attempt to simplify the data set for further analyses. From these analyses it was possible to show that there were certain factors common to all of the facilities we looked at, but that there were also some features unique to each facility. We also looked at the predictors of the behaviors we had examined.

Finally, we examined the sociometric choice data from observations, client choices and staff ratings and asked whether similarity choice and "mere exposure" principles accounted for certain of the social choice data.

Sociability

Table 3 describes the distribution of the behaviors we saw, and Table 4 portrays the degree to which people were seen alone and in groups of two, three or

Table 3

Percent Occurrence of Various Behavior by Facility and by Mode of Occurrence

	Facility					
	WE	WI	WH	WA_1	WA_2	H
Social Behaviors						
Verbalize	43	25	32	21	26	20
Gesture	1	1	1	2	2	1
Affection	3	3	3	1	3	3
Observation	2	2	3	5	5	2
Offer	0	2	1	1	2	0
Indefinite Social	2	2	2	6	3	2
Non-social						
Eat	19	23	16	17	20	13
Sleep	1	0	1	1	1	5
Work	0	0	4	2	2	0
Purchase	3	0	0	0	0	0
Body Care	0	0	0	4	0	0
TV	0	0	0	2	4	15
Stereotype	2	2	0	2	2	3
Other Non-social	16	29	25	22	20	25

Table 4

Percent of Observations in Groups of Various Size by Facility and Study

Facility	Alone	Dyad	Triad	Quartet
WE	38	42	15	5
WI	65	25	6	4
WH	49	37	7	6
WA_1	56	30	10	4
WA_2	58	35	5	2
H	70	25	4	1

more individuals. On the whole, the behavior during periods of relaxation was sociable. Most of the time was spent either sitting alone or in conversation with a single other person. There was a tendency for one of the workshops (WE) to be more sociable than the rest. But the differences in social behavior were not very dramatic. It should be pointed out that antisocial behaviors (annoyance, aggression, disruptive behavior) were very infrequent.

Although our research program is not concerned mainly with conversational analysis, the large amount of time people in our sample spent talking suggested that we look deeper into this aspect of their behavior. Therefore, Sue Eckel, a member of our team, explored this aspect further. In a first study, she measured the duration of conversational interactions of 20 normal people and 20 mentally retarded people while they ate in the cafeteria of the Illinois Institute for Developmental Disabilities. She also observed interactions of two subsets of 20 people each from our larger sample at WE and WI workshops. She found that normal people spent significantly more time in continuous conversation ($x = 4.63$ minutes) than did any of the three groups of retarded people ($x = 1.08$, 1.10, and 1.43 minutes). In the second study, she listened to what normal and mentally retarded people talked about. Table 5 shows frequency distributions of various topics of conversation among retarded and normal adults. The retarded people

Table 5

Percent Occurrence of Various Topics in Conversations of Mentally Retarded and Normal People

Topics	176 Observations Non-retarded People	262 Observations Retarded People
Work	18	6
Food	16	17
Entertainment	1	5
Gossip	34	17
Current Events	4	1
Money	10	6
Sports	2	0
Weather	1	2
Fashion	4	2
Other	0	8
Teasing	0	9
Activities	4	7
Neighborhoods	0	1
Health	2	4
Time	0	1
Vacation	0	1
Keys	0	1
Family/parents	1	3
Music	0	1
Cars	0	1
Cigarettes	0	1
Transportation	0	1
Kissing	0	1
Pills	0	1
School	1	0

talked about a greater range of topics, while the normal people gossiped more and spoke more about work. On the whole, however, the topics of conversation of these very different groups were remarkably similar.

The first phase of the analysis therefore showed that, on the whole, much of the activity in the workshops and home was social. Though there were differences between the workshops, the general pattern of distribution of the various behaviors was similar.

Predictors of Sociability

In the second section of the analysis, we looked into the relationships among the various measures of general sociability we had considered and then looked at the degree to which other measures predicted them. From the observation data, we first derived a score which consisted of the percent of all observations in which the person engaged in social behavior (% social). If the behavior had been a social interaction, we scored whether the person being observed had been the actor or recipient in the interaction. We could therefore also derive a score describing the percent of social behavior which was active (active ratio). If the behavior was not a social interaction, we noted whether it had been performed while the person was alone or was with others in a social aggregation. From this measure we derived the proportion of non-social behaviors which was done in an aggregation (aggregation ratio).

In principle, the percent-social score has two components. The first component is the number of unique groups the person is seen in. Most of the interactions were dyadic, this is a measure of the number of different people the subject was seen with (# groups). The percent-social score also reflects the amount of interaction or the intensity of the relationship with each unique group. We counted the number of times subjects were seen with each group they were in and calculated the mean of this number (average intensity) and also the number of times they were seen with their most frequent group (strongest relationship). Finally, from the observational data, we calculated the average distance between subjects and the person closest to them over all of the observations (distance).

We asked whether certain fairly obvious demographic and functional characteristics of individuals predicted these various measures of sociability. More particularly we wished to know whether it is possible to describe dimensions which characterize similarities and differences between the various facilities. It has by now become clear that facilities differ and that these differences need to be defined (Bjaanes & Butler, 1974). Previous efforts at defining these differences have relied heavily on staff interviews (Moos, 1974). Our view is that the staff perspective of how facilities work is only one aspect of the total picture. We believe that a more direct analysis of the ecology of these facilities is also possible. To demonstrate an example of this, we have looked at the correlates of our various measures of social behavior with seven other variables: two scores of the clients' general work productivity (hours worked and pay rate); the clients' own concept of their sociability; staff ratings of clients' physical attractiveness; and clients' age, sex, IQ and diagnosis (retarded vs. mentally ill).

Table 6 portrays the means of the various measures for the different facilities we looked at. Even a casual glance at these means reveals that the various facilities are different on almost all of these measures. Analyses of variance and a discriminant function analysis showed that all of these variables, except for perhaps sex ratio and diagnosis, discriminated between the facilities. We could also correctly place 77% of the cases in four workshops by taking these variables into consideration.

Table 6
Means and Tests of Various Measures in the Different Facilities

Measure	WA_1	WI	WH	WE	H	F ratio
	Facility					
Age (yrs)	46	40	45	33	44	14.91*
IQ	50	60	51	72	47	21.06*
Percent female	36	31	37	43	26	1.85
Percent social	38	32	45	54	29	21.20*
Percent dyads	30	28	38	42	24	19.40*
Number of groups	2.6	3.0	2.7	3.4	1.7	8.80*
Strongest relationship (%)	8	9	10	14	7	7.64*
Average distance (ft)	4.6	2.3	3.1	2.1	3.6	44.00*
Percent aggregate	74	85	87	92	69	54.77*
Percent active	87	76	81	86	79	6.18*
Self concept	–.43	–.27	–.21	.55		4.69*
Pay (dollars/hour)	.31	.41	.40	.49		5.83*
Hours worked	19.0	29.8	28.8	29.0		36.11*

*$p<.01$

Overall, and within facilities, the predictor variables mentioned above had varying success in predicting social behavior (cf. Table 7).

A multiple correlation of .64 was found between these predictors and percent social behavior, our most general measure of sociability. Multiple correlations for other behavior were moderate (.26-.57), and prediction varied both with respect to facility and social behavior analyzed. On the whole, age, diagnosis and hours worked were the best predictors. Sociability was positively related to youth and being retarded rather than mentally ill, and working more hours was associated with greater aggregative behavior.

Table 7
Predictions of Percent Social Behavior from Several Measures Overall and for Each Facility

	All Clients			Facility				
				WE	WI	WH	WA_1	H
Predictor	r	Beta	F	Significant Beta				
All predictors	.64		12.69*					
Age	–.40	–.19	7.75*			–.40		–.31
Diagnosis (retarded vs mentally ill)	–.37	–.37	27.06*	–.38		–.46	–.66	–.25
IQ	.24	.16	4.29				.55	.23
Sex	.17	.08	1.66					
Attractiveness	.12	.04	0.35					
Hours worked	.27	.04	0.14		.48			
Pay	.34	.20	3.13	.27				
Social self-concept	.35	.16	5.05		.53			

*$p<.01$

One of our major hypotheses was that brighter people would socialize more. There was some evidence for this in the correlations, but it was weak. This confirms a conclusion we have made from another study (Landesman-Dwyer, Berkson & Romer, 1979) that, within mentally disabled populations, intellectual level is not an important correlate of sociability. We also found no relationship between rated physical attractiveness and sociability. Other analyses we have conducted, however, indicate that attractiveness predicts sociability to a certain degree (Romer & Berkson, 1980). Let us summarize our results to this point. We have shown that mentally disabled people in community facilities are generally sociable. They interact mainly in dyads, and most of their social behavior with peers involves conversation. There are differences between facilities of the same type (e.g., sheltered workshops), and these differences are multidimensional. Social behavior varies between facilities, and so do its predictors. No single measure is a very good descriptor of the characteristics of facilities or of the people in them.

Social Choice

Our previous analyses dealt with the levels of various social behaviors. In this last section we will consider social choice factors. The guides to our analyses were related to both practical and theoretical considerations. In both educational and mental health settings, a traditional issue has had to do with whether people should be assigned to homogeneous or heterogeneous groups. That is, should people in the same program have similar characteristics. For example, should mentally retarded people of different levels of intelligence be assigned to the same or different residential placements.

One approach to answering this question is to assess the preferences of the people involved. Do people in mental health systems choose to be with others who are similar to themselves? Concepts of assortative mating assume similarity choice processes, and studies in social psychology have emphasized the existence of similarity choice for attitudes.

One feature of these studies is that they ordinarily confound other dimensions with the one they are testing. For instance, preference of children to be with others of approximately their same age may result simply from the fact that homogenous assignment for age is a characteristic of class placement in schools. That is, similarity choice may be a consequence of placement and therefore mediated by exposure.

In our study, it was possible for us to separate exposure from determinants of similarity choice. We did so for IQ, age and sex. We did this first by assessing whether clients' IQ, age and sex predicted the same characteristics of the people they were observed to associate with. These simple correlations shown in Table 8 all show strong similarity between clients and their associates. However, the table

Table 8

Measures of Similarity Choice for IQ, Age and Sex

Type of Relation	Similarity Characteristic		
	IQ	Age	Sex
Simple	.42*	.41*	.23*
Controlled	.19	.12	.36*

*p<.01

also shows the prediction of each characteristic within a multiple regression analysis in which we controlled the contribution of other person variables and of differences between facilities. Only in the case of sex does similarity-choice remain significant. Thus, a good deal of the apparent similarity choice for IQ and age was due to confounding with other variables and with homogenous placements in the various facilities. Our final analysis concerned the effects of "exposure." Recent research has suggested that being with other people is not only a necessary condition, but may also be sufficient for attraction between them. This principle may be useful in the design of mental health systems because it suggests that one can promote social integration among clients by taking into account the exposure principle. Stabilizing placements and moving people together when transfers are necessary might promote friendships. Moving people around a lot without maintaining the groups they have been in may contribute to superficiality of their relationships.

We tested whether exposure is a significant correlate of social choice by asking whether people choose to associate with those that they have been with most. We asked whether, in the workshops where they could freely interact with people from their own or from other residential facilities, they would interact more with the people they lived with. We also asked whether, in the residential facility, the clients tended to associate more with those individuals from the workshops they were assigned to. First, we adjusted the social choice scores so that they would take into account the proportion of people from own or other facilities who were available to interact with. If people interacted with others independent of whom they lived (or worked) with, they received a score of 1.0. Higher scores were expected from the exposure principle. In every facility studied, the average ratio exceeded 1.0, and in almost every case the effect was significant. Furthermore, the effect was evident from staff, client and observation data. These results may be seen in Table 9.

Table 9

Exposure Ratios for Staff, Client and Observation Measures of Social Choice

	WE	WI	WH	WA_1	WA_2	H
Staff	5.70*	4.72*	2.15	2.02*	2.03*	2.19*
Client	4.57*	3.82*	2.05*	1.38*	1.86*	1.95*
Observation	5.17*	2.38*	1.64	1.36*	1.80*	1.95*

$^*p<.05$

Conclusion

Well, this memo is even longer than usual for us, and we guess that you got more than you asked for. Let us summarize: despite the ideology which has motivated the deinstitutionalization movement, mental health facilities in which mentally disabled people live and work together are very much part of the current scene. We believe that the quality of life in these facilities is partly measureable by the nature of social interactions in them.

When we looked at these facilities, we found that much of the social behavior in them is normal. The things these people talk about are fairly normal, although the duration of the interactions tends to be short. Facilities differ along a number of dimensions. So when you establish guidelines for evaluation, you will want to be sure that they reflect the complexity of the differences between facilities. Certainly, we question whether the current classifications of facilities for funding purposes adequately describe the demographic or social characteristics of the people in them.

Social behavior is independently predictable from a number of variables, the most important of which seem to be age, diagnosis and hours worked. IQ is not a very good independent predictor. We wonder what is happening in these facilities to make older people less sociable. We would also like to see whether training programs which increase the amount of working time would also increase sociability.

With respect to social choice, it looks like people interact with individuals of similar age, sex, and IQ. However, it seems likely that these similarity choice effects may be attributable to homogeneous assignment to programs rather than to similarity choice per se. The issue for your guidelines then is to determine the extent to which similarity choice is a characteristic of the clients or of the attitudes of the staff who assign the clients to programs.

It seems clear that people generally choose to be with others that they have been with more. As long as the guidelines assume communal living for the mentally disabled and have as a goal the promotion of social integration in these communal settings, those programs which take note of the exposure principle probably should receive preferential funding. That is, those agencies which stabilize placements and, during referral, take into account the clients' informal associations are probably promoting the sociability of their clients.

We are finally ready to come to the point. We think, first of all, that the guidelines should include a statement about the importance of *informal* peer relationships in any programming for clients. Programming can assume that the characteristics of informal social behavior are essentially normal, although ways of promoting longer, more complex interactions should be encouraged. Facilities differ in the degree of peer social behavior, but how these differences are to be characterized needs more study. It might be useful to choose appropriate measures of social behavior from the goals of the specific workshop program and then ask what factors in the situation most clearly predict those measures.

More research is also needed before you include any definite statements about predictors of sociability. In general, IQ does not predict amount of social behavior very well, but age, diagnosis and hours worked seem promising. A further look into the source of the relationships between these factors and social behavior might ultimately help increase sociability. About all one can say now is that intellectual level is not an important predictor so IQ should not be used in too refined a way to design programs.

Perhaps more helpful are the principles of exposure and similarity choice. Our results suggest that, when given a choice, mentally retarded people choose to associate with people with whom they have had more contact and with people of their own cognitive level, age and sex. The guidelines might recognize that people be given the choice of associating with others who have common histories, age, cognitive level and sex. Since the relationships we have demonstrated are not very powerful, however, the guidelines should be written to *allow* access along these dimensions, certainly not to require them.

It seems to us that the guidelines should also recognize that knowledge about what happens in a facility cannot be obtained only by considering the perspective of the staff. Client opinions and outside observers provide additional supplementary information which seems useful in planning appropriate programs.

Finally, for now at least, it appears that for many mentally disabled adults "living in the community" means living in groups with other disabled people. A recognition of this fact, plus finding ways of making their lives productive and happy in this context, seem to be important emphases for the guidelines to establish. Perhaps with these emphases more "normalized" living will be possible.

With best wishes.

Sincerely,

Gershon Berkson
Daniel Romer

References

Bjaanes, A. T., & Butler, E. W. Environmental variation in community care facilities for mentally retarded persons. *American Journal of Mental Deficiency*, 1974, *78*, 429-439.

Heller, T., Romer, D., & Berkson, G. *Social interaction of mentally retarded and mentally ill clients in sheltered workshops*. Paper presented at the Annual Conference of the American Psychological Association, 1978.

Heller, T., Berkson, G., & Romer, D. Social ecology of supervised communal facilities for mentally disabled adults: V. Initial social adaptation. *American Journal of Mental Deficiency*, in press.

Landesman-Dwyer, S., Berkson, G., & Romer, D. Affiliation and friendship of mentally retarded residents in group homes. *American Journal of Mental Deficiency*, 1979, *83*, 571-580.

Moos, R. H. *Evaluating treatment environments: A social ecological approach*. New York: John Wiley & Sons, 1974.

Romer, D., & Berkson, G. Social ecology of supervised communal facilities for mentally disabled adults: II. Predictors of affiliation. *American Journal of Mental Deficiency*, in press.

Residential Placement and Adaptation of Severely and Profoundly Retarded Individuals

Sharon Landesman-Dwyer
Frederica MacL. Sulzbacher

University of Washington

Although severely and profoundly mentally retarded (SMR/PMP) individuals represent less than 5 percent of the mentally retarded population (Dingman & Tarjan, 1960; Mercer, 1973; Tarjan, Wright, Eyman, & Keeran, 1973), they constitute the majority of those needing lifelong residential services (Eyman & Miller, 1978). Over the past 15 years, professional and public concern about providing appropriate residential care for SMR/PMR persons has increased dramatically, reflecting changes in (1) demand for services, (2) treatment philosophy, and (3) knowledge about their behavioral potential.

With improved daily care, the use of antibiotics, and surgical intervention, the mortality rate for institutionalized SMR/PMR persons has declined steadily over the past 30 years (Conley, 1973). This longer lifespan, coupled with more active involvement of families and citizen advocate groups (Robinson & Robinson, 1976), and a decrease in the bed capacity of public institutions (Butterfield, 1976; Scheerenberger, 1979), has led to an increased demand for community-based services. Also, the prevailing treatment philosophy encourages keeping children in family-type settings and helping adults achieve their full developmental potential in "the least restrictive environment" possible (cf. Nirje, 1976). Finally, the behavioral potential of SMR/PMR people to acquire new skills and to respond adaptively to their environment has been well documented under experimental conditions (cf. Berkson & Landesman-Dwyer, 1977). This previously unrecognized capacity for growth and development in SMR/PMR individuals warrants study in the context of natural caregiving environments.

The bulk of the literature on deinstitutionalization and community adjustment concerns mildly and moderately retarded individuals. Unfortunately, a broad picture of where SMR/PMR persons are living and how they are adjusting has not been readily available. (Just how little information is available on this subject can be noted in scanning two bibliographies: *Alternatives in the Community for the Developmentally Disabled: A Bibliographic Index on Community-Based Alternatives to Institutionalization*, 1976 and *Reintegrating Mentally Retarded People into the Community: An Annotated Bibliography*, 1976.) As a beginning point, this paper provides a description of a statewide population of SMR/PMR people receiving services in a variety of residential settings.

Five major questions are addressed in this paper:

The authors express their gratitude to Judith Schuckit and Jody Stein Kleinman for supervising the research discussed in this chapter. Assistance in data collection came from Denise Boelens, Idamay Bunting, Renee Coppel, Renate Coulsen, Christine Curtis, Shelley Horst, L. Susanne Keller, Don Kay, Maureen Miltenberger, Debra Tombari, and Mary Weatherley. Timothy Brown, Irvin Emanuel, Richard Holm, and Gene P. Sackett provided assistance in planning, conducting, and anlyzing these studies.

1. Where are the SMR/PMR people living and what portion of the developmentallly disabled client population receiving residential services do they represent?
2. How many of the SMR/PMR persons living in community settings previously lived in state institutions?
3. Do the behavioral profiles of SMR/PMR persons living in community residential facilities differ significantly from those in public residential facilities (institutions)?
4. How many SMR/PMR individuals who had been placed in the community were subsequently returned to an institution? What were the reasons for these returns? Did the reasons differ from those for mildly and moderately retarded clients who also were returned to institutions from community placements?
5. In settings presumed the most "normalized," how are SMR/PMR persons adjusting? Do their daily activities differ from those of mildly and moderately retarded individuals living in the same places?

Methods

Subjects

In 1975 and 1976, the writers conducted a statewide survey of developmentally disabled individuals receiving social and health services in Washington State.[1] Table 1 summarizes the 8 types of residential settings studied and the sampling strategies used. There were 479 group residential facilities, from state institutions and nursing homes to group homes and licensed board-and-care facilities, and 1357 individual homes, including foster homes. The total population originally studied consisted of 6,952 developmentally disabled clients, of whom more than 95 percent were mentally retarded according to the criteria of the American Association of Mental Deficiency (Grossman, 1973).

Data Collection

Trained research analysts collected data related to (1) demographic and diagnostic characteristics, obtained primarily from central records for an individual client; (2) current functional and behavioral abilities, rated by a person who knew the client well; and (3) medical and nursing needs, also evaluated by someone familiar with the individual client. The majority of questionnaire items

[1]Detailed findings from this statewide survey are presented in the following reports, published by the State of Washington Department of Social and Health Services, Olympia, WA:

Landesman-Dwyer, S., & Brown, T. R. A method for subgrouping mentally retarded citizens on the basis of service needs, 1976.

Landesman-Dwyer, S., Keller, L. S., & Schuckit, J. J. Community training programs for developmentally disabled clients: Developmental centers and sheltered workshops, 1976.

Landesman-Dwyer, S., & Schuckit, J. J. Preliminary findings of the survey of state institutions for the mentally retarded, 1976.

Landesman-Dwyer, S., & Schuckit, J. J., & Keller, L. S. Survey of developmentally disabled individuals in nursing homes and congregate care facilities, 1976.

Landesman-Dwyer, S., Schuckit, J. J., & Keller, L. S. Family and foster care for developmentally disabled children and adults, 1977.

Landesman-Dwyer, S., Stein, J. G., & Sackett, G. P. Group homes for the metally retarded: An ecological and behavioral study, 1976.

Schuckit, J. J., & Landesman-Dwyer, S. Survey of the developmentally disabled in the Frances Haddon Morgan Children's Center and the Washington State School for the Blind, 1976.

Table 1

Residential Settings and Sampling Methods Used in a Statewide Survey of Developmentally Disabled Citizens

Residential Environments	Sampling Method	Total N Facilities
1. Public Residential Facilities (Institutions)	100% of residents were studied.	5
2. Specialized Institutions for Autistic, Blind, and Deaf Children	100% of residents were studied.	3
3. Group Homes for Developmentally Disabled Children and Adults	38% of residents, 45% of group homes.	48
4. Nursing Homes: Skilled Nursing Facilities (SNFs) Intermediate Care Facilities (ICFs)	a) 20% of generic SNFs and ICFs were selected on random, stratified basis. 100% of developmentally disabled clients were studied.	291
	b) 100% of residents in SNFs and ICFs *known* in advance to serve large groups of developmentally disabled clients.	18
5. Congregate Care Facilities and Boarding Homes	a) 20% of generic Congregate Care Facilities and Boarding Homes were selected on random stratified basis. 100% of developmentally disabled clients in these facilities were studied.	120
	b) 100% of residents in CCFs *known* in advance to serve large groups of developmentally disabled clients were studied.	12
6. Foster Care for Developmentally Disabled Children and Adults	100% of clients were included (60% response rate).	294[a]
7. Family Care, but receiving support services at home	35% of clients were included (60% response rate).	848[a]
8. Independent Living, but receiving some supervision or assistance	43% of clients were studied.	215[a]

[a] Number of clients

were from the AAMD *Manual on Terminology and Classification, 1973 Revision* (Grossman, 1973). In addition, descriptive data were collected on each community-based facility, including community and geographical location, building characteristics, staffing patterns, length of operation, percent of developmentally disabled clients, type of proprietorship, and administrative organization.

Reliabilities for extracting data from records and for the ratings by care providers were determined for each type of residential setting by replicating a random stratified 10 percent sample of the complete data set 4 to 8 weeks later. Items with test-retest reliability below 75 percent agreement were not used for further analyses.[2]

In this paper, data are also presented from two other studies conducted in Washington State. One was a detailed ethological study of 20 group homes, in which nearly 20 percent of the residents were severely or profoundly retarded. (For a complete description of the observational methods and subjects, see Landesman-Dwyer, Stein, & Sackett [1976, 1978].) The second study concerned 210 mentally retarded individuals who were returned to institutions after unsuccessful community placements; 118 (56%) of these residents were SMR/PMR persons. Retrospectively reviewed were the reasons for return, considering written documents from the institution, the community residences, families, and other service providers.

Results

The SMR/PMR clients comprised 40 percent of Washington State's 6,487 developmentally disabled population in the residential settings studied.[3] As Table 2 shows, the majority of SMR/PMR people (1,815) were living in state institutions, where they represented 79 percent of the institutional population. The remaining 792 SMR/PMR persons resided in community-based settings: 370 in nursing homes, 240 in group and boarding homes, and 184 in single family and foster homes. SMR/PMR individuals constituted 14 to 22 percent of the mentally retarded clients in these community-based residences, the lowest proportion in family home settings and the highest in foster care.

Sixty-six percent of the SMR/PMR people receiving community-based residential services previously had been institutionalized, as shown in Table 3. Nearly all of the SMR/PMR group home residents (96%) had a history of institutionalization as did approximately three-quarters of those in licensed board-and-care facilities (76%) and nursing homes (74%). A substantially smaller

[2]The reliability of the ratings varied significantly as a function of residential setting. We thus question the validity of studies that compare client adjustment to different environments using only adaptive behavior ratings by caretakers. The variation in reliability is attributable in part to differences across facilities in the following factors: (1) extent of experience with mentally retarded clients; (2) types of mentally retarded clients served; (3) familiarity with terms and concepts in the field of mental retardation; and (4) professional and paraprofessional training. In our opinion, the published reliability figures for the AAMD Adaptive Behavior Scales and for other similar rating instruments are not based on appropriate samples of clients across sufficient types of facilities. Accordingly, each study using such instruments needs to determine independently the reliability of data for its specific circumstances.

[3]For purposes of the analyses in this paper, the categories of "severe mental retardation" and "profound mental retardation" have been combined. The reason for this is that the accuracy of the label assigned to individuals was poor: 63 percent of the severely retarded were indistinguishable from the profoundly retarded in terms of our objective assessment of their self-help skills, productive and receptive language, and social and personal competence. Moreover, in the state institutions where standardized, periodic assessment of all residents is required, 35 percent received at least two different diagnoses as to their level of retardation.

Table 2

Residential Distribution of Severely and Profoundly Retarded Clients (SMR/PMR) in Washington State[a]

Residential Setting	SMR/PMR Clients (% of Total Population)		Total Population of Mentally Retarded Clients
State Institutions	1,815	(79%)	2,301
Nursing Homes:			
a) Skilled Nursing Facilities	273	(21%)	1,268
b) Intermediate Care Facilities	97	(20%)	467
Group Homes	132	(20%)	660
Licensed Board-and-Care Facilities	106	(16%)	649
Foster Homes	65	(22%)	294
At Home with Relatives	119	(14%)	848
Total	2,607		6,487

[a]School-aged children receiving only special education are not included.

Table 3

Institutionalization[a] History of SMR/PMR Clients in Community Residential Settings

Residential Setting	Previously Institutionalized		Never Institutionalized	
Nursing Homes	272	(73.5%)	98	(26.5%)
Group Homes	127	(96.2%)	5	(.8%)
Licensed Board-and-Care	80	(75.5%)	26	(24.5%)
Foster Homes	26	(40.0%)	69	(60.0%)
At Home with Relatives	14	(11.8%)	105	(88.2%)

[a]"Institutionalization" is defined as being a resident of a state institution for mentally retarded people for at least six months.

proportion of those in foster care (40%) and even fewer at home with relatives (12%) had ever been placed in public institutions.

Table 4 compares some of the demographic and behavioral characteristics of SMR/PMR clients in community versus institutional settings. For this analysis, only previously institutionalized individuals (N = 591) were included in the community sample to control for some of the variables associated with a history of institutionalization and to determine whether the deinstitutionalized sample was distinctly different from the currently institutionalized population. For 23 of the 27 characteristics the groups differed to a statistically significant degree ($p < .01$), regardless of whether univariate or multivariate analysis methods were used. Compared to the community sample, the institutionalized group was younger by an average of 11 years, and significantly more disabled in terms of level of retardation, motor functioning, hearing, self-help skills, and academic abilities. Severity of seizures and visual impairment were comparable for the groups. Generally, the institutional residents showed statistically significant higher rates of behavior problems although the magnitude of the differences was rather small.

Table 4

Comparison of SMR/PMR in Community (previously institutionalized) and Institution Settings

Client Characteristics	Community (N=591) $\overline{X}$	(sd)	Institution (N=1,815) $\overline{X}$	(sd)	F Ratio
1. Age	35.79 yrs.	(14.1)	24.77 yrs.	(11.4)	180.4**
2. AAMD level (4=SMR; 5=PMR)	4.21	(.4)	4.62	(.5)	154.4**
3. Seizures	1.21	(.5)	1.17	(.5)	1.05
4. Ambulation	1.09	(.3)	1.34	(.6)	32.8**
5. Vision	.27	(.6)	.35	(.8)	1.9
6. Hearing	.10	(.4)	.19	(.6)	5.1**
7. Arm-hand coordination	.24	(.7)	.42	(.8)	10.2**
Self-help skills					
8. eating	1.26	(.6)	1.40	(.9)	5.6**
9. dressing	1.48	(.7)	2.02	(1.1)	54.5**
10. toilet use	1.39	(.7)	1.71	(.8)	32.2**
11. Receptive language	1.71	(.5)	2.03	(1.3)	13.1**
12. Productive language	1.91	(.5)	2.26	(1.5)	13.7**
13. Reading	1.56	(.7)	2.11	(.6)	149.4**
14. Writing	1.54	(.9)	1.98	(.5)	147.3**
15. Numbers	1.67	(.8)	2.10	(.6)	106.1**
16. Time concept	1.43	(.5)	1.85	(.5)	124.5**
17. Sociability	1.68	(.6)	1.96	(.6)	43.2**
18. Initiative	1.72	(.7)	1.91	(1.4)	4.2**
19. Money skills	2.42	(.7)	1.86	(.5)	221.5**
Behavior problems					
20. physically aggressive	1.34	(.7)	1.38	(.8)	.6
21. self-abusive	1.16	(.5)	1.36	(.8)	13.7**
22. destroys property	1.27	(.7)	1.38	(.8)	3.9**
23. severely hyperactive	1.26	(.7)	1.39	(.8)	5.6**
24. extremely withdrawn	1.20	(.6)	1.17	(.5)	.6
25. stereotyped behaviors	1.23	(.6)	1.48	(.8)	18.7**
26. "bizarre, unacceptable"	1.15	(.5)	1.49	(.9)	32.9**
27. other problems	1.11	(.5)	1.48	(.8)	41.5**

Note: Scores on items 4-27 were converted to a three-point scale, where 3 represents the lowest degree of functioning or greatest degree of impairment and 1 indicates no impairment or problem or a high functional level.

$^{**}p < .01$

Somewhat surprisingly, the ratings on physical aggression toward others and on extremely withdrawn behavior were similar for community and institutional clients. (Note: the behavioral data for the entire institutional population revealed that mildly and moderately retarded individuals had significantly higher rates of aggression than did SMR/PMR clients.)

Given the dissimilarity between SMR/PMR persons in the community and the institution, a natural question is, "Were these groups different prior to deinstitutionalization or did community placement produce improvement?" Unfortunately, the retrospective data were inadequate to answer this question. However, another approach—looking at those SMR/PMR individuals who "failed" in their community placement and returned to the institution—provides some indirect clues. Table 5 compares SMR/PMR returnees with those never placed in the community. Unlike the comparison in Table 4, these two groups of residents did *not* differ on most variables. In fact, the largest and most significant difference was

Table 5

Comparison of SMR/PMR Institutional Residents Never Placed in the Community and Those Returned from Community Placements

Client Characteristics	Institution Residents Never Placed (N = 1,438) $\bar{X}$	(sd)	Placed & Returned (N = 252) $\bar{X}$	(sd)	F Ratio
1. Age	24.17 yrs.	(10.8)	28.18 yrs.	(14.0)	26.9**
2. AAMD level	4.62	(.5)	4.60	(.5)	.5
3. Seizures	1.18	(.4)	1.18	(.5)	0.0
4. Ambulation	1.36	(.7)	1.26	(.6)	5.3**
5. Vision	.33	(.8)	.43	(.9)	3.1**
6. Hearing	.19	(.6)	.21	(.6)	.3
7. Arm-hand coordination	.43	(.9)	.35	(.8)	1.9
Self-help skills					
8. eating	1.43	(.9)	1.26	(.6)	7.9**
9. dressing	2.03	(.8)	1.94	(2.0)	1.4
10. toilet use	1.74	(.8)	1.51	(.7)	16.3**
11. Receptive language	2.06	(1.4)	1.92	(.5)	2.1
12. Productive language	2.27	(1.5)	2.24	(1.5)	0.0
13. Reading	2.11	(.6)	2.09	(.6)	.4
14. Writing	1.99	(.5)	1.95	(.5)	1.7
15. Numbers	2.10	(.6)	2.09	(.6)	.1
16. Time concept	1.42	(.5)	1.54	(.6)	11.5**
17. Sociability	1.97	(.6)	1.90	(.6)	2.5**
18. Initiative	1.92	(1.4)	1.85	(1.6)	.5
19. Money skills	1.89	(.5)	1.80	(.6)	3.9**
Behavior problems					
20. physically aggressive	1.38	(.8)	1.43	(.8)	.9
21. self-abusive	1.36	(.8)	1.30	(.7)	1.4
22. destroys property	1.38	(.8)	1.39	(.8)	0.0
23. severely hyperactive	1.39	(.8)	1.35	(.8)	.6
24. extremely withdrawn	1.17	(.5)	1.17	(.5)	0.0
25. stereotyped behaviors	1.49	(.8)	1.46	(.8)	.2
26. "bizarre, unacceptable"	1.49	(.8)	1.48	(.8)	0.0
27. other problems	1.48	(.8)	1.47	(.8)	.1

Note: Scores on items 4-27 were converted to a three-point scale, where 3 represents the lowest degree of functioning or greatest degree of impairment and 1 indicates no impairment or problem, or a high functional level.

$^{**}p < .01$

that the returnees to the institutions were an average of 4 years older than those never placed outside the institution.

A separate study explored the reasons individuals returned to institutions. Of the 210 returnees for whom sufficient and reliable data were available, 56.1 percent were classified as SMR/PMR, as shown in Table 6. These SMR/PMR returnees were almost evenly divided between the categories of severe and profound mental retardation. The overall 6:4 ratio of male to female returnees parallels that in the institutional population in general although an interesting relationship was found between sex and level of intelligence. For residents functioning at the level of moderate retardation to borderline intelligence, more than twice as many males returned to the institution as did females (2.32:1.00) while the rates were nearly equal for males and females in the levels of severe and profound retardation (1.26:1.00).

Table 6

Returnees to Institutions by Intelligence Level and Sex

Intelligence Level	Males	Females	Row Totals
No diagnosis of mental retardation	5	4	9 4.3%
Borderline intelligence (1-2 sd below average)	8	2	10 4.8%
Mildly mentally retarded	19	10	29 13.8%
Moderately mentally retarded	31	13	44 21.0%
Severely mentally retarded	32	25	57 27.1%
Profoundly mentally retarded	34	27	61 29.0%
Column totals	129 61.4%	81 38.6%	210 100.0%

To understand why individuals do not adapt to new environments requires consideration of the types of environments they were placed in, as well as the individuals' characteristics. The majority of returnees in this study had been in nursing homes (51.3%) that had little or no prior experience with mentally retarded clients. Moreover, these returnees from nursing homes did not appear to have a substantial need for the specialized health care provided in such facilities. The clients' own families were the next most likely placement (20.8%), followed closely by group homes (18.7%). Only a small proportion of returnees had been in foster homes (4.0%), mental hospitals (3.5%), or board-and-care facilities (1.5%). The remaining clients (4.1%) were returned from a variety of private care settings. Somewhat surprisingly, the clients' level of retardation did *not* appear related to the type of placement. One exception was that there were no SMR/PMR returnees from board-and-care facilities in this sample.

Table 7 lists the major reasons clients were returned to the institutions. For some clients more than one reason was stated ($\overline{X} = 1.18$ reasons per client). Many reasons were given for the inadequate community adjustment of those SMR/PMR persons who were returned to institutions. The two most frequently mentioned reasons for return were inflicting physical harm on others (21.2%) and destroying objects, including firesetting (19.5%). These two reasons also were prominent ones for moderately and mildly retarded individuals. The SMR/PMR group differed notably from higher functioning returnees in the frequency of four types of behavior problems: self-abuse, constant masturbation, screaming uncontrollably, and loss of toileting skills or smearing feces. They also showed much lower rates of inappropriate sexual aggression toward others, police arrests, and having negative effects on others or failing to conform to group standards. It is noteworthy that 10 percent of the SMR/PMR clients were returned because their medical problems could not be handled by the care provider. Most often, the care provider for these returnees was a family or a group home.

Table 7

Reasons for Return to Institution by Level of Retardation[a]

Reason(s) Given	Not Retarded or Borderline Intelligence N=19		Mildly Retarded N=29		Moderately Retarded N=44		SMR/PMR N=118	
	f	%	f	%	f	%	f	%
Physically harmed others	2	10.5	7	24.1	11	25.0	25	21.2
Destroyed objects	1	5.3	8	27.6	7	15.9	23	19.5
Self-abusive	0		0		0		7	5.9
Inappropriate sexual aggression	4	21.1	5	17.2	5	11.4	3	2.5
Constant masturbation	0		0		0		4	3.4
Inappropriate nudity	1	5.3	0		1	2.3	4	3.4
Ran away or wandered	1	5.3	3	10.3	2	4.5	6	5.1
Severely hyperactive	0		2	6.9	2	4.5	5	4.2
Completely withdrawn	0		1	3.4	0		2	1.7
Screamed uncontrollably	0		0		1	2.3	6	5.1
Threw temper tantrums	0		1	3.4	5	11.4	4	3.4
Arrested by police	0		1	3.4	1	2.3	2	1.7
Psychotic episodes	3	15.8	0		1	2.3	0	
Resident's skill level regressed (excluding toileting skills)	2	10.5	1	3.4	3	6.8	6	5.1
Toileting skills lost and/or smeared feces	0		0		1	2.3	4	3.4
Medical problems of client could not be handled by care provider	3	15.8	2	6.9	5	11.4	12	10.2
Resident's presence had harmful effect on others; did not conform; had incompatible personality	6	31.6	11	37.9	7	15.9	12	10.2

[a]More than one reason was given for some clients accounting for column totals greater than 100%.

f = frequency; % = % of group

The group homes in Washington State collectively represent the most "normalized" out-of-home group settings available to mentally retarded clients, based on their licensing standards and commitment to active habilitation, participation in community programs, and provision of a home-like, personalized environment. Certainly there is a wide range of programs among these group homes (Landesman-Dwyer, Sackett, & Stein, 1976, 1978), and not all group homes provide optimal programs for their clients. In 1976, the writers conducted a detailed observational study of 240 residents in 23 group homes, selected on a random stratified basis. Nearly 18 percent of the subjects were SMR/PMR persons. (For details regarding the methodology and general findings of this research, refer to Landesman-Dwyer, Sackett, & Stein [1976, 1978].) In this paper, a highlighting of the observed behavioral differences related to clients' level of retardation will be presented.

The major observed behaviors that showed a statistically significant ($p < .01$) relationship to level of retardation are shown in Table 8. The data from this study showed that SMR/PMR residents spent significantly greater amounts of time engaged in "inactive behaviors" (usually sitting alone and doing nothing), "observing or imitating others," and "undesirable or bizarre behavior" than did more capable residents. They also were observed to be significantly less social and less helpful with household chores and to leave home less frequently compared to mildly and moderately retarded residents. For most of these behavioral categories, a linear relationship was detected between level of retardation and proportionate occurrence of the behaviors.

Table 8

Major Activity: Means and Standard Deviations for Significant Main Effects for Level of Retardation[a]

Major Activity Category	Mildly Retarded N=64	Mildly-Moderately Retarded[b] N=45	Moderately Retarded N=88	Severely-Profoundly Retarded N=43
Inactive Behaviors $F=6.91$ ($p < .001$)	14.7% (sd=8.3)	15.4% (sd=9.6)	17.9% (sd=11.5)	24.4% (sd=15.7)
Observing & Imitating $F=3.83$ ($p < .01$)	.2% (sd=.6)	.7% (sd=1.4)	.6% (sd=1.4)	.1% (sd=.4)
General Social Activities $F=6.17$ ($p < .001$)	15.4% (sd=10.0)	15.2% (sd=10.7)	12.9% (sd=8.9)	7.9% (sd=5.7)
Household Chores $F=5.79$ ($p < .001$)	12.7% (sd=9.2)	11.3% (sd=7.7)	11.1% (sd=8.3)	6.5% (sd=7.2)
Undesirable/Bizarre Behavior $F=12.74$ ($p < .001$)	.1% (sd=.5)	.4% (sd=1.9)	1.5% (sd=5.1)	5.1% (sd=8.8)
Leaving House $F=12.63$ ($p < .001$)	5.0% (sd=2.7)	5.8% (sd=4.0)	4.1% (sd=2.8)	2.1% (sd=1.8)

[a]All significant main effects were calculated by a stepdown multiple regression analysis and are reported only at the $p < .01$ significance level. All residents entering into the multiple regression analyses were observed for a minimum of 25 time periods.

[b]This intermediate category of mildly-moderately retarded was used for clients who had been assigned both labels at various periods and who currently were rated at the level intermediate to that of mildly or moderately retarded residents on their adaptive behavior skills.

The SMR/PMR group spent only 7.9 percent of its observed time in social interactions, about half the proportion observed for the mildly retarded group of residents. Further analyses of the actual nature of the residents' social interaction patterns showed additional differences related to level of intelligence (Landesman-Dwyer, Berkson, & Romer, 1979). Specifically, profoundly retarded clients were the only ones who failed to behave differently when they were in a social versus non-social situation. Nonetheless, some SMR/PMR clients were observed to have intense social relationships with others, predominantly with higher level individuals.

Discussion

Despite the large decline in the institutional population and significant growth in community-based residential alternatives in Washington State (Landesman-Dwyer, Stein, & Sackett, 1976), most SMR/PMR individuals receiving publicly subsidized care continue to live in large state institutions. Further, the majority of those in community residences live in nursing homes that tend to have much the same medical orientation, large size, lack of privacy, and routinized care schedules that characterize state institutions. It is important, however, to reiterate that school-aged children not receiving any social and health services from the state were *not* included in this survey. These data indicate that the impact of the "deinstitutionalization movement," as of 1976, on SMR/PMR persons was primarily (1) to provide more generic and less intense services to many placed in nursing homes, (2) to have proportionately more available resources to serve SMR/PMR clients who remain in state institutions—since staffing patterns have been enriched and training programs expanded at the same time the resident population declined, and (3) to have a relatively small number of previously institutionalized SMR/PMR people served in group homes and foster care. Given the comparisons of client profiles, it appears that those SMR/PMR persons who have left the institutions are a select group, at least to some degree. Despite the substantial range of abilities among SMR/PMR individuals in both institutional and community settings, those in the community had a higher average level of self-help, communication, and social skills and fewer severe medical and behavioral problems. Indeed, the SMR/PMR clients who failed to adapt to community residences were returned most often because of severe behavioral problems, notably physical aggression toward others or property.

The two major limitations in the descriptive data presented here are: (1) the lack of a longitudinal perspective and (2) the scant information on particular community residences. Often the case argued for community "failure" is that the facility is inadequate, which may have caused the client to act out. Another explanation is that these clients actually brought to the community residence more numerous problems or less general ability to adapt to a new setting than did those who remained. Probably an interaction between these two factors is the best retrospective explanation. There is no doubt that some SMR/PMR persons can fit very well into some community-based settings, as the behavioral observation study confirmed. Nonetheless, there continue to be some predicted behavioral differences related to the limited intelligence of these individuals. Such differences reinforce the professional view that specialized programs are needed to teach behaviors to SMR/PMR people that do not spontaneously occur or generalize appropriately for this population (Sackett, Landesman-Dwyer, & Morin, 1980). The social repertoire of SMR/PMR people is a prime example of this need.

Although SMR/PMR individuals often have the minimal necessary skills, they may not use these in the right situations or may fail to demonstrate enough of these behaviors to encourage the formation of meaningful relationships.

Initially, it was hoped this overview of SMR/PMR clients receiving residential care would lead to some recommendations about "matching" types of clients with types of settings. The historical facts associated with extremely unsystematic placement of clients into community settings prevented this. Moreover, the institutions continue to be the only sites with extensive experience serving SMR/PMR adults who have multiple and severe behavioral and/or medical problems. This does not imply that institutions necessarily are doing a good job; it does suggest that, *with the exceptions of families serving younger children and teenagers,* institutions are likely to remain a primary treatment site for this population. Caution is essential in developing new alternatives to provide long-term care and programming for the most dependent or most dangerous SMR/PMR clients. This caution applies equally to all settings. To answer the question of what types of residential settings promote the most effective habilitation for SMR/PMR people requires careful monitoring, and longitudinal studies are essential.

References

Alternatives in the community for the developmentally disabled: A bibliographic index on community-based alternatives to institutionalization. Life Project, Waisman Center on Mental Retardation and Human Development, University of Wisconsin, 1976.

Berkson, G., & Landesman-Dwyer, S. Behavioral research on severe and profound mental retardation (1955-1974). *American Journal of Mental Deficiency*, 1977, *82*, 428-454.

Butterfield, E. Some basic changes in residential facilities. In R. B. Kugel & A. Shearer (Eds.), *Changing patterns in residential services for the mentally retarded.* Washington, DC: President's Committee on Mental Retardation, 1976.

Conley, R. W. *The economics of mental retardation*. Baltimore: Johns Hopkins University Press, 1973.

Dingman, H. F., & Tarjan, G. Mental retardation and the normal distribution curve. *American Journal of Mental Deficiency*, 1960, *64*, 991-994.

Eyman, R. K., & Miller, C. A demographic overview of severe and profound mental retardation. In C. E. Meyers (Ed.), *Quality of life in severely and profoundly mentally retarded people: Research foundations for improvement*. Washington, DC: American Association on Mental Deficiency, 1978.

Grossman, H. J. (Ed.). *Manual on terminology and classification in mental retardation* (1973 revision). Washington, DC: American Association on Mental Deficiency, 1973.

Landesman-Dwyer, S., Berkson, G., & Romer, D. Affiliation and friendship of mentally retarded residents in group homes. *American Journal of Mental Deficiency*, 1979, *83*, 571-580.

Landesman-Dwyer, S., & Sackett, G. P. Behavioral changes in nonambulatory profoundly mentally retarded individuals. In C. E. Meyers (Ed.), *Quality of life in severely and profoundly people: Research foundation for improvement*. Washington, DC: American Association on Mental Deficiency, 1978.

Landesman-Dwyer, S., & Brown, T. R. A method for subgrouping mentally retarded citizens on the basis of service needs, 1976.

Landesman-Dwyer, S., Keller, L. S., & Schuckit, J. J. Community training programs for developmentally disabled clients: Developmental centers and sheltered workshops, 1976.

Landesman-Dwyer, S., & Schuckit, J. J. Preliminary findings of the survey of state institutions for the mentally retarded, 1976.

Landesman-Dwyer, S., & Schuckit, J. J., & Keller, L. S. Survey of developmentally disabled individuals in nursing homes and congregate care facilities, 1976.

Landesman-Dwyer, S., Schuckit, J. J., & Keller, L. S. Family and foster care for developmentally disabled children and adults, 1977.

Landesman-Dwyer, S., Stein, J. G., & Sackett, G. P. Group homes for the mentally retarded: An ecological and behavioral study, 1976.

Schuckit, J. J., & Landesman-Dwyer, S. Survey of the developmentally disabled in the Frances Haddon Morgan Children's Center and the Washington State School for the Blind, 1976.

Landesman-Dwyer, S., Stein, J. G., & Sackett, G. P. Group homes for the mentally retarded: An ecological and behavioral study. Olympia: State of Washington Department of Social and Health Services, Division of Planning and Research, 1976.

Landesman-Dwyer, S., Stein, J. G., & Sackett, G. P. A behavioral and ecological study of group homes. In G. P. Sackett (Ed.), *Observing behavior* (Vol. 1): *Theory and application in mental retardation*. Baltimore: University Park Press, 1978.

Mercer, J. R. *Labeling the mentally retarded*. Berkeley: University of California Press, 1973.

Nirje, B. The normalization principle. In R. B. Kugel & A. Shearer (Eds.), *Changing patterns in residential services for the mentally retarded* (Rev. ed.). Washington, DC: President's Committee on Mental Retardation, 1976.

Reintegrating mentally retarded people into the community: An annotated bibliography. Reston, VA: Program for the Analysis of Deinstitutionalization Resources, The Council for Exceptional Children, 1976.

Robinson, N. M., & Robinson, H. B. *The mentally retarded child: A psychological approach*. New York: McGraw-Hill, 1976.

Sackett, G. P., & Landesman-Dwyer, S. Toward an ethology of mental retardation: Quantitative behavioral observation in residential settings. In P. Mittler (Ed.), *Research to practice in mental retardation* (Vol. 2): *Education and training*. Baltimore: University Park Press, 1977.

Sackett, G. P., Landesman-Dwyer, S., & Morin, V. Naturalistic observation in design and evaluation of special education programs. In T. R. Kratochwill (Ed.), *Advances in school psychology*. Hillsdale, NJ: Lawrence Erlbaum Associates, in press.

Scheerenberger, R. C. *Public residential services for the mentally retarded, 1979*. Madison, WI: National Association of Superintendents of Public Residential Services for the Mentally Retarded, Central Wisconsin Center for Developmentally Disabled, 1979.

Tarjan, G., Wright, S. W., Eyman, R. K., & Keeran, C. V. Natural history of mental retardation: Some aspects of epidemiology. *American Journal of Mental Deficiency*, 1973, *77*, 369-379.

Change Over Time in the Community: Findings of a Longitudinal Study

Nancy J. Bell
Department of Child Development
and Family Studies

Carol Schoenrock
Gerard Bensberg

Research and Training Center in
Mental Retardation
Texas Tech University

Comprehensive follow-up studies of recent years have contributed substantially to information regarding factors associated with community functioning of retarded persons following release from an institution. Unlike former studies which typically employed the single success criterion of remaining in the community, recent studies have involved more elaborate evaluations of community functioning, whether intensively focused on selected aspects of community life (Clark, Kivitz, & Rosen, 1968) or broader in scope (Gollay, 1976). A wide range of predictor variables has been examined, including background and institution-related factors (Bowman & Hoffman, 1967) and community environment variables (Gollay, 1976). Complementing these studies are the detailed descriptions of daily life in the community provided by Edgerton (1967).

The primary question in research on community adjustment is no longer whether the majority of former institution residents can remain successfully in the community, but rather whether factors can be identified which affect community living in areas such as specific skills, degree of independence, and life satisfaction. The above studies have addressed this issue, but there is a related aspect of deinstitutionalization about which little is known: how community living changes over time and how various individual and environmental factors are related to these changes in functioning. This information is needed for several reasons. First, the results of previous studies have not always been consistent. One reason for this may be that different factors affect community functioning at various points in time. Second, it may be that there are certain time periods during which environmental factors have the most impact, with associated implications for increased attention to these factors during those times. Finally, the availability of descriptive information on the factors which do or do not change over time is basic to both future program development and research efforts.

Some longitudinal studies have been reported in the literature, but most have involved two or three contacts separated by many years (Baller, Charles, & Miller, 1966; Edgerton & Bercovici, 1976; Kennedy, 1966). More relevant to the present study are investigations of changes in skills over shorter intervals, such as those of Aanes and Moen (1976) and Yaron (1974) in group home settings. Both reported essentially positive results in that a number of skills did improve over time (5-12 months). Both investigators noted the greatest weaknesses in kitchen duties and

---

This project was supported by Grant No. 56-P-30318 from the Department of Health, Education, and Welfare, Social and Rehabilitation Services.

other chores, and Aanes and Moen also pointed to problems in money handling, shopping skills, and number/time concepts.

The present study was designed to examine multiple aspects of community functioning across time among people with different characteristics living in different types of environmental settings. Projects of this scope have disadvantages as well as advantages. Compared with more limited investigations of change in one type of residential setting, large-scale studies have the advantage of generalizability and permit comparisons among groups of individuals and among settings. However, they do not permit the in-depth skills assessment possible in smaller studies. Consequently, both types of investigations are clearly needed, and one cannot substitute for the other.

This longitudinal study involved gathering interview and questionnaire information in the community from former institution residents and from parents or residential staff. The data were collected over a two-year period from the time of entry into the community. This report includes only a portion of the data from the study—information from client interviews—and focuses upon change over time.

Method

The sample for the longitudinal study consisted of individuals furloughed from all state schools for the retarded in Texas over a 14-month period, with the exception of those leaving on short-term furloughs. Characteristics of these 582 individuals are presented in Table 1. Two to three years after entering the community, 327 (56.2%) were known to be living in the community and 68 (11.7%) had returned to the state school. Others were located in nursing homes (3.6%), prisons (.7%), psychiatric hospitals (1.2%), or were deceased (1.2%). The circumstances of the remainder of the original sample were not known because of refusals to participate in the study (7.2%), unknown locations (6.9%), moving from the state (3.2%), or for other reasons (8.1%).

Table 1
Sample Characteristics

Gender:		Male 297 (51%)		Female 285 (49%)	
IQ[a]:	Under 20 45 (7.7%)	20-35 94 (16.2%)	36-51 121 (20.8%)	52-68 227 (39.1%)	69+ 94 (16.2%)
Age[b]:	Under 11 19 (3.3%)	11-17 103 (17.8%)	18-30 314 (54.1%)	31-49 102 (17.6%)	50+ 42 (7.2%)
Furlough Location:	Residential Facility—MR 180 (30.9%)	Residential Facility—other 16 (2.8%)	Nursing Home 6 (1.0%)	Parent or Guardian 330 (56.7%)	Child Welfare 6 (1.0%)
	With Employer 17 (2.9%)	Independent Living 27 (4.6%)			

[a]One IQ score unavailable from records.
[b]Two birthdates unavailable from records.

Community data were obtained from all but 179 individuals in the sample. Of the remaining 403, 90 received one contact, and 313 received from two to five contacts during the course of the study. Approximately 75% of the contacts were made by field interviewers and 25% were made by project staff. A contact typically consisted of an interview of approximately one hour with the former state school resident, questionnaire information from parents or staff of community facilities, and ratings completed by the interviewer. There were a number of occasions in which only a portion of this information could be obtained, and thus either completed interviews or completed parent questionnaires constituted contact.

Field interviewers throughout the state were recruited through contacts with Mental Health and Mental Retardation Centers, local chapters of the Texas Association for Retarded Citizens, colleges and universities, and individual sources. During the course of the project, 130 persons were trained as interviewers, with approximately 25 actively involved at any one point in time. For prospective interviewers, training consisted of: a) review of procedures as specified in a detailed field manual; b) familiarization with interview forms; c) taping one or more practice interviews; and d) receiving feedback on the practice interviews from project staff.

Longitudinal Analysis of Interview Data

Sample and design. For purposes of examining trends over time, periods of five months were established, beginning with the first month after entry into the community and ending with the 25th month. Four groups were then designated, composed of people with interviews conducted in adjacent time periods (cf. Table 2). Thus, although it was not possible to analyze data from the same group of

Table 2

Longitudinal Sample Constitution and Characteristics

Group Constitution

Group	n	Time Periods of Interviews (months since furlough)	
1	66	1-5 (Time 1)	6-10 (Time 2)
2	87	6-10 (Time 2)	11-15 (Time 3)
3	92	11-15 (Time 3)	16-20 (Time 4)
4	64	16-20 (Time 4)	21-25 (Time 5)

Group Characteristics

	Groups 1		2		3		4	
Gender								
1 (male)	33	(50%)	43	(49.4%)	44	(47.8%)	25	(39%)
2 (female)	33	(50%)	44	(50.6%)	48	(52.2%)	39	(61%)
IQ								
1 (35 & under)	1	(1.5%)	11	(12.6%)	9	(9.8%)	6	(9.4%)
2 (36-51)	14	(21.2%)	21	(24.1%)	16	(17.4%)	11	(17.2%)
3 (52+)	51	(77.3%)	55	(63.3%)	67	(72.8%)	47	(73.4%)
Age								
1 (17 & under)	6	(9.1%)	9	(10.3%)	6	(6.5%)	11	(17.2%)
2 (18-30)	41	(62.1%)	46	(52.9%)	58	(63.0%)	32	(50.0%)
3 (31+)	19	(28.8%)	32	(36.8%)	28	(30.5%)	21	(32.8%)

individuals across all time periods, it was possible to examine change within each group and also trends across groups for the entire 25-month period. It should be emphasized that within each group the same individuals are represented in the first and second time period for that group; but across groups the membership overlaps but is not identical.

Two sets of analyses are presented in this report. The first involves change over time in community functioning for those respondents who remained in the community during the course of the study (i.e., excluding those who returned to the state school). Differences between returnees and nonreturnees are presented elsewhere (Bell & Schoenrock, 1979). The second set of analyses examines factors related to community functioning for each of the five time periods. The independent variables included in these analyses are: a) gender of interviewee; b) age (17 and under, 18-30, 31 and above), c) IQ (35 and under, 36-51, 52 and above), d) residence type (with parents or guardian, half-way house, group home), e) population of town (under 100,000, 100,000-399,000, 400,000 and over), and f) distance from services of Mental Health and Mental Retardation Centers (in excess of 30 miles, within 30 miles). Additional distinctions have been made within these variables for other aspects of this project, but the sample sizes for the longitudinal analysis required broader categories and the omission of one residential group (those living independently) because it was represented by very few people.

Community lifestyle variables. The dependent variables used in the analyses are presented in Table 3. These were taken from the interviews to represent dimensions of community functioning. The items consisted of structured responses where the interviewee was required to choose between two or three alternatives, open-ended responses involving frequencies of activities within a given time period, and items designed to test basic skills.

One additional item, self-esteem, was measured by a 24-item scale, each item requiring a yes/no response. Direction of wording was reversed for half of the items. Aspects of self-esteem included in the scale were relationships outside the home, family relationships, physical appearance, and general emotional state (e.g., "I am often unhappy"). Items were selected, and in some cases slightly modified, from those included in the Self Appraisal Inventory (Instructional Objectives Exchange, UCLA, 1972).

Results

Change Over Time

For the analysis of change over time, repeated measures analysis of variance was used for within group comparisons. Means for each time period (maintaining group distinctions) were plotted for each of the variables listed in Table 3. With the exception of three variables mentioned below, if there were no statistically significant ($p < .05$) increases or decreases within any of the groups, even though a slight trend upward or downward was observed from Time Period 1 through 5 (T 1-5), it was concluded that no significant change had occurred for that variable. There were three instances in which significant change did occur within one of the groups, but the variable was classified as stable since a) trends for the other groups revealed little change and b) means for T-1 and T-5 were similar.

Of the 24 variables listed in Table 3, 15 did not change over the 25 months according to the above criteria. Means (or percentages where appropriate) for T-1 and T-5 are presented in Table 4. Subsequent analyses were also done of the

Table 3

Dependent Variables

Category	Variable
Basic Skills	1. Total of 8 basic skill items assessed during interview (e.g. write name, give address, range 0-24)
Employment	2. Have job now
	3. Hours work/week
	4. Job satisfaction (total of 5 items, range 5-15)
Home and Family	5. Homemaking: number of activities performed (7 items, range 0-7)
	6. Degree of independent homemaking: e.g. cook full meals (total of 4 items, range 4-12)
	7. Marital status
	8. Bank accounts & insurance (4 items, range 0-4)
Community Interaction	9. Number of places visited in community (22 items, range 0-22)
	10. Frequency of church attendance/month
	11. Frequency of movie attendance/month
	12. Frequency eat in restaurants/month
	13. Frequency of YMCA-type activities/month
Relationships	14. Number of close friends
	15. Number of times telephone friends/week
	16. Frequency friends come to home/month
	17. Frequency visit friends/month
	18. Whether date
	19. Frequency visit neighbors/month
	20. Friendliness of neighbors (range 1-3)
Citizen	21. Whether arrested
Helpers	22. Whether person to help when needed
Problems	23. Total number of problems (15 items, range 0-15)
Self-Esteem	24. Self-esteem scale (24 items, range 0-24)

individual problem items to determine if there were shifting patterns of problems over time. No consistent upward or downward trends were detected for any of these items. Things that were reported most frequently as problems during the first five months after entry into the community persisted as the most frequent problems after two years, and these were: a) finding a job you like (57%), b) handling money (49%), and c) fixing things that break (44%). Least frequent problems were: a) transportation (26%), b) knowing what to do when sick (33%), and c) keeping the place you live clean (34%).

Patterns of change. Nine of the variables included in these analyses did exhibit some signs of change across time although in no instance was the change dramatic and in some cases it is questionable whether the trends should be interpreted as real change. They are discussed in some detail because they are aspects of community functioning which should be considered in future studies of change.

Table 4
Variables Which Did Not Change Over Time

Variable No. (see Table 3)	Description	Time 1 Value	n	Time 5 Value	n
2[a]	Employed (% yes)	72.9%	48	72.5%	51
3[a]	Employed full time	52.1%	48	56.9%	51
4[a]	Job satisfaction (low score = more satisfied)	5.8	32	6.2	36
5	No. homemaking activities	5.4	55	5.5	62
7[a]	Married (% yes)	2.1%	48	3.9%	51
9	No. places visited	12.9	51	13.4	59
12	Restaurant visits/month	1.5	49	1.3	52
15	Call friends/week	.8	36	1.7	33
16	Visits from friends/month	1.3	48	1.5	53
17	Visit friends/month	1.3	46	1.7	50
18[a]	Dating (% yes)	33.3%	45	29.8%	47
20	How neighbors act (low score = most friendly)	1.5	39	1.5	43
21[a]	Arrested (% yes)	14.9%	47	12.2%	49
22[a]	Helper (% yes)	95.6%	45	85.4%	48
23	Problem total	5.8	45	6.6	44

[a]Excludes children

Two patterns of change were identified which describe seven of the nine variables (cf. Table 5). The first was a gradual decline across time which occurred for three of the community interaction variables following the first five months in the community. These variables involved attendance in church, movies, and YMCA-type organizations. There was a significant within-group change only for movie attendance, but for all variables there was a downward trend across group over time and a significant difference in the percentage attendance between T-1 and T-5 for YMCA-type activities (chi-square, $p < .05$).

The second pattern of change involved an increase which began to occur sometime during the second year after entry into the community. Basic skills, as measured during the interview (e.g., write name, give address), did not change from T-1 to T-4, but did increase significantly between T-4 and T-5. There was also evidence of an increase in the degree of independence in homemaking skills beginning at T-3. This variable dealt with items such as cooking full meals rather than simply fixing snacks, doing a complete grocery shopping rather than buying a few items, and so forth. Finally, there was some increased involvement in relationships. An increase at T-4 was observed for the item regarding number of close friends, and an increase at T-3 occurred for frequency of visiting neighbors. For neighbor contact, there were no significant within-group changes; the increase at T-3 was a between-groups difference. However, the increase was not unique to Group 3 but was maintained by Group 4, so may in fact reflect a real change at about that point in time. Also, it may be worth noting that number of phone calls made to friends each week, listed in Table 4, did increase somewhat over the two years.

Table 5
Variables Which Did Change Over Time

Variable No. (see Table 3)	Description	Time 1 Value	Time 1 n	Time 5 Value	Time 5 n
Pattern I: Gradual Decline					
10	Church attendance/month	2.4	51	1.9	50
	4+times	43.8%		34.7%	
11	Movie attendance/month	1.4	50	.6	53
	4+times	20.8%		2.1%	
	Decrease, Time 3-4 $p < .02$				
13	YMCA, etc. attendance/mo	.39	49	.10	38
	1+times	19.0%		2.0%	
	Decrease, Time 4-5 $p < .08$				
Pattern II: Increase, Time 3 or 4					
1	Basic skills	14.34	47	15.34	56
	Increase, Time 4-5, $p < .006$				
6	Independent homemaking	5.4	55	8.6	42
	Increase, Time 3-4 $p < .03$				
	Increase, Time 4-5 $p < .06$				
14	Number close friends	3.3	23	4.1	30
	Increase, Time 4-5 $p < .03$				
19	Visit neighbors/month	1.9	36	3.9	29
Other Patterns					
8[a]	Banks accounts	1.3	40	1.9	45
	Increase, Time 1-2 $p < .005$				
24	Self-esteem	17.5	48	17.4	51
	Decrease, Time 2-3 $p < .008$				
	Increase, Time 4-5 $p < .08$				

[a]Excludes children

Finally, two variables which did not fit either of the above patterns are financial affairs and self-esteem. The first involved the existence of bank accounts and insurance. There was a significant increase in this variable between T-1 and T-2, after which it did not change. Self-esteem decreased significantly from T-2 to T-3, then began a gradual increase from T-3 to T-5.

Factors Related to Community Functioning by Time Periods

The analysis procedures for determining factors which related to the dependent variables for each time period consisted of: a) analyses of variance for each of the dependent variables with the six independent variables described previously, and

b) a comparison of significant effects between groups for each time period. Only the significant effects which were replicated across the two groups for a given time period and dependent variable are considered here, consequently reducing the possibility that these effects are chance occurrences. Effects for T-1 and T-5 are also reported even though in these instances the results are based upon only one group. The original intent of this analysis procedure was to permit an analysis of interactions, particularly between respondent and environmental characteristics. However, the sample size within each group permitted only an analysis of main effects. Such interactions are being examined in the project, but not in conjunction with the longitudinal analysis.

Environmental characteristics. Of the three environmental variables included in these analyses, distance from a Mental Health and Mental Retardation Center did not relate to any of the community functioning variables. Community functioning was affected to some extent by both size of town and type of residential unit (cf. Table 6). During T-1, those in or near large cities (400,000+) attended church less frequently and movies more frequently than did those living in less populated areas. In contacting friends, those from the largest cities called friends on the phone more frequently than did the other groups, while those from the least populated areas visited friends more frequently during T-3.

Type of residential unit was statistically related to employment status; but since this difference was mainly between those living with parents and those in residential units and is strongly affected by the large number of children in the former setting, it is not included in Table 6. Differences during T-1 for number of homemaking activities were of the same kind and may be for the same reason.

Table 6

Factors Related to Community Functioning

Variable No. (see Table 3)	Description	Factors Related at Each Time Period[a] 1	2	3	4	5
1	Basic skills	IQ	IQ	IQ		IQ
2	Employed		IQ	IQ	IQ	BSk[b]
5	Homemaking	SX,R	BSk	BSk	BSk	BSk
9	Places visited			BSk	BSk	BSk
10	Church	SX,P				
11	Movies	A,P		BSk		
12	Restaurants		BSk	R		
14	No. close friends				SX	
15	Call friends			BSk,P		BSk
17	Visit friends			P	SX	
22	Helper					BSk
23	Problems	BSk (neg., .08)				
24	Self-esteem	BSk				

[a]$p < .05$; SX = sex, P = population, R = residence type, A = age, BSk = basic skills.
[b]All relationships with BSk positive unless noted otherwise.

Residential unit was also related to the type of community activities in one analysis—those living in halfway houses ate in restaurants more frequently during T-3 than did the other groups.

Respondent characteristics. Of the respondent variables, gender and age had minimal impact upon the aspects of community functioning included in this investigation. During T-1, women engaged in a greater number of homemaking activities and went to church more frequently than did men, but these differences did not persist past the first five months. During T-4, men reported having a greater number of close friends and visited friends more frequently than did women (men averaged over two visits per month, women less than one). Aside from the obvious relationships of age to employment status (not included in Table 6), age was related only to movie attendance during T-1: the middle age group (18-30) attended most frequently.

Intelligence was strongly related to ability to perform basic skills (as measured during the interview) and upon employment status. Considering employment, those with IQs under 35 were less likely to be employed than others in the sample. In regard to basic skills, there were clear distinctions between all IQ groups which were significant for all comparisons except one (Group 4, T-4). Averaged over all time periods, the means for the IQ categories 35 and below, 36-51, and 52 and above were 4.85, 9.68, and 15.77, respectively.

Since the basic skills variable was strongly related to IQ but to no other independent variables, a correlational analysis was conducted with the other dependent variables. Its appearance in Table 6 indicates that there was a statistically significant ($p < .05$) correlation between basic skills and at least two dependent variables for each of the time periods. The greater number of corelationships between basic skills and other dependent variables than was found with IQ may be due to the differences in analysis procedures, the fact that the basic skills score is a more recent measure, or that it is composed of items directly relevant to community functioning.

There was only one dependent variable to which basic skill level was consistently related across time, and that was number of homemaking activities performed. Beginning at T-2, those demonstrating a higher level of basic skills during the interview also reported performing more homemaking activities.

Among community interaction and relationship variables, basic skill level was more of a factor during the middle and toward the end of the two-year period than at the beginning. The number of places visited in the community was related to basic skills at T-3 through T-5, movie and restaurant attendance was related to basic skills during T-3 and T-2, respectively, and telephone contact with friends was correlated with basic skills during T-3 and T-5.

Finally, basic skill level was positively related to having a helper during T-5 and to self-esteem during T-1. Although there were no relationships between total problems and basic skills which met the standard significance criteria, the pattern of relationships between skills and problems across time may be important to an understanding of some of the other findings. Correlations between skills and total problems were negative during T-1 ($-.28$, $p < .08$) and T-2 for Group 1 ($-.35$, $p < .05$). By T-3, they were positive, although not high in magnitude. Examining individual problems, 14 of 15 were negatively correlated with skills during T-1, while the majority were positive during T-3. For Group 1, five of the individual problems had a statistically significant, negative relationship to skills; for the rest of the groups, there was one such negative relationship (during T-2) and four significant positive relationships (during T-3 and T-4). Two of the problem areas having substantial negative relationships with skills during T-1 and T-2 were positively and significantly correlated with skills during T-3. These dealt with problems finding friends of the same sex, and problems deciding what food to buy.

Discussion

General Issues

It is well known that interview responses, particularly from retarded persons, are of questionable validity. Recent analyses done to determine the extent of the problem are not encouraging (Sigelman et al., this volume). One way of dealing with validity issues in the future is to employ alternative methods as a substitution for, or in addition to, interviews. However, this does not mean that there is no valid information obtainable from interviews; rather that caution must be exercised in the interpretation of data gathered in this way. This discussion deals with validity issues only in those instances where they appear to be plausible alternatives to other interpretations although it is recognized that this factor may have a more general influence upon the results of a study such as the one reported here.

The sample for the longitudinal study was selective in that it included only those having two or more interviews while residing in the community. It could be argued that these were the more accessible and cooperative people, and to some extent, that is probably true. On the other hand, the completion and timing of interviews in this study was largely determined by the scheduling and general dependability of field interviewers, and this factor likely contributed more to the composition of the longitudinal sample than did characteristics of the interviewees. It is true that, compared to the original sample, the mean IQ of the longitudinal subsample was higher as reflected in a comparison of Tables 1 and 2. This IQ difference was not restricted to the longitudinal sample but occurred for the entire sample of interviewees compared with non-interviewees due to inaccessibility or nonresponsiveness of the lower IQ individuals. Since many previous community adjustment studies have included only the mildly retarded in the sample, it is helpful to have even a 30% representation of lower ability respondents (i.e., IQ below 52) for purposes of making comparisons.

Change Over Time

Lack of change over a two-year period was not unexpected for some variables, particularly in the case of marital and employment status. This expectation was based upon the fact that the majority of the sample was in a sheltered living situation or at home for the duration of the study. For a second set of variables, there was no body of research on which to formulate expectations, but change in a specified direction would have been viewed as positive in the sense of increased integration into the community (e.g., more community interaction, a larger social network, fewer problems in community living). Finally, change was expected, based upon the literature, for basic skills including homemaking activities.

The overall impression gained from an examination of community functioning over time is that there was very little change in this sample during the two-year period. As mentioned earlier, even the variables which did change over time changed only slightly in most cases. In one instance (number of homemaking activities) the lack of change may have been due to a limited scale range. For the majority of variables, however, a ceiling effect cannot account for the findings.

A more optimistic interpretation of the results is possible if the Pattern II changes in Table 5 are viewed as the beginning of a continuing upward trend. It may be that more than two years is required for substantial change in these aspects of community functioning. If this is the case, then basic skills, degree of independence in homemaking activities, and social network show signs of positive change, and the results for self-esteem are also encouraging. Community interaction variables decreased rather than increased over time, but if going places in the community is gradually replaced by getting together with friends, this may also be a positive trend.

Factors Related to Community Functioning

Of the independent variables examined, ability level (IQ and basic skill level) had the most frequent statistically significant relationship with community functioning. The relatively minor impact of environmental factors upon community functioning should probably be attributed to the nature of the environmental variables included in these analyses rather than to a lack of importance of this category of variable. It is important to document any differences which may exist between residential circumstances and location as categorized here, but these are not otherwise meaningful variables. In future analyses of these data, more detailed environmental information obtained from sources other than interviews with retarded persons will be examined.

There are two interesting aspects to the relationships found between dependent variables and basic skills (subsequently referred to as ability). First, relationships between community functioning and ability occurred most frequently after 10 months in the community and almost never during the first five months. This was true for homemaking activities, community interaction, phone contacts with friends, and helpers. The finding is not attributable to the uniqueness of any one group since the relationships were replicated across groups for each time period. Nor is there reason to expect that inaccurate reporting of activities, varying with ability, began at this time. It may be that the residential settings begin to permit or encourage more activities after a certain period of time in the community, and the higher ability individuals are better able to take advantage of these opportunities. However, the correlations between ability and functioning during these periods do not necessarily represent improvements for those of higher ability across time. Such patterns are yet to be determined through analyses of subgroup changes.

With respect to helpers, the positive relationship between ability and helpers is similar to the findings of Lambert (1976), but it is not clear why this occurred only at the end of the two-year period. Perhaps helpers begin to respond differentially to those of higher ability at this time because they perceive improvements and wish to reinforce the trends.

Second, as previously described, the direction of relationships between ability and problems changed over time. Initially, those with higher ability acknowledged fewer problems. After about 10 months in the community, relationships between ability and number of problems tended to be positive. Also, the positive relationship between ability and self-esteem occurred only during the first five months. It may be that these results for both problems and self-esteem are a first interview phenomenon in that fear of being returned to the institution produces less truthful responses during the first time period, and those with more ability are better able to give socially desirable answers. It is equally possible, however, that the responses were truthful and that increased problems for the higher ability individuals after a period of time in the community correspond to a time when more demands are being placed upon them and life becomes more complicated. Future studies might examine the period from eight to twelve months after entry into the community to determine the nature of demands placed upon individuals and to explore the extent to which adequate preparation has occurred and support is available.

Summary

The findings of this study indicated that: a) the aspects of community functioning included in this study were relatively stable over a two-year period; b) when change did occur, it tended to be toward the end of the two-year period; c) ability level (basic skills) was related to community functioning more consistently than age, gender, or the environmental variables included in these analyses; d) relationships with ability were more frequent following approximately 10 months in the community than prior to that time; and e) there is a possibility that the time period around 10 months after entry into the community is a particularly difficult time and warrants further investigation.

References

Aanes, D., & Moen, M. Adaptive behavior changes of group home residents. *Mental Retardation*, 1976, *14*(4), 36-40.

Baller, W., Charles, D., & Miller, E. Mid-life attainment of the mentally retarded: A longitudinal study. *Genetic Psychology Monographs*, 1967, *75*, 235-329.

Bell, N. J., & Schoenrock, C. Factors associated with reinstitutionalization of retarded persons following community placement. Manuscript submitted for publication, 1980.

Bowman, P. S., & Hoffman, J. L. *An investigation of factors contributing to successful and non-successful adjustment of discharged retardates*. Pownal, ME: Pineland Hospital and Training Center, 1969.

Clark, G. R., Kivitz, M. S., & Rosen, M. *A transitional program for institutionalized adult retarded*. Elwyn, PA: Elwyn Institute, 1968.

Edgerton, R. B. *The cloak of competence: Stigma in the lives of the mentally retarded*. Berkeley: University of California Press, 1967.

Edgerton, R. B., & Bercovici, S. M. The cloak of competence: Years later. *American Journal of Mental Deficiency*, 1976, *80*, 485-497.

Gollay, E. *A study of the community adjustment of deinstitutionalized mentally retarded persons* (Vol. 5). Cambridge, MA: Abt Associates, 1976.

Instructional Objectives Exchange. Self Appraisal Inventory. In *Measures of self-concept, K-12*. Los Angeles: College of Education, University of California at Los Angeles, 1972.

Kennedy, R. A. *A Connecticut community revisited: A study of the social adjustment of a group of mentally deficient adults in 1948 and 1960*. Hartford: Connecticut State Department of Health, Office of Mental Retardation, 1966.

Lambert, C., Jr. *Retarded adults: Their adjustment and community milieu*. Toronto: Ministry of Community and Social Services, 1976.

Yaron, A. *Final report: A project to evaluate the effectiveness of resocialization for mentally retarded discharged from institutions and other segregated environments. July, 1971-June, 1974*. Denver: State of Colorado Division of Developmental Disabilities, 1974.

Return of Retarded Adults to Natural Families: Issues and Results

Barry Willer
James Intagliata
Nancy Wicks

Division of Community Psychiatry
State University of New York at Buffalo

Whenever there is discussion of retarded people leaving institutions to live in alternate settings, there frequently is little or no mention of returning them to their natural families. It is interesting that institutionalization in the past was frequently recommended because of the expected benefits to the family. The current trends in discharge patterns suggest that while there is interest in providing the retarded with renewed opportunity to live in less restrictive settings, return to the natural family is not very common. It is also not commonly recommended. Even though attitudes about institutionalization have changed many have still, it seems, continued to view the retarded living with their natural families as a less than desirable outcome.

In a national survey on deinstitutionalization (Wyngaarden & Gollay, 1976) it was found that approximately 40% of discharges from public institutions were returns to the natural family. However, this figure was found to vary considerably across the United States. In the more intense follow-up study of Gollay, Freedman, Wyngaarden and Kurtz (1978) only 14% of individuals studied were returned to their own home. The author's study of discharge patterns in New York State suggest that even this figure may be an overestimate, at least for New York.

Lack of interest in returning the retarded to their natural home is reflected also in the limited amount of research on what happens to the retarded when they return home and how the family reacts. In this paper the writers intend to present some preliminary results of a New York State investigation in order to examine the effects of discharge to the natural home on the discharged individual and his family. In general, the natural families are compared with foster family care families, the natural families of individuals who were placed in alternate settings, and group home "parents."

Study Procedures

This investigation involved a questionnaire survey of all individuals, institutionalized for at least one year, and released from one of six institutions across New York State. Release had occurred from 1972 to 1976. This presentation only includes the results of the follow-up of individuals released from four institutions. Individuals from one of the institutions not included were followed up using personal interviews, and much of the data compiled was not compatible with the questionnaire data. Data on releases from the sixth institution are only now being prepared for analysis.

This study was assisted under the Department of Health, Education, and Welfare, Region II, Office of Human Development, Developmental Disabilities Office, Grant No. 50P10568/2.

Total number of returned questionnaires was 31 from natural families, 140 from family care families, 165 from group home parents, and 104 from natural families of individuals placed in alternate settings. Return rates were 31 percent for natural families, 71 percent for family care families, 76 percent for group home parents and 35 percent for natural families of individuals in alternative settings. The percentage of families returning the questionnaire was noticeably lower for natural families, and follow-up phone calls revealed that there was considerable resentment toward the institution which accounted for much of the noncooperation.

Data compiled on each individual released included pre-release behavior characteristics, degree of retardation and basic descriptive information such as age and length of institutionalization. Post-release data included specific client behaviors, ratings of behavior characteristics using the Devereux Adolescent Behavior Rating Scale (Spivack, Haines & Spotts, 1967), perceived burden of care, use of services, basic descriptors of the home environment, and the number of persons in the home.

Results

Gollay, Freedman, Wyngaarden and Kurtz (1978) reported that retarded individuals who return home are likely to be younger and more severely retarded than individuals being placed in other settings. The study reported here found similar patterns. These are shown in Table 1.

Table 1

Intellectual Functioning Level by Type of Placement

Functional Level	Percent of Individuals Released to		
	Natural Home	Family Care	Group Home
Mild +	—	24.4	42.2
Moderate	30.8	20.5	26.7
Severe	61.5	44.9	29.6
Profound	7.7	10.3	1.5
	100.0	100.0	100.0

The data in Table 1 are based on intellectual assessments conducted while the individuals were still in the institutions, and they have since been found to be somewhat unreliable. Although it is clear, from these and other data on pre-release behavior characteristics that those individuals released to group homes and other community residential facilities are generally of a much higher level of intellectual functioning, very little difference has been found between individuals placed in their natural homes or in family care. A close analysis of behavior problems of the individuals released to either the natural home or family care indicates that they were much more likely to have problems of speech, ambulation, self-care, and to throw tantrums. Individuals placed in group homes were more likely to have problems of anxiety, hyperactivity, and relating to peers and authorities. The differences in the types of problems perceived by caretakers appear strongly related to the differences in intellectual functioning among the groups.

Differences exist also between the families of individuals returned home and the families of individuals placed elsewhere, and these offer some clues to why many families reject return to the natural home as an alternative. For example, families of mentally retarded persons placed outside their natural home were on the average slightly better educated, of higher average income, and of higher average age. However, the relationship of each of these variables is not strong enough to explain adequately why so many families reject return of the retarded relative.

A strong relationship was found between the reason for original institutionalization and the likelihood of return. Individuals who returned to their natural home were much more likely to have been institutionalized because of behavior problems. The reason for institutionalization of individuals placed outside their natural home was much more likely to have been that "it was recommended by a physician." This finding is supported by previous research (Mercer, 1966), but there is no clear explanation of the relationship. It is possible that families who so willingly follow the advice of professionals are also more influenced by the social norm which today, at least in the United States, suggests that retarded adults should not return to their natural home. It is also possible that the reason for admission was not simply the advice of the physician but may be subtle and less attractive to state, such as the family not being able to cope with the stigma and guilt of having a retarded child.

Another factor related to likelihood of return to one's natural family was length of institutionalization. Individuals who returned home, on the average, spent less time in the institution. Returning home may relate to the age of the individual, the age of the parent, or the length of institutionalization (since these factors are all related), or length of institutionalization may relate to a third factor, namely the effect of institutionalization on the natural bond between the family and the retarded family member. There is considerable evidence that institutional practices tend to discourage family involvement and support and frequently lead to reduction in the frequency of family visits. It seems reasonable to expect that families who have less attachment to the individual will be less likely to have their retarded family member return home.

Impact on the Family

The reasons for retarded persons returning home are many and varied. Nevertheless, regardless of the reason, the individual's return home appears to have a significant impact on the family. In an earlier report on this study it was pointed out that families frequently endure a crisis at the time of release. This crisis is related to fears about their ability to deal effectively with possible behavior problems of the retarded individual (Willer, Intagliata & Atkinson, in press). However, these families generally overcame their initial fears and most indicated later that they accepted deinstitutionalization as necessary and that return home was beneficial for the family as a whole and for the retarded member. This same study found that many families of individuals placed outside the natural home also experience crisis, although the crisis was more likely to be extreme guilt—guilt over the original decision to institutionalize and the decision not to have the family member return home. This guilt did not disappear as readily as the anxiety experienced by natural families who did encourage their family member to return home.

Return of the retarded individual to his natural family does present some long term burden of care problems for the family, particularly on the female head of household. These women indicated that care for the family member generally was their responsibility (75%). Although most families indicated the individual was, in general, easy to manage (79%), most also indicated burden of care difficulties similar to those experienced by families of individuals who were returned from psychiatric institutions (Doll, 1976). The burden of care items and corresponding percentages are presented in Table 2 for both natural families and family care families.

Table 2
Problems of Caring for Retarded Persons in the Home: Percentage of Female Head of Household Agreement

Problem Types	Home Placement Families	Family Care Families
Difficult to get free time	46%	23%*
More supervision than expected	24%	21%
Caused relatives to react	16%	3%*
Neglect of family members	13%	9%
Caused neighbors to react	12%	8%
Unwilling to invite friends	1%	8%
Disagreements about care	8%	9%

*p <.10

The primary difficulties for the women who cared for the retarded individuals in the home relate to the retarded persons' needs for supervision and the caretakers' inability to get relief, even for brief periods. One respondent noted, "It is very difficult to get a 'baby sitter' for a retarded adult." Added to this is the fact that about a third of the natural family homes were made up of the retarded individual and only one other person, invariably the mother. The relatively low percentage of women reporting that relatives, friends or neighbors have behaved differently since the retarded person rejoined the family suggests that while stigma may remain somewhat of a problem, it does not necessarily affect social relationships.

Another factor which has an important impact on the natural family is the financial burden of maintaining the handicapped family member. In discussions with professionals who argue against return to the natural family, the financial burden is frequently mentioned. The argument is that the family should not be expected to endure a financial burden simply because they have a retarded family member.

It has already been pointed out that families that return their retarded family member to their home tend to be of the lower income group. The fact is, about 45 percent of these families were below $6,000 annual income, usually on a fixed income pension. This does not argue against the possibility of financial burden, but it does suggest that financial burden may not be the primary consideration in making the decision to reaccept the retarded person into his natural home. However, it was also found that about one-quarter of the female heads of household of families who rejected return were employed full time and felt they would have to give up their job and the associated income and life style in order to accommodate a retarded family member.

In a separate study of costs of community based care, Intagliata, Willer and Cooley (in press) indicate that the board and care costs of having an adult live in the home is about $2100. In New York State the family with a retarded adult has access to a number of sources of financial aid. The social security benefit is $1500 which is a little less than the expected costs. As well, the retarded individual is eligible for medicaid, to cover medical costs, and most community services are available at no expense. Even with this assistance, however, families are able to identify certain services which are unavailable because of cost (cf. Table 3).

Table 3

Percent of Families Indicating Services Unavailable Because of Cost

Service Type	Percent
Physical therapy	30.0
Counseling-Individual	15.8
Speech Therapy	21.1
Transportation Services	21.1
Recreational Services	10.5

There is some truth to the argument that some services are unavailable because of cost, but it appears that financial burden may not be as serious a problem as some professionals would suggest. On the other hand, it is important to note that New York State, which provides a state supplement to social security benefits, provides a smaller supplement to individuals placed within the natural family than that given to individuals in family care or group homes.

Despite the burden the family endures when a retarded family member returns home, families were also able to identify benefits gained as a result of having the member return. The benefits ranged from an enrichment of family life (72%), to the member's assistance in the upkeep of the home (60%), increased understanding of mental retardation (72%), and relief from feelings of loneliness (76%).

Restrictiveness of the Home Environment

Another common argument against return of the retarded adult to the natural home is that natural families tend to be overprotective and provide a restrictive environment for the individual. Overprotectiveness is generally defined as encouraging dependency behaviors and preventing the development of normalized behavior patterns. One subscale of the Devereux Behavior Scale deals specifically with dependency, defined as "seeking adult approval and attention" and "clinging" to adults inappropriately. Table 4 presents the percentage of individuals rated as abnormally high (more than one standard deviation above the average) on dependency in each of the placement categories. The differences are not statistically significant, suggesting that natural homes are not as overprotective as is often believed.

Table 4

Percent of Individuals by Placement Exhibiting Above Normal Dependency Behavior

Placement Type	Percent Dependent
Home-Placed	43
Family Care	42
Group Home	38

The extent to which natural families encourage normalized behavior is difficult to ascertain. A comparison of individuals in natural families with those in family care indicates that there is a slightly higher percentage who are capable of unsupervised travel on public transportation (30% versus 22%). Both groups are significantly lower than group home residents (53%), although, as has been noted, group home residents tend to be far more often in the mild/moderate range of retardation. At least with respect to independent travel, natural families appear to have encouraged normalized behavior as much or more than family care families.

As a final test of the effects of family and family care environments, the individuals placed in them were compared on *below* average scores on a variety of subscales of the Devereux Behavior Scale. Below average, that is greater than one standard deviation below the norm, on any subscale was assumed to reflect *repression* or *stunting* of the behavior represented in the subscale. Table 5 presents the percent of individuals scoring below average in family care and natural family placements. No differences were statistically significant, using chi-square analysis, except that on the emotional control subscale. Emotional control refers to appropriate expression of anger and being able to respond effectively to frustration. Being below average would suggest that the individual represses anger and feelings excessively. Individuals in family care were considerably more often rated as being overly repressive of anger and personal feelings.

Table 5

Percent of Individuals Displaying Below Average Scores on Devereux Subscales

Subscale	Home Placement	Family Care Placement
Inability to delay gratification	29%	36%
Defiant-Resistive	58%	56%
Domineering-Sadistic	48%	53%
Heterosexual interest	39%	49%
Hyperactive-Expansive	42%	38%
Emotional control	32%	50%*

*p <.05

In short, the evidence would suggest that natural families are no more restrictive than family care families, although it seems that both types of families are more restrictive than they might ideally be. The writers experience is that normalization and dignity of risk are often foreign terms and foreign concepts to both natural and family care families and that both family types have operated with essentially no training and relatively little assistance. Training and assistance might lead to vastly reduced levels of restrictiveness.

Impact on the Individual

Assessment of individual gains as a result of deinstitutionalization is a complex process especially when inadequate data are provided on pre-release behavior patterns. In this study there were three outcome measures and individuals in natural family and family care homes can be compared on these, if the assumption is made that the individuals do not differ in some critical factors directly related to successful outcome. The three measures used are the Institutional Scale, a scale used to assess behavior in the institution (readministered at follow-up), the Devereux Adolescent Behavior Scale and a series of questions identifying specific problem areas at the time of release and again at follow-up.

The Institutional Scale was used to assess behavior patterns at follow-up because it was the only scale administered to all subjects prior to release from the institution. The scale has not been carefully assessed for reliability and, as mentioned earlier, the institutional data show signs of relatively low reliability. The best the scale data can provide is some indications of trends. Table 6 presents the percentage of individuals exhibiting problems for each item on the scale. These data suggest that individuals placed at home were more likely to have sexual behavior problems and to exhibit self-abusive behavior. Individuals in family care were more likely to exhibit withdrawal. As previously mentioned, individuals released to the natural home were more likely to exhibit peer relationship problems and tantrum behavior prior to release, and both these factors were more prevalent in natural families at follow-up, although the differences only approach statistical significance.

Table 6

Percent of Individuals Exhibiting Problems by Placement Type

Problem Area	Natural Family	Family Care
Relationships		
Peers	19.3	12.1
Authority	22.6	16.9
Sexual	16.6	5.7*
Behavior Problems		
Assaultive	13.0	8.7
Self Abuse	19.4	5.8*
Tantrum	38.7	25.0
Destructive	13.3	20.0
Hyperactive	25.8	20.1
Withdrawal	32.2	18.1
Anxiety	29.0	28.6
Self Care		
Toilet Training	19.4	21.6
Eating	12.9	29.3
Dressing	16.2	25.2
Speech		
Speech	67.8	58.6
Comprehension	58.1	49.7
Ambulation	19.3	29.5

*$p < .05$

The second source of outcome data is the Devereux Behavior Scale administered only at follow-up. Results are presented in Table 7 as the percent of individuals scoring one standard deviation above the norm on each of the subscales. The results indicate that individuals in the natural home tend to be less defiant but also less able to handle frustration (to delay gratification) and more likely to get angry and lose (emotional) control. These data may suggest that, indeed, natural families tend to be more indulging of their mentally retarded member, often allowing the individual to have his own way and enduring more frequent and/or stronger emotional outbursts when the member is not indulged.

Table 7

Percent of Individuals Displaying Above Average Scores on Devereux Scales

Subscale	Home Placement	Family Care Placement
Inability to delay gratification	39%	19%*
Defiant-Resistive	3%	14%*
Domineering-Sadistic	29%	19%
Heterosexual interest	13%	7%
Hyperactive-Expansive	26%	13%
Emotional control	39%	17%

*$p < .05$

The third outcome compared was the extent to which individuals overcome problems presented at the time of placement. Table 8 presents these data as a success rate, the percent of individuals who improved in each of the problem areas.

Table 8

Comparison of Living Alternatives on Success Rates with Initial Placement Problems[a]

Problem Category	Natural Family	Family Care
Money management	11.8	25.3*
Handling emergencies	23.5	23.2
Shopping	26.7	35.4
Meal preparation	28.6	33.3
Use of telephone	38.5	38.4
Travel skills	28.6	41.8
Disobedience	18.2	44.7*
Self cleaning	33.3	61.5*
Destructive behavior	–25.0	53.6*
Bathroom behavior	33.0	61.8*

[a]Problems are presented in order of decreasing frequency of problem occurring initially upon placement.

*$p < .05$

Some problem areas such as destructive behavior and bathroom behavior were infrequent to begin with so the success rate percentages are less meaningful. However, on the whole it appears that family care clients were more often perceived as overcoming initial placement problems than individuals in the natural home. Individuals in family care were significantly more likely to show gains in money management, obedience and self care. A comparison between family care and group home clients found nearly equal rates of success in these two placement alternatives although clients in group homes were clearly different to begin with.

Finally, natural family and family care placements were compared regarding rates of reinstitutionalization. Of the total sample of individuals placed in natural homes, only 4% returned to the institutions for periods longer than 30 days compared with 11% for family care and 21% for group homes. It should be mentioned that a sizeable percentage of group home clients previously had lived in family care. Thus, although the return rate percentage for group homes was 21%, it likely would have been somewhat smaller if only direct placements from institutions were considered. Similarly, if only direct placements to family care were considered, the 11% probably would have been slightly higher. There were few such movements prior to placement in natural homes so that the 4% return rate probably reflects accurately the rate of reinstitutionalization within this group.

Discussion

There are a variety of reasons why families of the mentally retarded generally reject the idea of having their relative return home following release from the institution. Obvious reasons are the age of the parents and financial constraints. However, there are also reasons relating to parent attitudes and institutional practices. Parents who are both working or are of higher socioeconomic status are the least likely to accept return. There is a strong possibility that parents are concerned about the stigma of having a retarded son or daughter in the home again. Although not reflected in the data, many single mothers (widowed or divorced) who encouraged the return home of their son or daughter indicated that this would not have been possible had their husband still lived there. On the other hand, many single mothers who rejected return, indicated that because they were single they could not handle the behavior of the individual.

Institutional practices seem particularly important to placement of the individual in settings other than the natural home. Institutional staff generally regarded the natural family as having made the decision to "give up" their family member when he was institutionalized. Families indicated they were made to feel uncomfortable about even making visits to the institutions, and were discouraged from participation in decisions about programming or release from the institution. Also, when release was mentioned, most families were extremely anxious and many opposed the move. Any resistance was generally treated by placement staff as rejection of return to the natural home. In short, it seemed that placements in group homes and family care were perceived as more convenient for all concerned.

The results of placement in any community-based residential setting was found to be, in general, successful for the individual. The data suggest that individuals adjusted fairly well, and a sizeable proportion showed significant gains in daily living skills, self-care and behavioral functioning. Individuals placed with natural families did not do as well, it seems, as individuals placed in family care even though there appeared to be few differences between the two groups at the time of the initial placement. It should be pointed out, however, that natural families received far less follow-up and assistance from community service staff of the institution than did foster families. Furthermore, it seems that natural families have less access to community support services such as respite care, day programming, and recreation. Finally, because of the interference of institutional practices and parent attitudes, it seems that some families who may be better equipped to deal effectively with the retarded family member are discouraged from having the member return.

It seems reasonable to infer that if natural families could be provided with training, better support services and better financial assistance, they could become a viable placement option for retarded persons now in institutions. The relatively low cost of care in the natural family is one important motivation for the reconsideration of this option. The current changes in services to the mentally retarded call for increased releases from institutions, major improvements in the quality of institutions and development of alternatives to institutions. All of these elements of the deinstitutionalization movement are extremely expensive. Return to the natural family, even considering the cost of appropriate services and financial supports, may be the least expensive alternative available. Because of cost factors, it is possible that placement options such as family care and group homes eventually will come to be seen as alternatives to the natural family (as opposed to alternatives to institutions) to be used only when the family cannot cope effectively because of age or family difficulties. It is only current social beliefs and attitudes toward families of the mentally retarded which prevent this from happening.

References

Doll, W. Family coping with the mentally ill: An unanticipated problem of deinstitutionalization. *Hospital and Community Psychiatry,* 1976, *27,* 183-185.

Gollay, E., Freedman, R., Wyngaarden, M., & Kurtz, N. R. *Coming back.* Cambridge, MA: Abt Books, 1978.

Intagliata, J. C., Willer, B. S., & Cooley, F. Cost comparison of institutional and community based alternatives for mentally retarded persons. *Mental Retardation,* in press.

Mercer, J. R. Patterns of family crisis related to reacceptance of the retardate. *American Journal of Mental Deficiency,* 1966, *71,* 19-32.

Spivack, G., Haines, P. E., & Spotts, J. *Devereux Adolescent Behavior Rating Scale manual.* Devon, PA: The Devereux Foundation, 1967.

Willer, B. S., Intagliata, J. C., & Atkinson, A. C. The crisis of deinstitutionalization for families of the mentally retarded. *Mental Retardation,* in press.

Wyngaarden, M. & Gollay, E. A. *A study of the community adjustment of deinstitutionalized mentally retarded persons* (Vol. 4). Cambridge, MA: Abt Publications, 1976.

Factors Related to the Quality of Community Adjustment in Family Care Homes

James Intagliata
Barry Willer
Nancy Wicks

Division of Community Psychiatry
State University of New York at Buffalo

The current literature on community adjustment of formerly institutionalized mentally retarded persons is comprised of more than 175 studies spanning the last five decades. However, in spite of the fact that this topic has been the focus of so much study, the most recent review of this literature (Heal, Sigelman & Switzky, 1978) reports few, if any, agreed upon predictors of successful community adjustment. While the failure of this literature to identify the "recipe" for success has been attributed to a host of methodological inadequacies (Heal et al., 1978; McCarver & Craig, 1974), the present study will address just two of these problems.

First, while a number of researchers (Freedman, 1976; Sigelman, Bell, Schroenrock, Elias & Danker-Brown, 1978) have noted the need to approach community adjustment as having a variety of possible levels, the literature continues to be dominated almost exclusively by studies attempting to predict it as a dichotomous phenomenon. More specifically, the dichotomy defines success as tenure in the community and failure as reinstitutionalization. Thus, most of the currently available predictors of success, in fact, are just factors associated with a person's being able to remain in the community when placed there. Whether or not these same variables can predict the quality of life experienced by persons in the community, however, remains to be demonstrated.

A second major problem in the literature is that the typical approach taken by those conducting community placement studies has been to generate and compare aggregate descriptions of broad classes of community residential alternatives (e.g., family care homes, group homes) in an apparent effort to identify which is the "best" for mentally retarded persons. The meaning of "best" varies from one study to another but typically includes comparisons on such factors as recidivism rates, degree of client independence and reported client satisfaction.

While there is a need for these kinds of aggregate descriptions and broad comparisons, there are both limitations and problems with this approach. First, assignment of clients to the various placement types is generally non-random. In most cases, subjects assigned to the various facility types differ widely on factors relevant for adjustment, even from the point of their release from institutions. To the extent that the types of clients assigned to different residential alternatives vary, it might prove a more useful strategy to study what factors lead to successful adjustment within rather than across these residential types.

A second and perhaps more important issue is that the strategy of comparing across residential types implies that there is more variation between different types

---

This study was assisted under the Department of Health, Education, and Welfare, Region II, Office of Human Development, Developmental Disabilities Office, Grant No. 50P10568/2.

of settings than within a given setting type. Family care homes are treated as if they were a homogeneous class, as are group homes, or hostels. What research in New York State has led the writers to believe, however, is that there is a great variation in the environments provided by any given class of residences. In other words, once you have seen one family care home, you have *not* seen them all.

Finally, the strategy of comparing different placement types with each other suggests that the objectives of community placement are similar, if not identical, regardless of the setting. While there are clearly some general goals that should be common to any community placement, not enough has been done to highlight the fact that different settings provide different opportunities and experiences. The goals of placing someone in an independent apartment may not be the same as those for placement into a hostel. Moreover, placement into one type of family care home may have objectives different from those of another family care placement. This is not to suggest that comparisons between broad classes of placement types have no value, but rather, that too little attention has been given to documenting the variation of settings within these classes.

The study described here attempts to respond to some of the issues just raised. First of all, unlike most other studies of community placement, the sample for the present research excludes reinstitutionalized persons. Thus, by standards employed in previous studies all subjects could be assumed to have adjusted successfully to the community. This study, however, rejects this assumption and instead focuses on identifying those factors which account for variation in the level of adjustment of persons who have remained in the community.

Second, this study focuses on placements made to a single type of community residence, the family care home. In New York State, where the study was conducted, these homes have been the most frequently utilized community placement. At present there are over 1,600 such homes in the state serving over 4,800 mentally retarded residents. Similar foster or family care homes are provided for mentally retarded persons in 35 states (Hill, Sather, Kudla & Bruininks, 1978).

Focusing on family care homes the following important questions were addressed: 1) How can the quality of a family care home be conceptualized and measured? 2) Are there different ways to define quality and, if so, how do these definitions relate to each other? 3) What characteristics of care providers, clients and the community in which they live contribute to making some family care homes of higher quality than others?

Method

Subjects

A sample of subjects released from four developmental centers in New York State and placed into family care homes was selected for the present study. The following criteria were used for selecting this sample: 1) Subjects must have been placed into family care homes during the period from January 1, 1974 through December 31, 1976; 2) subjects had to have been institutionalized for one continuous year prior to their release; 3) subjects had to be 13 years or older at the time of release; and 4) subjects had to have remained in the community at least one continuous month following release. A total of 197 subjects from these centers met the criteria. Questionnaires were then mailed to the family care providers for each of these subjects. Of the 197 mailed, 141 (71%) were completed and returned. These returned forms provided information on 141 subjects who were cared for by

87 different providers. Following the return of these questionnaires, a care provider assessment scale was mailed to each social worker assigned to one of the 87 providers in the sample. These scales were completed on 77 (89%) of the providers who served 128 of the retarded residents in the study sample.

Residents. Of the 128 residents in these 77 homes, 33% were 30 years old or younger, 48% were from 31 to 60 years old, and 19% were older than 60. Their average age was 43. With respect to intellectual functioning 25% were mildly retarded, 21% moderately retarded, 45% severely retarded and 9% profoundly retarded. In regard to daily activities, 86% took part in structured programs outside of the home, with 19% attending school, 61% sheltered workshops or jobs, and 6% some combination of both.

Care Providers. All of the 77 care providers in the sample were female. Their average age was 55 with 70% of providers between the age of 40 and 60. Sixty-nine percent were married and, of the remaining single providers, 61% were widows. Of the care providers, 43% had less than a high school diploma while 14% were college graduates. Twenty-eight percent lived in urban-suburban areas, 38% in small towns, and 34% in rural areas. With respect to family income, the majority (55%) earned less than $12,000 annually, and only 9% earned more than $20,000. Further, 36% of respondents indicated that they and not their husbands were the primary family wage earner. With respect to the number of mentally retarded residents in each home, 38% had 1-2, 27% had 3-4, and 27% had 5 or more.

Raters. Social workers participating in the rating had worked with care providers for an average of six years with the range being from three months to 18 years.

Measures

There were two measurement instruments employed in this study. The first was a comprehensive questionnaire mailed to all family care providers in the sample. This questionnaire dealt with the following subject areas: 1) demographic information on providers; 2) residents' daily and leisure time activities; 3) changes in residents' self-care and social skill competency levels; 4) impact of the residents on care providers' home life and psychological well-being; and 5) the use of, obstacles to obtaining, and future needs for community-based support services.

The other instrument utilized in the study was a family care provider assessment scale. This scale was used to evaluate the care providers on nine facets of their performance as well as to provide a judgment regarding the overall quality of their work. The nine facets included in this scale deal with the following areas: 1) participating in the development and implementation of resident treatment plans; 2) encouraging client growth, independence and use of community resources; 3) relating to clients in a warm and caring manner; 4) the care provider's level of emotional stability and organization; and 5) her abilities in coping with both routine and non-routine client problems. This assessment scale was sent to the social workers assigned to each family care home in the study as well as to a smaller sample of nurses assigned to the homes attached to one institution.

The quality assessment scale was used for several purposes: 1) to identify social workers' views of what particular aspects of care provider performance contribute most significantly to overall quality; 2) to determine how, if at all, nurses' views on care provider quality differed from those of social workers; and 3) to determine if professionals' ratings of care provider quality were consistent with other commonly accepted approaches to assessing quality (e.g. amount of positive behavioral change in residents).

Together the comprehensive questionnaire and care provider assessment scale were used 1) to determine the extent and nature of variability within family care home environments and 2) to identify which factors (resident, care provider, community), if any, could discriminate between family care homes of varying quality.

Results

Family Care Provider Assessment Scale

Reliability of ratings. In order to determine the reliability of the quality assessment scale used, the independent ratings of nurses and social workers on 24 family care homes were compared. Results demonstrated substantial agreement on all aspects of the scale. The correlations of ratings for the nine individual scale items ranged from .66 to .80. The correlation between the two groups on the overall rating of the quality of the provider was .84.

Different views of quality. In order to assess the relative importance attached by social workers to each item in their overall perception of care provider quality, correlations of individual items with the overall rating were rank-ordered. The same procedure was followed with respect to the nurses' assessment scale ratings. The results of this comparison are presented in Table 1.

Table 1

Rank-Orders of Individual Items Correlation with Raters' Overall Assessment of Quality

Item	Social Workers (n = 77)	Nurses (n = 24)
Encouraging independence	9 (.51)	1 (.82)
Supporting new behaviors	8 (.59)	2 (.80)
Stability-organization	1 (.72)	4 (.77)
Knowledge of client needs	2 (.70)	7 (.71)
Warmth-caring	3 (.66)	3 (.77)
Coping with problems	4 (.63)	5 (.76)
Implementing treatment plans	6 (.62)	6 (.73)
Contributing to treatment plans	5 (.63)	9 (.61)
Encouraging use of community	7 (.60)	8 (.71)

This analysis suggests a number of thoughts for consideration. First, the correlations of individual items with the overall ratings of each group are consistently quite high. It would seem then that both social workers and nurses agree that all scale items represent important aspects of care provider quality. Second, while there are no startling differences between the groups with respect to the strength of correlations for particular items, there are some notable differences in the rank-orderings. The most striking differences are on the items "encouraging independence" and "supporting new behaviors." While the nurses apparently considered these the most important items in contributing to care provider quality, the social workers considered them the least important.

This difference, however, does not mean that social workers feel that it is unimportant for care providers to encourage new behaviors and independence in their clients. Rather, what it suggests is that while both social workers and nurses rate each item as important to overall quality, there may be real differences in the priorities the two groups assign to specific components of quality. Whether these differences are due to different professional training, the different roles played by nurses and social workers in monitoring these homes, or other factors cannot be determined here.

Differences According to Quality Measures

It was decided to divide the 77 providers into two groups based on the social workers' rating of their overall quality. Group one, "Lower Quality" (LQ) was comprised of those providers whose performance was rated as average or below average (n = 37). Group two, "High Quality" (HQ) were those providers who were rated as above or considerably above average in their performance (n = 40). Following the assignment of all providers, the two groups of providers were compared to determine 1) if there were any significant differences in the growth, activities, independence and social support of their residents and 2) which factors, if any, discriminated between lower and high quality family care environments.

Initial comparability of residents. Before proceeding with comparisons of the two groups on resident related characteristics, it is essential to address some basic aspects of their initial comparability. With respect to level of retardation there were no significant differences between the clients in HQ and LQ homes. In HQ homes 44% of clients were in the mild-moderate range and 56% in the severe and profound categories. In LQ homes it was essentially the same distribution with 47% of residents in the mild-moderate range and 53% in the severe-profound categories.

Comparisons were also made on a number of measures of client functioning which were administered to clients prior to the time of their release from the institutions. There were no statistically significant differences between the residents in HQ and LQ homes with respect to levels of skill in ambulation, speech, toileting, eating or dressing. Ratings of resident behavior problems (assaultive behavior, self-abuse, tantrums, destruction of property, running away, withdrawal, anxiety, stealing, sexual behavior, relating to peers and relating to authority) at the time of release were also compared. Again, no statistically significant differences were found.

Ratings of resident behavior made by care providers were also compared. Providers were asked to rate retrospectively the clients' problems at the time they first entered the home. Again there were no statistically significant differences between the two groups of providers in reports of client difficulties in either the basic areas of self-care, destruction of property, and disobedience, or in the higher skill areas of telephone use, meal preparation, money management or shopping. Although they were not statistically significant differences, LQ care providers were somewhat more likely to report resident problems in toileting (30% vs. 23%) while HQ providers were more likely to report difficulties in residents' travel behavior (60% vs. 44%).

In general, it appears that with respect to initial levels of functioning the clients placed into LQ homes were substantially similar to those placed in HQ homes. This similarity was borne out both by ratings administered by institutional personnel near the time of placement and by retrospective reports of the care providers themselves.

Resident behavioral change. Since improvement in client functioning is a readily accepted index of quality, it seemed essential to determine whether the two groups of homes identified by social worker ratings could be similarly discriminated by comparing client behavioral changes. Change in client functioning was assessed in two different ways. First of all, providers were asked to rate clients' level of difficulty in various behavioral areas both at the time the resident entered their home (retrospective) and at the point the questionnaire was completed (generally a period of two years). Table 2 presents a chi-quare comparison of the proportion of residents in lower vs. high quality homes whose functioning was reported to have improved in various behavioral areas.

Table 2

Comparison of Proportion of Residents with Initial Functioning Problems Who Improved

Behavior	Lower Quality	n	High Quality	n	p
Self-Care Skills					
Personal hygiene	66%	24	48%	21	.21
Toileting	53%	19	73%	11	.30
Behavior Control					
Disobedience	52%	21	37%	16	.41
Destructive behavior	57%	13	46%	14	.58
Community Skills					
Telephone use	20%	41	61%	36	.001*
Travel	24%	29	55%	29	.02 *
Meal preparation	24%	37	44%	25	.10 *
Shopping	35%	40	31%	32	.30
Money management	20%	41	29%	31	.27

*$p < .10$

First of all, this analysis suggests that significant numbers of clients in both lower and high quality family care homes are making improvements in levels of functioning. Second, and more important, however, there seem to be differences in the types of changes reported. In general, LQ providers are more likely to report resident improvement in behavioral control while HQ providers are consistently more likely to report improvement in residents' community living skills. However, the differences between the two groups are statistically significant only for the community living skills of telephone use ($p < .001$), travel ($p < .02$) and meal preparation ($p < .10$).

A second comparison of resident change in the two groups of homes was based primarily on differences in residents' Devereux Behavior Rating Scale scores. This scale was included in the comprehensive questionnaire and was completed by providers on all residents in the sample. The behavior ratings of residents in LQ homes were then compared with those in HQ homes. The results of this analysis are presented in Table 3.

Table 3

Comparison of Proportion of Residents with Abnormal Devereux Behavior Ratings

Subscale	Lower Quality (n=66)	High Quality (n=62)	p
Overcontrol			
Heterosexual interest	53%	42%	.25
Ability to delay	23%	13%	.20
Lack of Control			
Heterosexual interest	14%	2%	.02*
Bizarre actions	50%	29%	.03*
Hyperactivity	17%	7%	.08*
Domineer-sadistic	26%	10%	.02*
Defiant-resistive	18%	10%	.20

*p <.10

This table demonstrates that residents in LQ homes consistently show more inappropriate behavior than do residents in HQ homes. This inappropriate behavior manifests itself on both ends of the scale. On one end, residents of LQ care homes were more likely, though not significantly so, to show abnormal overcontrol of certain behaviors (heterosexual interest, ability to delay) than were residents in HQ homes. On the other end, residents in the LQ homes were significantly more likely to show abnormal lack of control of certain behaviors. These included heterosexual interest ($p = .02$), domineering-sadistic behavior ($p = .02$), bizarre action ($p = .02$) and hyperactivity ($p = .08$). Further, it should be noted that with respect to heterosexual interest, residents of lower quality homes were significantly more likely to show both abnormal overcontrol and lack of control.

One conclusion suggested by this analysis is that clients in HQ homes are significantly more likely to display *normal* behavior in a number of areas than are the residents of LQ homes. Unfortunately, since there were no Devereux rating on residents at the initial point of their placement, it is not known for sure whether these differences existed from the point they entered these homes or whether they developed over time in the community. However, according to behavioral ratings made by institutional personnel just prior to placement, the two groups of residents displayed an equal frequency of problems in areas (anxiety, hyperactivity, tantrums, sexual behavior and relating to others) which seem closely related to those on which they are now seen to differ consistently. While the ratings administered by institutional personnel by no means establish the behavioral equivalence of the two groups in a precise fashion, it would seem that the differences in normal behavior between the residents of lower and high quality homes may be at least, in part, a result of the style with which care providers manage their residents.

Residents' use of time. Another area of quality on which the two groups of homes was compared relates to residents' use of time. First of all, residents of lower and high quality care homes were compared with respect to how they regularly spent daytime hours during the week. Results of this comparison showed that residents of LQ homes are more likely to spend their day at home and not participate in structural day programs than are residents of HQ homes (27% vs. 3%, $\chi^2 = 9.4$, $p < .005$). Consistent with this finding is the care providers' report that significantly more residents in LQ homes than HQ homes have too much time on their hands (36% vs. 3%, $\chi^2 = 8.02$, $p < .005$). Residents of both types of homes, however, were equally likely to perform routine chores around the home.

With respect to use of leisure time, a comparison of residents' activities appears in Table 4. First of all, this table shows that regardless of the overall quality of the home, residents in family care are getting out into the community for a significant number of activities. In fact, the rates of activity participation reported for these residents of family care homes is much higher for all types of activity than those reported by Scheerenberger and Felsenthal (1976) for residents of other types of community-based facilities.

Table 4

Comparison of Residents' Activities

Activity	Lower Quality (n = 66)	High Quality (n = 62)	p
Restaurant	89%	97%	
Barber/beauty shop	86%	95%	
Church	71%	93%	.002*
Party	83%	90%	
Park	78%	70%	
Movie	43%	61%	.07 *
Amusement park	56%	61%	
Swimming	34%	46%	
Zoo	46%	44%	
Camp	33%	38%	
Ballgame	9%	31%	.005*
Museum	15%	30%	
Library	13%	23%	
Bar	3%	5%	

*p <.10

With respect to the present sample, however, this table shows that while residents of HQ homes are consistently more likely to engage in almost every activity, these differences are only statistically significant for attending church ($p = .002$), ballgames ($p = .005$), and movies ($p = .007$).

Level of independence. Another aspect of quality on which the two groups of homes were compared related to residents' level of independence. One measure dealing with independence was the question asking providers to indicate the highest level at which their residents could travel without supervision. There was no significant difference in the independence levels of the two groups of residents. While 47% of residents in LQ homes were restricted to house or yard, 37% of HQ residents were similarly constrained. With respect to use of public transportation, 22% of residents in LQ homes were able to do so without supervision as were 26% of HQ residents. The fact that relatively few residents in either group of homes are able to travel independently suggests that it is the care providers themselves who are responsible for arranging for resident transportation to the multitude of activities that were reported in Table 4.

The other measure relating to independence asked providers to indicate whether they often do things for residents that they could do on their own. Providers in LQ homes were more likely (24% vs. 12%) to report doing so although this was not a statistically significant difference ($\chi^2=1.7$, $p=.19$).

Social support. A final way to compare the quality of environments is to examine the type and degree of social support available to residents. It was found that residents of HQ homes had considerably more visits from parents or relatives within the last month (.84 vs. .42, $F=3.67$, $p < .01$). Further, although not significantly different statistically, it was found that while 42% of LQ residents had friends visit in the care home, 60% of HQ residents had similar visits.

Summary of relationships between quality measures. In general, it appears that the social workers' discrimination of quality in family care homes is both a reliable and valid measure. Its reliability is supported by the substantial agreement with independent ratings made by nurses. Its validity is supported by the fact that those homes rated as high quality are consistently superior to lower quality homes on other quality measures including ratings of residents' behavioral changes, use of time, level of independence, and social support. While differences between these two groups of homes on these measures are not always statistically significant, they consistently favor the high quality homes.

With respect to the specific behaviors which differentiate the two groups of providers, social workers' ratings suggest that high quality care providers when compared to lower quality providers are more likely to 1) be active in treatment planning, 2) be encouraging of clients' independence and use of services, 3) have residents improve in levels of behavioral functioning, 4) have residents actively using community resources, and 5) allow residents to behave as independently as they are capable.

Correlates of Family Care Home Quality

Resident factors. As already discussed, there were no significant differences between residents in LQ and HQ homes in level of intelligence, initial level of behavioral skills, or initial frequency of behavior problems. The only resident factor on which the two groups were significantly different was age. Residents of LQ homes were significantly older (average age 48) than residents of HQ homes (average age 38) ($F=2.15$, $df=69$, $p<.04$). More specifically, 32% of residents in LQ homes compared with 10% of HQ residents were 60 years of age or older.

Since there was a significant age difference between the residents in the two groups of homes, further analyses were conducted to determine if previously reported differences between HQ and LQ homes in client growth and living were due to the resident age differential. Results of these analyses showed that client age could not in itself account for differences between the two groups in the amount or type of behavior change reported. Further, it did not account for observed differences in level of independence or degree of social support available to the residents of the two groups of homes. The only difference between the LQ and HQ residents which may have been due to age was the degree of their participation in structured day programs outside of the home. Older residents ($>$ 40 years of age) were much more likely than younger ones ($\leq$ 40 years of age) to stay at home during the day ($\chi^2 = 4.87$, $p < .05$).

In general, it would appear that the differences observed between HQ and LQ homes in residents' behavior change, and overall quality of life cannot be attributed to differences in the residents themselves. Thus, to explain the differences care provider and community characteristics must be examined.

Care provider characteristics. There was no significant difference in the average age of LQ care providers and HQ providers. However, HQ care providers were somewhat more likely (25%) to be 61 or older than were LQ providers (10%). With respect to marital status, again the groups do not differ significantly. However, HQ providers are somewhat more likely to be single than are LQ providers (38% vs. 28%). A comparison of income levels shows the two groups to be almost identical with average income for LQ providers being $12,000 and for HQ providers $11,400.

Notable differences between the two groups of providers begin to emerge, however, when education level, experience and motivation for their role are examined. With respect to education HQ providers attended school longer than did LQ providers. More specifically, HQ providers were significantly more likely to have finished high school than were LQ providers (69% vs. 47%, $\chi^2 = 3.8$, $p = .05$). In addition, HQ providers were significantly more likely to have attended college (32% vs. 11%, $\chi^2 = 5.3$, $p < .025$).

With respect to experience which they felt prepared them for their role, there were no significant differences between the two groups. However, HQ providers were more likely than LQ providers to have had health related training (45% vs. 30%).

Although not significant, differences were also found between the two groups in their reasons for becoming a provider, Table 5 demonstrates that LQ providers were more likely than HQ providers to report their need for money (28% vs. 15%) or their desire to just take care of someone (43% vs. 28%) as major motivating factors. On the other hand, HQ providers were more likely to indicate their past experience in working with the mentally retarded (33% vs. 19%) or having had a mentally retarded relative (23% vs. 9%) as major motivating factors.

Table 5

Reasons for Becoming a Family Care Provider

Reason	Lower Quality (n=37)	High Quality (n=40)
Have worked with the mentally retarded	19%	33%
Wanted someone to care for	44%	28%
Have or had mentally retarded relative	9%	23%
Needed extra money	28%	15%

A final area in which lower and high quality providers were compared relates to the burdens and benefits which they have felt with their job. The comparison between the two groups on reported burden is presented in Table 6. Results of this analysis showed that while none of the differences for specific items was statistically significant, LQ care providers were more likely than HQ providers to report most types of burdens. More specifically, LQ providers are more likely to report difficulties in managing the resident, being solely responsible for caring for residents and neglecting responsibilities to other family members. On the other hand, HQ providers are somewhat more likely to report difficulties with getting free time away from residents.

Table 6

Resident Burden in Family Care

Burden	Lower Quality (n=37)	High Quality (n=31)
Resident care falls on me alone	76%	61%
More supervision than expected	32%	21%
It's difficult to go out alone	28%	35%
Resident is difficult to manage	24%	7%
Neglectful of responsibilities to family	18%	3%
Neighbors make remarks	14%	9%
Have to do without because of money	16%	19%
Caring for resident has been financial burden	12%	7%
Disagreement about caring for resident	12%	7%
Difficulties with relatives	8%	3%
Family members are less willing to invite others home	4%	0%

With respect to reported benefits there are no major differences between LQ and HQ providers. The majority of both groups reported that living with residents had increased their understanding of mental retardation (96%) and had enriched their family life (78%). However, LQ providers were more likely than HQ providers (71% vs. 58%) to report that residents help keep them from being lonely.

Community characteristics. Though not a statistically significant difference, LQ providers are somewhat more likely to live in rural areas than are HQ providers (46% vs. 26%). Given this fact it was expected that LQ providers might tend to report that support services were less often available or more difficult to obtain. However, when reports of service unavailability from LQ and HQ providers are compared, there were no significant differences between the two groups in the availability of physical therapy, speech therapy, recreational activities, special bus service or counseling services. However, LQ providers are more likely to report that speech therapy and physical therapy are unavailable to residents while HQ providers are more likely to report recreational activities as unavailable.

In addition to availability, service use was also reported by providers. Just as with availability, there are no significant differences between the two groups of providers with respect to their use of services. However, HQ providers are more likely than LQ providers (71% vs. 50%) to report use of recreational services even though HQ providers had indicated that such services were less likely to be available to their residents. The only service which LQ providers reported using more frequently than HQ providers was counseling for the residents in their home (36% vs. 16%).

A final area of service use on which providers were compared is respite care. Results of questions in this area showed that HQ providers are significantly more likely to have taken a respite from their residents than are LQ providers (97% vs. 80%, $\chi^2 = 3.89$, $p = .05$). The reasons given by LQ providers for not taking respite included difficulty in finding someone both qualified and willing as well as the cost of such respite care. Consistent with these reports, when asked if they would consider leaving their residents at the institutions if respite beds were provided there, LQ providers were significantly more likely to respond affirmatively than were HQ providers (38% vs. 18%, $\chi^2 = 3.93$, $p = .05$).

Summary of correlates with care provider quality. In this study a number of differences were found between high quality and lower quality providers. In general, high quality providers were more likely to 1) be better educated, 2) have had health related training, 3) be motivated to take the job because of past experiences in relating to or working with the mentally retarded, 4) to live in urban areas, 5) more readily seek out services and activities for their residents, 6) actively involve themselves in resident treatment planning, 7) establish a stable, well-organized home, 8) establish warm, supportive, but not dependent relationships with residents, and 9) encourage residents to use community resources and develop new skills.

Conversely, lower quality care providers are more likely to 1) be less educated, 2) have only the experience of raising their own children as background, 3) be motivated to take the job because of wanting someone to care for or as a means of extra income, 4) live in rural areas, 5) be less likely to use services for residents, even when available, 6) be less involved in resident treatment planning, 7) have a more unstable, less organized home, 8) establish dependent relationships with clients to avoid loneliness, and 9) be less concerned with residents' developing new living skills and more concerned that residents' unruly behavior is managed.

Discussion

The goals of the present study were to begin to explore the concept of successful adjustment in a more qualitative fashion and to identify and attempt to explain variation in the quality of a single placement type, the family care home. In general, these objectives were achieved.

Perhaps the most important component of the study was the family care provider assessment scale which was completed by the caseworkers assigned to each home in the study. The use of this scale demonstrated two important points. First of all, it provided an opportunity to demonstrate that the concept of quality in a family care home may be viewed in different ways by different groups. While the quality ratings of social workers gave strongest weighting to provider involvement in treatment planning and organization, nurses gave highest priority to providers' activities to facilitate client growth and independence. If the views of still other groups were sought (e.g., parents of residents, care providers themselves), it is likely that new and different orderings of priorities would emerge. However, while the different priorities reflect various perspectives on what components are most essential to quality, the results of this study demonstrated that even groups with somewhat different perspectives substantially agree in their discrimination of lower and high quality family care homes.

A second point which became clear was that it is possible not only to develop a reliable measure of family care provider quality but a measure that seems quite valid as well. Using social workers' judgments based on this scale, it was possible to identify successfully those homes in which 1) more resident growth took place, 2) more normal resident behavior was exhibited, 3) more residents used available community resources, 4) more client independence was fostered, and 5) more social support was available to residents. Thus, this study demonstrates the convergence of five separate indices of quality in the homes judged superior by social workers' assessment scale ratings.

Perhaps even more important than the success in designing a reliable, valid measure of quality, however, is the fact that a set of predictors of genuine success in family care has begun to emerge. The majority of studies of family care to date have utilized community tenure as the criterion for success (Bishop, 1957; Brown, Windle & Stewart, 1959; Gray & Parr, 1957; Meyer, 1951; Sternlicht, 1978; Windle, 1962). Results of their studies suggest that success in family care is most likely to be achieved with older clients (Hiatt, 1957; Sternlicht, 1978; Windle, 1962) and when care homes are located in rural areas (Jackson & Butler, 1963; Krishef, 1959).

However, in the present study in which success was defined in terms of normalization and the developmental model, rather than as mere community tenure, quite different results were found for these two predictors. With respect to age, although younger clients were reported to present more management problems, they seemed to be living a more active and perhaps more satisfying life than older clients. More specifically, they were more likely to participate in day programs and leisure-time activities outside the home as well as have more friendships. With respect to location of care provider homes, rural locations were associated with *less* not more community involvement. Together, these findings show that the factors identified as predictive of successful placement depend greatly on the way in which success itself is defined.

While there was an indication that resident and community variables had some impact on quality, it appears that characteristics of the care providers themselves play a more crucial role in determining the adjustment made by family care residents. This is not a startling finding when one thinks about it, but unfortunately, the care provider has not been treated as a major factor in most previous work. Interestingly, the only previous follow-up study (Windle, Sabagh, Brown & Dingman, 1961) assessing the impact of care provider characteristics on success in family care found no significant relationships. However, again, success was defined as community tenure rather than in the more qualitative fashion used in this study. Hopefully, future research into family care placement will continue to use both qualitative measures of success as well as attend to the impact of care provider characteristics.

The suggestions made here regarding the focus of future studies of family care home placement should also be applied to research on the adjustment of mentally retarded persons living in other residential settings. There is, in fact, already evidence which indicates that the substantial variation observed in family care home environments is also present within other types of community residential facilities (Bjaanes & Butler, 1974; Butler & Bjaanes, 1977). What is needed then, are studies which will identify those particular facets of each type of setting that seem to facilitate the community adjustment of its residents. Indeed, it is possible that the particular environmental factors which facilitate adjustment will vary from one type of setting to another. However, if future research takes a more setting-specific focus, it is likely that a more complex but consistent picture of the community adjustment process will emerge.

References

Bishop, E. G. Family care: The patients. *American Journal of Mental Deficiency*, 1957, *61*, 583-591.

Bjaanes, A. T. & Butler, E. W. Environmental variation in community care facilities for mentally retarded persons. *American Journal of Mental Deficiency*, 1974, *78*, 429-439.

Brown, S. J., Windle, C., & Stewart, E. Statistics on a family care program. *American Journal of Mental Deficiency*, 1959, *64*, 535-542.

Butler, E. W. & Bjaanes, A. T. A typology of community care facilities and differential normalization outcomes. In P. Mittler (Ed.), *Research to practice in mental retardation: Care and intervention* (Vol. 1). Baltimore, MD: University Park Press, 1977.

Freedman, R. *Approaches to defining and measuring the community adjustment of mentally retarded persons: A review of the literature*. Cambridge, MA: Abt Associates Inc., September 1976. (Project report)

Gray, P. A. & Parr, E. A. *Children in care and the recruitment of foster parents*. Social Survey, S. S. 249, London, 1957.

Heal, L. W., Sigelman, C. K., & Switzky, H. N. Research on community residential alternatives for the mentally retarded. In N. R. Ellis (Ed.), *International review of research in mental retardation* (Vol. 9). New York: Academic Press, 1978.

Hiatt, M. S. Casework services in community placement of defectives. *American Journal of Mental Deficiency*, 1951, *56*, 204-211.

Hill, B. K., Sather, L. B., Kudla, M. J., & Bruininks, R. H. A survey of the types of residential programs for mentally retarded people in the United States in 1978. Unpublished paper of the Developmental Disabilities Project on Residential Services and Community Adjustment, University of Minnesota, September, 1978.

Jackson, S. K. & Butler, A. J. Prediction of successful community placement of institutionalized retardates. *American Journal of Mental Deficiency*, 1973, *68*, 211-2117.

Krishef, C. H. The influence of rural-urban environment upon the adjustment of discharges from Owatonna State School. *American Journal of Mental Deficiency*, 1959, *63*, 860-865.

McCarver, R. B. & Craig, E. M. Placement of the retarded in the community: Prognosis and outcome. In N. R. Ellis (Ed.), *International review of research in mental retardation* (Vol. 7). New York: Academic Press, 1974.

Meyer, G. A. Twelve years of family care at Belchertown State School. *American Journal of Mental Deficiency*, 1951, *55*, 414-417.

Scheerenberger, R. C. & Felsenthal, P. *A study of alternative community placements*. Madison, WI: Central Center for the Developmentally Disabled, September, 1976. (Project report)

Sigelman, C., Bell, N., Schoenrock, C., Elias, S., & Danker-Brown, P. Alternative community placements and outcomes. Paper presented at the annual meeting of the American Association on Mental Deficiency, Denver, Colorado, May 19, 1978.

Sternlicht, M. Variables affecting foster care placement of institutionalized retarded residents. *Mental Retardation*, 1978, *16*(1), 25-28.

Windle, C. Prognosis of mental subnormals. *American Journal of Mental Deficiency Monograph Supplement*, 1962, *66*, 1-180.

Windle, C. D., Sabagh, G., Brown, S. J. & Dingman, H. F. Caretaker characteristics and placement success. *American Journal of Mental Deficiency*, 1961, *65*, 739-743.

IV. Research on Providing and Evaluating Community Placements

Foster Family Care for Mentally Retarded People: A Qualitative Review

James Intagliata

Nancy Crosby

Linda Neider

Division of Community Psychiatry
State University of New York at Buffalo

Foster family care homes are currently one of the most widely used alternatives to institutional placement for mentally retarded persons. However, despite the expanded use and changing nature of this residential alternative, as well as the increased research attention it has received, there have been no recent efforts to integrate and review the growing literature on family care. The present paper provides such a review. Specifically, the authors (1) briefly review the history and rationale for the use of foster family care, (2) describe the characteristics of foster family care providers and the mentally retarded persons living in their homes, (3) review the research on the quality of life for mentally retarded residents living in foster family care and the factors related to this quality, and (4) discuss recent developments as well as future directions in the use of this important residential alternative for mentally retarded persons.

"Family care" as used in this review, generally refers to a program administered by a state's department of mental hygiene, mental retardation, or health (or an equivalent department) which involves the placement of mentally retarded persons into specially licensed or approved private homes. Typically, the number of residents in any given home does not exceed six. Although a large number of mentally retarded persons are served in generic foster care programs, such programs will not be considered in this paper.

History of Family Care Placement

The use of private family homes for the foster care of mentally disabled persons was begun in the sixth century in the city of Geel, Belgium (Caplan, 1969; Smitson, 1970). However, family care homes were not used for the mentally disabled in the United States until the late 19th century. While these homes served mental patients in Massachusetts as early as 1885 (Vaux, 1935) it was not until 1931 in New York that they were used as an alternative to institutions for mentally retarded persons (Heal, Sigelman & Switzky, 1978). Early family care programs typically involved a selected group of high functioning residents of institutions who were placed with rural families to share their home and assist in their farming chores. As suggested by Pollock (1940, 1947), these programs had a number of benefits. First, family care homes were thought to provide a more natural and congenial life for retarded persons. In addition, family care placements offered a means of providing socially beneficial employment to families in the community and a lessened need for institutions, thus reducing costs to the state.

Interest in and use of family care placement for mentally retarded persons declined somewhat during the 1940s and 1950s. A number of factors were probably responsible. Adams (1971) suggested that the country's preoccupation with the problems of World War II and unemployment drew national attention away from retarded people. Kraus (1978) noted that the increasing mechanization of farm work may have made placement of retarded persons less desirable for rural families. In addition, during this period there was a backlash against community placement among professionals who felt that the lack of available facilities, adequate supervision and sufficient state and local funding made continued community placement unwise (Doll, 1962).

A number of social forces came together in the 1960s to set the stage for widespread deinstitutionalization of mentally disabled individuals in this country. Though this trend was initiated earlier and more extensively for the mentally ill (Conroy, 1977), significant numbers of mentally retarded persons were also released from institutions and placed in the community. Once again, family care homes became a popular placement alternative for mentally retarded persons. Between 1960 and 1966 alone, nine states established family care programs for mentally retarded residents. By 1966 more than 5,700 mentally retarded persons in 26 states were living in family care homes (Morissey, 1966).

In the 1970s the number of mentally retarded persons leaving institutions continued to increase at a steady rate. This continued deinstitutionalization effort led to the accelerated use of family care homes throughout the country. In New York State, for example, the number of family care residents increased almost 300% between 1970 (1,259) and 1975 (3,694) (New York State Plans of Compliance, 1975). According to a recent national survey (Bruininks, Hill & Thorsheim, 1980) an estimated 8,600 mentally retarded persons were living in family care homes in 21 states as of 1977. Further, the authors reported that by the end of 1978 the number of states making use of specially licensed foster care homes for mentally retarded persons had reached 32.

The current rationale for utilizing family care homes is not unlike that offered by Pollock (1947) more than 30 years ago. Family care is seen as the most normalized placement for an individual who is capable of living in a home-like setting, but whose own family cannot provide it (Adams, 1970; Nirje, 1969). It is also felt that family care offers retarded individuals an important opportunity to become integrated within a family and a community (Adams, 1975; Birch & Belmont, 1961; Garrett, 1966, 1970; Stedman & Eichorn, 1964). Further, it has been suggested that placement into family care homes rather than institutions may make it easier for natural family members to keep in contact and perhaps eventually reunite with their mentally retarded relative (Adams, 1970; Garrett, 1970). Finally, when compared with other community-based residential alternatives, family care homes represent a relatively inexpensive option (Baker, Seltzer & Seltzer, 1974; Bruininks et al., 1980; Gardner, 1977; Heal & Daniels, 1978; Intagliata, Willer & Cooley, 1979).

While the current rationale for using family care is generally consistent with that of the past, there is some indication that changes are occurring within the family care model. In the early years, family care programs generally had a custodial orientation. Placements were primarily made in rural areas that did not allow residents any significant amount of community participation. Such an approach was consistent with the prevailing treatment philosophies of the times.

With the recent deinstitutionalization movement and widespread acceptance of the normalization principle, however, the emphases within family care programs have begun to shift. A number of family care programs have begun actively to develop the habilitative potential of family care home environments for their residents (Adams, 1975; Baker et al., 1974; Willer & Intagliata, 1979). In some cases, these homes are now intended to serve as transitional settings in which residents can acquire the self-care and community living skills necessary for moving on to more independent living situations within the community. For other residents who may not move to other settings, the habilitative emphasis is intended to make family care homes less restrictive environments.

Thus, family care is a community residential model in transition. As a model that has been used for almost 50 years, it is currently staffed by care providers who have begun their work at different points in time, with different treatment philosophies to guide them. Accordingly, there is presently wide variation in the purpose, character and quality of family care home environments.

Care Providers

A general profile of foster family care providers who serve the mentally retarded can be drawn from existing research. While the majority of family care providers are married couples, it is usually the female head of household who has assumed the major responsibility for care. As a result, most of the research describing care providers has focused on the characteristics of the female care provider. Characteristics reviewed here include age, marital/parental status, education, motivation, background/training, and location of home.

Age

The majority of studies report providers to be middle-aged or older (Smitson, 1970). More specifically, Parks (1959) reported the average age of his care provider sample as 49, while the average age reported in a recent study of New York State care providers (Intagliata, Willer & Wicks, 1979) was 55. Other studies (Intagliata, 1978; Meyers, Lei, Nihira & Eyman, 1979; Windle, Sabagh, Brown & Dingman, 1961) have consistently reported that most care providers are 50 years of age or older. Meyers et al. (1979) reported that two-thirds of their sample of California family care providers were at least 50 and almost all were over 30.

While there is an extensive literature reporting the characteristics of generic foster care providers the present review focuses exclusively on the characteristics of providers who serve the mentally retarded. In one of the few studies comparing different groups of providers, Rich (1965) found that foster care providers for mentally retarded persons were somewhat older than those caring for normal children and were typically part of well-settled family units rather than young couples.

Marital/Parental Status

The majority of care providers are reported to be married. Specifically, Lei, Sheehy and Wilson (1980) reported that 80% of their care provider sample were married. Similarly, Intagliata, Willer and Wicks (1979) reported that 69% of their sample were married, with the majority of single care providers being widows. With regard to parental status, Justice, Bradley and O'Connor (1971) reported that 93% of their foster care provider sample had raised their own children. Other studies (Intagliata, Willer & Cooley, 1979; Meyers et al., 1979) support this finding by reporting that the majority of their care providers in their samples had families of their own.

Education

Earlier studies typically reported that foster care providers had limited educations, often below that of the general population (Fanshel, 1961; Gray & Paar, 1957; Maas & Engler, 1959; Parks, 1959). More recently, it has been reported that the majority of providers have completed high school (Rich, 1965; Windle et al., 1961). The most recent studies have indicated that 12th grade is the average or the median education level of foster care provider samples (Gollay, Freedman, Wyngaarden & Kurtz, 1978; Meyers et al., 1979), with Intagliata (1978) reporting that 18% of providers he studied were college graduates.

The trend of these reports indicates that the education level of foster care providers is shifting gradually upward. Further, providers as a group now vary widely in their education level, including persons who never finished high school as well as those with four-year college or even graduate degrees. As indicated by Adams (1975), current trends suggest that the number of old style foster parents (i.e., little education, lower socioeconomic status) may be decreasing while a more intellectually sophisticated population of foster care providers is developing. This shift coincides with a much broader trend toward greater professionalization within foster care programs. This trend will be discussed at greater length later in this paper.

Motivation

Generally, the motivations that family care providers have most frequently identified for taking the job have been altruistic ones. Specific examples include wanting the personal satisfaction that comes from caring for someone (Culley, Settles & Van Name, 1975; Fanshel, 1966; Intagliata, 1978; Intagliata, Willer & Wicks, 1979; Jaffee, 1970; Mamula & Newman, 1973; Scheerenberger, 1976) or from knowing that you are doing something useful for the community (Culley et al., 1975; Fanshel, 1966; Jaffee, 1970; Madison & Schapiro, 1969). Public attitudes about foster care providers seem to be in agreement with these reports. Dick (1961) reported that most people believe that altruistic motives (e.g., love of children) more so than financial ones lead people to become care providers.

An additional factor that may motivate individuals to become care providers specifically for the mentally retarded is having had prior direct experience with the mentally retarded. Justice et al. (1971) reported that 32% of their foster care provider sample had a mentally retarded family member, while Rich (1965) noted that one-third of her sample had their own retarded child already living with them. Other studies report that many foster care providers for mentally retarded persons have either had close contact (Garrett, 1970) or had previously worked with mentally retarded persons before becoming a care provider (Intagliata, 1978; Intagliata, Willer & Wicks, 1979).

Other motivations attributed to foster care providers for taking their role suggest that the work may provide a special opportunity for caretakers to meet some of their own personal needs. For example, some authors (Fanshel, 1960; Kay, 1966) have suggested that many providers take on the caring role in order to undo the deprivation that they themselves experienced in childhood. In support of this explanation, Rich (1965) found that in 75% of foster care homes studies, at least one foster care provider had been raised in a single parent home. Another possible personal motivation identified by many professional staff who recruit and supervise providers is that older married couples may take the job in order to re-experience the parenthood role in which they have found great satisfaction. There is some research evidence to support this assertion, albeit indirectly. Babcock (1965) in a further analysis of 50 foster families from Fanshel's (1960) study sample, noted that the couples had typically married at a young age, had their own children early, and that their marriage had strongly emphasized the parental role. Further, Justice et al. (1971) noted that the majority of the foster care providers in their sample had come from large families. One additional personal factor that may motivate some providers to take on the role is the desire for companionship. A number of foster care providers, especially widows, have reported that one benefit they have received is being able to share their home with another person without whom they might otherwise feel lonely (Intagliata, Willer & Wicks, 1979; Mamula & Newman, 1973).

It is not surprising that the family care literature identifies altruism as the primary motivation of most care providers, given that they have traditionally received only reimbursement for the room and board costs of their residents. However, the recent shift of orientation in some family care programs may begin to alter the motivations of individuals electing to become care providers. Specifically, a number of programs have begun to take steps to make family care homes a more active treatment setting by paying trained providers a salary (in addition to resident room/board costs) for providing intensive, individualized training activities for their residents (Baker et al., 1974; Lei, Sheehy & Wilson, 1979; Willer & Intagliata, 1979). As a result, care providers may receive a salary ranging from $150-$300 a month per resident for providing services, depending on the level of resident need. These changes clearly give foster family care a more professional image as well as make it more financially rewarding. Thus it may gradually begin to attract a pool of new providers with different motivations than have traditionally been reported.

Background/Training

Providing foster family care has frequently been viewed as an intuitive activity which draws upon the kinds of skills developed in raising one's own children. Indeed, in a number of studies family care providers have reported that their own experience as parents was their major preparation for the care provider role (Intagliata, 1978; Scheerenberger, 1976). Nevertheless, a significant number of providers in most studies have reported more specialized preparation. Most frequently they report the experience of having worked in health related institutions that serve the kinds of disabled persons for whom they later provide foster family care. The proportion of family care providers for mentally retarded persons who have reported such prior experience has varied from 18% (Scheerenberger, 1976) to 26% (Intagliata, Willer & Wicks, 1979) to 36% (Windle et al., 1961) to 71% (Justice et al., 1971). Generally, however, while some providers have had health-related care experience, few have had any formal training to prepare them for their role.

The need to develop specialized training for foster care providers serving the mentally retarded has been acknowledged repeatedly (Dick, 1961; Garrett, 1966; Guerny, 1977; Intagliata, 1978; Mamula, 1970; Mamula & Newman, 1973). This need has become even more pressing as ongoing deinstitutionalization has resulted in widespread use of these homes for formerly institutionalized mentally retarded persons of all ages and levels of disability (Baker et al., 1974; Gollay, Friedman, Wyngaarden & Kurtz, 1978; Willer, Intagliata & Wicks, 1979).

In response to the need, a number of training programs have been developed to assist providers in preparing for the demands of their role. Further, recent reports

(Baker et al., 1974; Meyers et al., 1979; Willer & Intagliata, 1979) suggest that family care providers are increasingly likely to be offered such training. While these programs will not be discussed in detail in this paper, a thorough review of currently available training packages is presented elsewhere in this monograph.

Location of Homes

As described previously, in earlier years almost all family care placements were made in rural areas. Such a practice was consistent with the then prevailing institutional model of care which, among other purposes, sought to segregate mentally retarded persons from the mainstream of community life. However, following the shift in service ideology there is evidence that family care homes are now more evenly distributed among communities of varying size.

Two states that have made quite extensive use of family care homes illustrate this point. In New York, which has the largest family care program for mentally retarded persons in this country, 44% of the homes are still located in rural areas or small towns. However, 29% are in small cities (2,500-50,000), 9% in somewhat larger cities (50,000-250,000) and 18% in major urban/suburban centers (>250,000) (Bruininks et al., 1980). In California, which has also made widespread use of family care homes, Eyman and Begab (1979) indicated that the majority of the homes they studied were located in suburban areas. Nationwide, while more foster care homes tend to be located in smaller communities, a significant proportion are now distributed among cities of intermediate and large size (Bruininks et al., 1980). Though they are much more likely to be located in rural areas, the diversity in the size of the communities in which family care homes are now located is similar to that reported for other community residential facilities (O'Connor, 1976).

These findings reflect the changing orientation within family care programs to locate new homes so as to facilitate participation of the residents in community life (Lei et al., 1980; NYS Department of Mental Hygiene, 1976). Hence, just as family care philosophy once reflected the prevailing institutional model of care it has now begun to shift to become more consistent with the current model of community based care.

Residents

Until recently there had been no reliable estimates of either the number or personal characteristics of the large number of mentally retarded persons living in family care homes in this country. However, a recently completed survey (Bruininks et al., 1980)[1] fills this void and provides the most comprehensive national data available. As noted earlier, this survey indicated that as of 1977 there were more than 8,600 mentally retarded persons living in specially licensed family care homes in 21 states. Based on the responses of those providers who returned the survey it is possible to construct a basic profile of these residents' characteristics.

Age

Because generic foster care programs have traditionally served children, many persons have assumed that family care homes for mentally retarded persons also serve a similar age group. The data provided by Bruininks et al. (1980) clearly indicate that this assumption is inaccurate. Specifically, of the more than 5,700 family care residents surveyed, 36% are 40 years of age or older, 25.3% are 22-39 years of age, 17.9% are 15-21 years old and just 20.9% are younger than 15.

These data reflect the fact that while family care homes have been used as a residential alternative for children and adolescents unable to remain with their natural families, they have increasingly served as a community placement for formerly institutionalized mentally retarded adults. This is particularly true in New York State where family care homes have been used as placements for formerly institutionalized persons to such an extent that 54% of mentally retarded family care residents are 40 years of age or older.

When these data on family care residents' age are compared with those of mentally retarded persons living in other community residential alternatives, they suggest that family care has been more widely used as a placement for older individuals. Specifically, O'Connor (1976) reported that the vast majority (75%) of mentally retarded persons living in community residences (group homes, hostels, boarding and halfway houses) were 17-34 years of age. Only 17% of persons in community residences were 40 years of age or older (O'Connor, 1976) compared with 36% of family care residents (Bruininks et al., 1980). Given that family care homes are also widely used for children and adolescents, these data reaffirm the observation of McCarver and Craig (1974) that family care placements have typically involved the extremes in terms of resident age.

Level of Retardation

Morissey (1966) reported that mildly and moderately retarded persons were given placement preference in the majority of family care programs. This is understandable given that there were a large number of higher functioning persons being released from public institutions at the time his survey was conducted. As deinstitutionalization has proceeded, however, the proportion of severely and profoundly retarded persons being placed in the community has increased. Consequently, the proportion of more severely retarded persons living in family care homes has also increased. According to Bruininks, Hill and Thorsheim (1980), 35.1% of mentally retarded persons living in family care homes in 1977 were severely or profoundly retarded, 37.9% were moderately retarded and only 26.7% were in the mild or borderline category.

The comparison of these results with data on the level of retardation of persons placed into the other small community residences surveyed by O'Connor (1976) suggest that severely and profoundly impaired individuals are more likely to have been placed in family care homes. Specifically, the severely and profoundly retarded comprised 35.2% of family care residents (Bruininks et al., 1980) as compared with only 19.2% of those in other small community residences (O'Connor, 1976). At the upper level of intellectual functioning, 52.8% of persons in community residences were reportedly in the mild, borderline or normal categories (O'Connor, 1976) compared with just 26.7% of family care residents (Bruininks et al., 1980).

Together, the data on age and level of retardation suggest that while family care homes serve a diverse resident population they are much more likely to serve older and more severely retarded persons that are other small group residential alternatives. Unfortunately, comparisons between family care homes and other community residential alternatives have frequently been made without adequate attention being given to differences in the resident populations served.

Additional Physical and Behavioral Characteristics

Bruininks et al. (1980) also describe selected physical and behavioral characteristics of family care residents. According to their survey, 15.4% could not talk, 5.9% were not toilet trained and 4.8% were non-ambulatory. In addition, behavior problems were reported for 10.6% of all residents. Further, a significant proportion reportedly had secondary handicaps including deafness (3.9%), blindness (2.7%), epilepsy (8.4%), cerebral palsy (4.3%) or autistic traits (2.9%). The proportions of family care residents with these behavior deficits and additional handicaps are similar to those reported for persons in other small community residences (O'Connor, 1976).

Quality of Life in Family Care

The research on the community adjustment of mentally retarded persons has focused on a number of different aspects of residents' lives. The concerns regarding resident adjustment relate to aspects of normalization and the developmental model as well as general client satisfaction. More specifically, studies have explored the degree to which mentally retarded persons in the community (1) live, work and recreate in a fashion consistent with the rest of the community, (2) progress in the development of adaptive behavior (self-care, community living skills) that will enable them to live as independently as they are capable and (3) are personally satisfied with their lives. In a more general sense, these aspects can be considered to define the quality of life for mentally retarded persons living in the community.

This section will review research findings regarding the quality of life of mentally retarded persons living in family care homes. The particular aspects that will be discussed include (1) life within the family care home, (2) the extent of residents' interaction/integration with the community, (3) changes in resident adaptive behavior, and (4) recidivism and movement of residents. Findings regarding residents' own reports of satisfaction in family care homes will be presented when available.

Life Within the Home

Based on their study of 55 homes Baker et al. (1974) concluded that most residents had been well-integrated and accepted into the family units. However, they also reported that many residents had assumed dependent childlike roles within the family and that most lived passively within the home rarely assuming any responsibilities for even routine household chores. In general, relative to other community residential alternatives examined, the authors concluded that family care offered a passive and overprotective community living environment. However, the authors noted that the greater degree of protection reported may, in part, have been a reasonable reflection of the fact that more severely retarded persons were placed in family care homes than in any other type of setting studied.

Bjaanes and Butler (1974) conducted an intensive study of resident and care provider behavior in two family care homes. While they found that residents in both homes routinely had assigned household chores, they reported that the homes differed significantly on a number of other dimensions. One such dimension was the proportion of resident behavior that was spent in passive leisure or other isolating activities versus the proportion spent in active, interactive activities. In one home 89% of all resident behavior was found to be active-interactive while just 6% was passive-isolating. In the other home, however, only 38% of resident behavior was active-interactive, while 44% was passive-isolating. Another behavior dimension studied was the degree to which residents behaved independently (acting without relying on others for cues and assistance). Again, results showed significant differences between the behavior of residents in the two homes. In both cases, the authors attributed these results to specific differences in the styles of the care providers in the two homes.

The work of Butler and Bjaanes (1974, 1977) highlighted the wide variation that exists in the environments of family care homes as well as other community residential settings. Their findings suggest that broad statements intended to characterize all settings within a given residential type are likely to be misleading. Thus, there is a need for research efforts which focus on determining the extent of environmental variation and how it relates to effectiveness.

Willer and Intagliata (1980) studied a sample of 229 residents in 140 different family care homes throughout New York State. Consistent with other studies (Baker et al., 1974; Newman & Sherman, 1979) they found evidence that the residents were generally well integrated into the care providers' family units. Specifically, the vast majority of residents reportedly join the family in social activities all or most of the time and a number of providers reported routinely taking their residents with them on family vacations.

This study also assessed the social environment of family care homes using the Family Environment Scale developed by Moos (1974). This scale focuses on the measurement and description of the relative emphases placed on interpersonal relationships, personal growth and organizational structure within the family. The results showed that, relative to the norm, family care homes place greater emphasis on interpersonal relationships and organizational structure and about average emphasis on personal growth dimensions. More specifically, family care providers place great emphasis on togetherness and cohesion in their homes. Further, although activities in family care homes are generally structured, providers did not appear to be excessively rigid or controlling in managing residents. Finally, relative to other environmental dimensions, providers placed less, but still considerable, emphasis on personal growth dimensions of independence and achievement.

With respect to resident activities within the home, 87% of family care residents surveyed by Willer and Intagliata (1980) had assigned household chores. These chores included making their bed, cleaning the house, doing the dishes, mowing the lawn and shoveling snow. As reported by the residents themselves, having household responsibilities gave them a sense of their importance and contribution within the home. Residents' free time around the home was most frequently spent watching T.V. (not unlike many non-retarded persons). However, other free-time activities reported included listening to the radio, taking walks, bike riding, playing cards, doing household chores and reading. Only 13% of residents were reported to have too little to occupy their time. In summary, while the authors found a great deal of variation within family care home environments, the results of their study suggest that the majority of residents live as integrated members of family units, assume regularly assigned household chores and enjoy typical leisure activities in and around their homes.

Scheerenberger and Felsenthal (1976) also studied a variety of aspects of resident life within family care homes. In general, all residents interviewed reported enjoying living in their residence. More specifically, 94% of residents reported enjoying their food and all felt they were getting enough to eat and drink. In addition, most residents (83%) had their own bedrooms and were allowed to decorate them as they wished. Trained interviewers also made independent judgments regarding the homes and indicated that all family care residents seemed happy, had personal possessions and a place to keep them, lived in homelike environments, and had good personal hygiene. Further, they reported that residents were dressed and generally treated by care providers in an individualized, age-appropriate manner.

Scheerenberger and Felsenthal (1976) also examined the degree of independence given to family care residents. They reported that 94% of residents indicated they could go outside whenever they wanted. Most, however, did not leave their neighborhood without supervision. With respect to conformity within the home, only one-third of residents reported having fixed times to get up and go to bed (i.e., being required to get up/go to bed at the same time, 7 days a week). By comparison, the majority of group home and adult home residents reported fixed schedules. Further, interviewers independently judged the conformity of homes visited and found that residents of group and adult homes were much more likely than family care residents to attend recreational activities in groups and to live by fixed bedtime and eating schedules. The authors concluded that increasing the number of persons in any home setting is likely to result in increased "scheduling" of events for sake of convenience.

In general, the authors felt that results regarding the personal adjustment and in-home normalization of family care residents were quite positive. For the most part, they compared quite favorably with residents in other settings studied. The only noticeable exception was that family care residents were significantly less free to engage in normal sexual conduct than were persons living in group homes.

In summary, the studies reviewed indicate that family care residents are well integrated into the family units within their homes. However, findings regarding the activities and responsibilities of family care residents were somewhat mixed. The evidence suggests that while many residents live active, normalized lives within family care homes, a number of others live with care providers who encourage resident passivity with their overprotective style. Consequently, the quality of residents' lives within family care homes is likely to depend greatly on the way in which particular family care programs are managed as well as on the particular attitudes and skills of individual care providers.

Interaction/Integration With the Community

Programs. Involvement of a mentally retarded person in meaningful daytime activity, generally outside the living residence, has to be a significant consideration in assessing the quality of life. Such activities would include school, competitive employment, sheltered workshop programs, or other types of structured programs (e.g., day care or recreational programs). Of course, the type of activities that are appropriate vary depending on the individual's age, capabilities and preferences. Some residents may, in fact, prefer not to be heavily involved in regular structured programs outside of their residence and, of course, should have the option not to participate in all but the mandated programs.

The day activities of family care residents have been examined in a number of different studies. Some authors have reported little resident interaction with community programs (Butler & Bjaanes, 1977) and the widespread absence of out-of-house programming (Baker et al., 1974). Others, however, suggest a far more optimistic picture. In studies involving samples of children and adolescents living in family care, Justice et al. (1971) found that 85% of the residents attended school while Scheerenberger and Felsenthal (1976) reported that all of their sample were enrolled in formal educational programs. However, Justice et al. (1971) indicated that day care services and prevocational programs needed for some residents were virtually nonexistent.

In a study of 229 adolescents and adults (13-81 years of age) living in family care homes in New York, Willer and Intagliata (1980) found that 91% were involved in structured activity programs outside of their home. Specifically, 74% were attending sheltered workshops and 17% school. Moreover, 97% of these individuals were involved in programs five or more hours each day, five days a week. The only individuals not attending programs were generally quite elderly.

The differences in the results of these studies further illustrate the wide variation in the character and quality of family care homes within this county. However, unlike differences in residents' activities within the homes, variation in the use of external day programs is more likely due to poor planning and administration of family care programs rather than individual care provider characteristics. If family care programs are to provide their residents with quality community care, those responsible for administering them must make a commitment to ensure that residents and providers receive the necessary supportive services. While structured day programs are only one component of such supportive services, it is obvious that some family care programs have made a strong commitment to providing these services while others have not.

Generic community resources. An important aspect of normalized life in the community is the degree to which mentally retarded persons make use of a variety of community resources commonly frequented by others. Examples of these resources would include stores, restaurants, movies, church/temple, parks, and zoos.

Butler and Bjaanes (1977) reported that family care residents have little interaction with external settings and rarely utilize community opportunities. Similarly, other studies have reported that family care residents are generally geographically and socially isolated from the community (Baker et al., 1974; Bjaanes & Butler, 1974).

As with the findings regarding programs, however, there have been more optimistic reports regarding family care residents' use of community resources. Scheerenberger and Felsenthal (1976) reported that the majority of family care residents made use of such community resources as stores (100%), park/zoo (94%), church (88%), movies (75%), and restaurants (69%). In fact, residents in family care homes were more likely to report use of community resources than were residents in group homes or adult homes. Willer and Intagliata (1980) found similar results with the majority of family care residents reportedly using restaurants (96%), barber/beauty shop (91%), church/temple (77%), movies (66%), community centers (62%) and parks (60%). Other community resources used by residents included amusement parks, zoos, ballgames, libraries, museums and bars.

However, though there is evidence that family care residents make use of a wide range of community activities, it appears that they are typically accompanied by their care providers or other supervising adults. Specifically, Scheerenberger and Felsenthal (1976) reported that only 21% of family care residents venture into the community alone. While this proportion was relatively comparable to that reported for group home and adult home residents, the authors felt that the degree of independent use of the community by residents was disappointingly low. They speculated that two factors: (1) living apart from the community and (2) the absence of convenient transportation, explained why most residents were usually accompanied by an adult during community outings.

Other studies (Bjaanes & Butler, 1974; Willer & Intagliata, 1980) have also indicated problems with independent use of the community by family care residents. Specifically, Willer and Intagliata (1980) reported that while family care residents used community resources as frequently as did group home residents, they were less likely to do so independently. The major reason was that only 22% of family care residents reportedly traveled outside of their immediate neighborhood without provider supervision. Similarly, though Butler and Bjaanes (1974) did not indicate the actual level of independent use of community resources by family care residents, they reported that it was markedly less than that of board and care residents.

Results comparing family care residents' use of the community with that of individuals in other types of facilities must be interpreted cautiously given that the characteristics of the clients placed in different types of community settings cannot be assumed equivalent. Nevertheless, the absolute levels of independent use of the community reported for family care residents (Bjaanes & Butler, 1974; Scheerenberger & Felsenthal, 1976; Willer & Intagliata, 1980) are low enough to raise concern. At this point, the extent to which these findings can be accounted for by limiting characteristics of the residents (age extremes, level of retardation), overprotective styles of care providers, the isolated location of homes or some combination of related factors is not clear. Further study of this important area of concern is needed.

Social support. In recent years increasing attention has been given in the health, mental health and mental retardation literatures to the concept of social support networks (Caplan, 1974; Heal et al., 1978; Kaplan, Cassel & Gove, 1977). Simply defined, such networks are comprised of persons (e.g., friends, relatives, service providers) with whom one has an ongoing supportive relationship or to whom one can turn in times of need or crisis. The importance of such networks for the successful community adjustment of mentally retarded persons living in the community has been highlighted in a number of studies (Edgerton, 1967; Gollay et al., 1978; Sigelman, Bell, Schoenrock, Elias & Danker-Brown, 1978).

The research regarding the degree and type of social support available to persons in family care homes has focused on the roles played by various individuals including care providers, friends, neighbors and residents' own relatives. As discussed earlier, there are consistent reports that residents are well integrated into the family unit within the residence itself (Baker et al., 1974; Edgerton, 1967; Newman & Sherman, 1979; Scheerenberger & Felsenthal, 1976; Willer & Intagliata, 1980). More specifically, there is evidence that residents participate actively in the life of the family and rely on their fellow residents and care providers for needed support.

These reports are encouraging given that the close personal relationships that develop between residents and their care providers are an important strength of the family care model. According to Willer and Intagliata (1980), interviews with deinstitutionalized mentally retarded persons indicated that their satisfaction with life in the community was drawn, in great part, from their relationships with other people. Further, residents reported not only appreciating having someone on whom they could depend but took great personal pride in feeling that this individual also depended on and needed them. This suggests that the most positive and effective social support is offered by care providers who actively seek to establish mutuality in their relationships with residents.

There is evidence, however, that many residents in family care homes, as well as other community residential settings, are caught up in elaborate one-way dependency relationships with care providers. Such relationships are likely to inhibit residents' growth in adaptive behavior and independence (Baker et al., 1974; Edgerton, 1967). This is a matter of concern and suggests that many care providers could benefit from training regarding interpersonal relationships with their mentally retarded residents. Effective training in this area could thus serve to enhance one of the most potentially positive aspects of the family care model.

The nature of family care residents' relationships with friends and neighbors has also been explored. Scheerenberger and Felsenthal (1976) reported that almost all (94%) residents interviewed indicated that they had "a special friend." By comparison, 25% of group home residents and 20% of adult home residents reported that they had no such friends. In addition the authors reported 72% of family care residents indicated that they had a boyfriend or girlfriend.

Willer and Intagliata (1980) also interviewed a sample of family care residents regarding friendships. All respondents named at least one particular person with whom they enjoyed getting together, and on whom they felt they could depend. Most respondents, in fact, named more than one such person. While in many cases the individuals named were mentally retarded peers in the same home, the network of identified friends frequently included mentally retarded peers living elsewhere, as well as non-retarded neighbors. Regarding the peers who lived elsewhere, 52% of residents reportedly spent time with them during the evening or weekends while the remainder interacted with such friends only at their day program sites (school, sheltered workshop). A number of residents also indicated that they considered particular neighbors to be their friends. When interviewers explored how residents had established these friendships, it became clear that they were at least initially mediated by the residents' care providers. Interestingly, none of the group home residents interviewed in the study identified any neighbors among their friends.

One possible explanation of this finding is that family care providers, who are already an integral part of their neighborhoods, are typically in a much better position to facilitate resident interaction with neighbors than are the staff of group homes who may often be viewed more as "outsiders" than community residents. Consistent with this interpretation Baker et al. (1974) reported that family care residences met relatively less opposition from the community than did other types of residential facilities, primarily because the individual care providers already lived in the community.

The degree of community acceptance of family care homes has been examined in a number of studies. Justice et al. (1971) noted that a significant number of care providers (34%) reported a problem with antagonistic neighbors. Lack of community acceptance, in fact, was the problem most frequently cited by their provider sample. However, the proportion of providers reporting problems with neighbors has been noticeably lower in more recent studies, specifically 16% (Bruininks et al., 1980) and 8% (Willer & Intagliata, 1980). In general, most studies reviewed (Baker et al., 1974; Bruininks et al., 1980; Mamula & Newman, 1973; Scheerenberger & Felsenthal, 1976; Willer & Intagliata, 1980) seem to indicate that the attitudes of neighbors toward family care homes are generally positive and supportive.

Another important aspect of resident social support is contact with natural family members. One advantage often cited for placement of mentally retarded persons in the community, in fact, is that it can facilitate contact between residents and their relatives. Only two of the studies reviewed reported on the degree of contact that family care residents have with their own relatives. Bruininks et al. (1980) reported that only 36% of all residents surveyed received parental visits at least annually. As pointed out by the authors, this relatively low percentage may be accounted for by the fact that many family care residents have been placed from institutions and may have had little or no contact with their families for some time. However, in their study of New York State family care residents (many of whom were elderly and previously institutionalized for years), Willer and Intagliata (1980) reported that 60% were visited at least annually by their relatives and 21% within the previous month.

This suggests that the degree of natural family contact with family care residents may depend on factors other than the characteristics of the residents (age, length of institutionalization). Possible contributing factors may include the extent to which relatives are informed of or involved in the family care placement of the resident, the attitudes of care providers toward parental visits, as well as the general policies that guide the operation of a given family care program. While the role played by these or other related factors is not presently clear, it is evident that the simple act of placing individuals out of an institution and into the community is not, by itself, sufficient to create or re-establish their supportive ties with family members.

Availability and use of support services. In addition to having an informal network of persons who provide personal and social support, mentally retarded persons living in the community must also have access to a broad network of more formal support services. In order to match the coverage of services provided by large institutions, this network must be comprised of a large and varied group of individual service providers. Further, it must include services designed to meet not only the support needs of residents, but also those of their care providers.

A number of studies have examined the availability and use of support services by residents and providers in family care. The findings with regard to one important aspect of such services, namely structured out-of-home activity programs (e.g., school, sheltered workshops) for residents, have already been discussed. However, a variety of other service components are also essential. These include medical and dental care, physical therapy, speech therapy, recreation programs, counseling for residents, as well as training and respite services for care providers.

Although neither Baker et al. (1974) nor Bjaanes and Butler (1974) included specific data on the availability or use of support services by family care providers, both studies reported that providers and residents made relatively little use of existing community resources or facilities. On the other hand, Justice et al. (1971) reported that existing medical, educational, and recreational services were heavily used by family care providers. In fact, 80% of providers reportedly used planned activity programs (outside of the home) for their residents. However, while available services were widely used, the authors reported that 27% of care providers felt that existing programs were either inadequate or insufficient. Specifically, they identified needs for medical and dental care, day care services for young residents ineligible for school, prevocational training programs, sheltered workshops, and vocational relief (respite) services.

Browder, Ellis and Neal (1974) reported that the majority of care providers were able to meet most or all of their residents' out-of-home needs. However, they noted that the lack of transportation and the cost of some services were obstacles for a number of providers. In general, the authors concluded that the quality of care being provided in family care homes could be improved by providing caretakers with better transportation services, increased funding, respite services and training. Bruininks et al. (1980) reported that inadequate funding (58%) and the lack of support services (31%) were the two problems most frequently cited by family care providers. Only 4% of providers in this nationwide study identified the lack of transportation or training as problems.

Two recent studies (Intagliata et al., 1979; Willer & Intagliata, 1980) explored the availability, accessibility and actual use of specific community support services by family care providers. Medical and dental care were reported to be available and accessible for all residents. Further, 98% of residents receiving medical care were served by community-based physicians, with most individuals (75%) being cared for by the providers' own family physician. Among other services, respite and recreational services were reported to be the most available (90%, 85%) and the most heavily utilized (90%, 76%). Counseling, physical therapy and speech therapy services were reportedly available to 70% to 80% of providers and were utilized as needed. When services were available, cost was rarely identified as an obstacle to utilization, but transportation difficulties were noted by many providers (43%). With respect to ongoing support provided by family care program agencies, 92% of providers reported being visited on a regular monthly basis by case managers. Lei (1979) also reported that family care homes in California are routinely provided with case management services.

In summary, these studies suggest that while a wide range of services are available and routinely used by family care providers, a number of service gaps and problems with service accessibility continue to exist. While the nature and extent of such gaps vary from one area to another, most studies report that transportation for family care residents is inadequate. This is a signfiicant problem area since lack of transportation reportedly affects (1) the level of absolute and independent use of community resources and (2) the use of more formal support services. If family care homes are to serve their residents effectively, those managing programs must respond more adequately to this area of provider and resident need.

Changes in Resident Adaptive Behavior

One objective of the deinstitutionalization movement has been to give mentally retarded persons an opportunity to exercise their legal right to live in the "least restrictive environment" possible (Willer, Scheerenberger & Intagliata, 1978). In addition, the movement of persons into community residential settings has been linked with the expectation or assumption that these more normalized, less restrictive environments would be more likely to facilitate the growth of a wide variety of adaptive, independent resident behaviors. However, while many studies have explored the degree to which community settings have incorporated normalization principles, it is only recently that researchers have begun to examine the type and degree of changes which occur in the adaptive behaviors of mentally retarded persons living in these settings.

Eyman et al. (1979), for example, asserted that while it is important to assess the degree to which environments are normalized, evaluations of the effectiveness of community residential settings must ultimately take their behavioral impact into account. Bjaanes, Butler and Kelley (in this volume) have taken a similar perspective and, in fact, have offered a distinction between residential settings that emphasize "environmental normalization" (i.e., culturally appropriate physical settings and staff behavior) and those that aim for "client normalization" (i.e., growth in behavior adaptive for living in the community). According to the authors, environmental normalization is a necessary but not sufficient condition for client normalization. Specifically, client normalization depends on structural habilitation as well as environmental normalization.

The results of studies examining a variety of aspects of normalization in family care home environments have already been discussed in this section of the review. Studies focusing on changes in the adaptive behavior of family care residents have also appeared in the literature. Some of these (Baker et al., 1974; Bjaanes & Butler, 1974; Browder et al., 1974; Murphy, Rennee & Luchins, 1972) have implied that mentally retarded persons are likely to make little, if any, positive change in adaptive behavior while living in family care homes. Specifically, they characterized the family care environments studied as unnecessarily restrictive (Bjaanes & Butler, 1974), overprotective and custodial (Baker et al., 1974), and perhaps the community equivalent of an institution (Browder et al., 1974; Murphy et al., 1972). However, none of these studies actually assessed changes in resident adaptive behavior over time. Instead, based on what they found at a given point in time they made the judgment that family care home environments were generally not conducive to resident behavioral progress.

More recent studies (Eyman & Begab, 1979; Eyman, Silverstein, McLain & Miller, 1977; Eyman et al., 1979; Intagliata et al., 1979; Scheerenberger & Felsenthal, 1976; Willer & Intagliata, 1980), however, have specifically examined longitudinal changes in the adaptive behavior of family care residents and report consistently positive results. In general, residents living in family care homes are reportedly progressing significantly in self-care skills, community living skills, personal adjustment, and social behavior.

Typically, the greatest degree of positive change has taken place with residents' self-care skills (e.g., personal hygiene, eating, dressing) (Eyman & Begab, 1979; Eyman et al., 1979; Intagliata et al., 1979). However, there is also evidence of resident progress in community living skills. Eyman et al. (1979) reported that the average score of 245 community residents (75% living in family care) on the community self-sufficiency skills domain (e.g., money management, shopping, meal preparation, household chores) of the *Adaptive Behavior Scale* nearly doubled over a three-year period. Positive change on this domain was independent of resident age and was reported for residents of all levels of retardation. Intagliata et al. (1979) also reported that family care residents were making significant progress in community living skills, though the likelihood of such positive change varied significantly depending on characteristics of the particular family care home environment. However, Willer and Intagliata (1980) reported that, in general, family care residents were significantly less likely to show progress in community living skills than were group home residents.

Freeman (1978) also examined the use of foster home care, especially with regard to mentally retarded children. As a group, the residents studied had a high degree of emotional disturbance, numerous behavior problems and physical limitations in addition to mental retardation. Results of the study indicated that most of the children showed significant improvement in a variety of areas including I.Q. scores, socialization skills, and even physical functioning (attributed to exercises foster parents learned and used with the children).

In summary, there seems to be consistent evidence that many residents in family care homes make positive changes in adaptive behavior over time. Moreover, the magnitude of this change has been reported to exceed that found for individuals of similar age and level of retardation who live in institutional settings (Eyman et al., 1977). However, while it is encouraging to know that many family care residents are making behavioral progress it is even more important to identify why some types of gains are more likely than others and why the type and extent of resident progress varies significantly from one home to another.

Recidivism/Movement

While they are not a direct measure of the quality of life in community residential setting, rates of recidivism and general client movement reflect on the stability and general effectiveness of the setting. The recidivism rate (return to the institution), for example, is frequently treated as an index of the quality of a particular community setting. Unfortunately, such rates are routinely reported without the reasons for the recidivism actually being understood. Generally, recidivism rates are the result of a complex interaction of such factors as client preparation for the community, the compatability between clients and the particular settings into which they are placed, the competence and tolerance of care providers, the availability of support services for clients and care providers as well as the institution's policy regarding accepting readmissions. Thus, while high recidivism rates generally reflect significant problems, it is impossible to identify their specific nature unless a great deal of contextual information about placement failures has been collected.

A number of studies have reported on recidivism rates for family care residents. McCarver and Craig (1974) concluded that the 39.5% rate of placement failure (return to the institution) was no worse than that reported for other community residential settings. The authors, however, did not indicate over what time period these rates were calculated. Baker et al. (1974) reported that 17.3% of the residents living in the family care homes they studied had returned to institutional settings over a one-year period. However, they did not indicate the average time lapse between these residents' community placement and their return. Gollay et al. (1978) studied a sample of 78 persons who had been placed into family care homes over a two year period (1972-1974). They found that 32% were living back in the institution at the time of their follow-up.

Given the different ways in which each of these studies has calculated recidivism rates, it is difficult to compare them in any meaningful fashion. What is clear is that some significant number of persons placed into family care homes return to institutions at some point in time. However, the reasons for placement failure in family care are varied and not particularly well understood. Various researchers have identified client, care provider, and community variables associated with recidivism. Those studies that have attempted to identify factors associated with community adjustment in family care placement will be discussed in the next section of this review.

An important aspect generally ignored in recidivism studies is the degree of permanence associated with institutional returns. The importance of this information is illustrated by Willer and Intagliata (1980). They found that 20% of a sample of 657 persons released to the community during 1973-1976 were living back in institutions at the time of follow-up (1977-1978). However, of the 522 persons living in the community, 14.9% had at least one non-respite return to an institution since their release. Thus, many returnees are likely to be given repeated opportunities to "make it" in the community and some number are likely to succeed in spite of previous failures or problems.

While recidivism rates have received a great deal of attention in the literature, returns to an institution are only one component of overall rates of movement out of community residential settings. For example, if a particular community residential setting is intended to be a transitional step to more independent living, there ought to be a significant rate of resident movement into less restrictive settings. Since some placements inevitably fail (i.e., clients move to more restricted settings) there is thus likely to be both positive and negative movements from such a transitional setting. As with recidivism rates, however, client movement rates may be difficult to interpret without sufficient contextual information.

A number of studies have examined the rates of movement (from one community setting to another) for family care residents. For example, Baker et al. (1974) reported that 51% of the residents in the family care homes they studied had moved elsewhere within the previous year. Of those who left, 34% returned to an institution or hospital, 23% returned to live with their natural families, 7% moved to another family care home, 22% transferred to a community residence, and 11% moved to their own apartments. In general, these figures illustrate a great deal of variation in the impact of family care home environments on residents. Approximately one-third of those leaving returned to a more restrictive living environment (i.e., institution) while an equal number moved on to more independent living settings (i.e., community residences, apartments).

Bruininks et al. (1980) also reported on resident movement from family care homes. Their results indicated that 20% returned to an institution, 22% moved to another family care home, 7% returned to live with their natural families, 31% moved to group homes and 7% moved to apartment or independent living. While the level of restrictiveness found in these alternative settings was not assessed by the authors it would appear that 22% of residents moved to more restrictive environments (i.e., institution, nursing home) while 37% moved on to more independent settings (i.e., group homes, supervised apartments, independent living).

The results of these studies, showing that family care homes serve as a positive transitional placement for many clients, are consistent with the evidence that many family care residents are making positive adaptive behavior changes in self-care and community living skills. On the other hand, a number of residents do not fare as well in family care homes and are returned to more restrictive settings. This would suggest that the positive behavior changes reported for family care residents, in general, do not take place for all residents. Thus, it is important to attempt to identify those factors associated with success in family care placements.

In addition to movement out of family care homes to more or less restrictive living settings, there is also evidence of considerable movement of residents from one family care home to another. Willer and Intagliata (1980) report that 55% of their sample of 229 family care residents have lived in at least two different family care homes since their release from the institution. Similarly, Bruininks et al. (1980) reported that 32% of the residents entering the family care homes in their sample during a one year period had come from other family care homes. Movements from one foster care home to another would seem likely to disrupt the elements of familial relationships that are viewed as an essential strength of this placement type (Bruininks et al., 1980). On the other hand, they may indicate that the agencies arranging such placements are actively monitoring the effectiveness of the client-home match and do not hesitate to shift clients when appropriate. Clearly, this inter-home movement merits further study.

Summary on Quality of Life

The major conclusion regarding the quality of life of mentally retarded persons living in family care homes is that it varies a great deal. In some cases, residents live active normalized lives both within the home and the community, make significant progress in adaptive behavior skills and even move to more independent living situations. In other instances, however, family care residents live passively in unnecessarily restrictive situations, perhaps deteriorate in their behavioral functioning and are sometimes returned to more restrictive living settings. Given this variation it is essential to identify the client, care provider and environmental factors that are related to the effectiveness of family care home environments.

Factors Associated With Effectiveness in Family Care Homes

Sternlicht (1978) reviewed a set of studies that had examined factors associated with the community adjustment of family care residents. Two characteristics of these studies, however, limit their contribution to our understanding of family care home effectiveness. First, they focused primarily on resident characteristics with relatively little attention given to care provider or community variables. Second, these studies equated successful community adjustment with a resident's simply remaining in the community. Thus, the identified predictors of community "success" are merely factors associated with community tenure. Whether or not those same factors are associated with the quality of adjustment made by residents who remained in the community was never demonstrated. Nevertheless, Sternlicht's (1978) review of these studies can be briefly summarized here.

While a variety of resident characteristics were examined in these studies, few were found to be significantly related to resident adjustment. Specifically, resident age, sex, level of functioning and length of institutionalization were not found to be consistently related to placement success. However, "unacceptable" resident behavior (Bishop, 1957; Brown, Windle & Stewart, 1959; Eagle, 1967; Nihira & Nihira, 1975; Windle, Stewart & Brown, 1961) and poor health (Eagle, 1967; Justice et al., 1971; Windle et al., 1961) were found to be related to placement failure. Regarding care provider factors, there was some evidence that providers' emotional stability and maturity were related to resident placement success (Penniman, 1974; Windle, 1962). Finally, though environmental factors were given almost no attention in the studies reviewed, Eagle (1967) reported that adverse environmental conditions account for a large number of community placement failures.

Clearly, these studies give us limited insight into the factors associated with success in family care placement. Further, they tell us little or nothing about the complex interplay of resident, care provider and environmental factors associated with the varying levels of community adjustment attained by those persons who successfully remain in family care homes.

The inadequacies of much of the previous research have begun to be identified and addressed in some more recent work (Bjaanes & Butler, 1974; Butler & Bjaanes, 1977; Eyman & Begab, 1979; Eyman, DeMaine & Lei, 1979; Intagliata & Willer, 1980; Intagliata, Willer & Wicks, this volume; Lei, 1979; Meyers et al., 1979). The most important characteristic shared by these studies is that each was designed to identify factors that contribute to the adjustment rather than mere community tenure of family care residents. That is, these studies establish residents' normalized use of the community or change in adaptive behavior as the target to be predicted. Further, unlike many previous studies, they give attention to care provider and community variables in addition to resident characteristics. With this more comprehensive approach they provide an opportunity to determine how each group of factors acts alone and/or in interaction with others to affect the course of resident adjustment in family care homes.

Bjaanes and Butler (1974) found that the degree of family care provider involvement with residents was positively related to the proportion of resident behavior judged to be independent and interactive. In their later work (Butler & Bjaanes, 1977), these same authors reported that providers who had a higher therapeutic orientation (i.e., confidence in clients' abilities accompanied by specific activities for helping them to develop) tended to spend more time interacting with clients in their homes as well as to make greater use of outside activities for residents. These studies are particularly important because they direct attention to the wide variation in the specific characteristics of family care and other community residential environments. Further, they begin to demonstrate that care provider style has significant effects on resident behavior and development.

Subsequent studies have refined this approach and have focused on explaining how resident, care provider and environmental factors contribute to specific areas of resident adaptive behavior including self-care skills, community living skills and personal-social responsibility. In general, they have reported that individual resident characteristics play a significant role in determining the level of adjustment achieved by residents. Specifically, the family care residents who make the greatest degree of positive adaptive behavior change in the community tend to be those who were at a higher level of intellectual and behavioral functioning when initially placed (Eyman & Begab, 1979; Eyman et al., 1979; Eyman et al., 1977; Intagliata & Willer, 1980). However, though resident factors account for the majority of variance in adjustment these studies have provided evidence that the socio-psychological characteristics of family care home environments play an additional and significant contributing role in resident adaptive behavior change.

Though the specific measures used in each study vary to some degree the study results are generally consistent. For example, using *PASS 3* (Wolfensberger & Glenn, 1975) ratings, Eyman et al. (1979) found that the factors (1) location and proximity of services, (2) facility comfort and appearance, and (3) facility openness and blending with the neighborhood were positively associated with resident progress in adaptive behavior regardless of age or level of retardation of the residents. The authors explained that each of the identified facility characteristics was indicative of settings that facilitate assimilation of the residents into the community through supportive encounters with adult or non-retarded persons. As noted by Eyman et al. (1979) these results are consistent with other studies (Eyman et al., 1977; Zigler & Balla, 1977) that have found a positive relationship between resident-oriented care practices and the behavioral development of mentally retarded persons living in both institutional and community settings.

Using another measure of family care home environment (Family Environment Scale, Moos, 1974), Intagliata and Willer (1980) also found a number of home characteristics to be related to resident development. Specifically, they reported that residents living in homes where moral, ethical and religious values are emphasized made greater progress in self-care and community living skills. On the other hand, they found that residents living in homes that are managed with rigid rules and procedures tend to make significantly less progress in these areas. The nature of the relationship between the moral-religious orientation of care providers and the behavioral development of their residents remains to be explained. However, the findings of a negative relationship between environmental rigidity and resident development is consistent with those studies that have highlighted the importance of flexible, resident-oriented care practices for behavioral growth (Eyman et al., 1977; Eyman et al., 1979; Zigler & Balla, 1977).

Other aspects of care provider style have also been found to have a significant impact on residents' development. For example, both Eyman and Begab (1979) and Intagliata and Willer (1980) reported that family care providers who encourage resident autonomy and are tolerant rather than overprotective in their caring styles facilitate significantly greater positive adaptive behavior change in their residents. Further, these same two studies reported that while care provider style has an impact on all residents some are affected more than others. Specifically, while higher functioning residents are more likely to progress regardless of where they are placed, the progress of more severely retarded residents seems even more dependent on the caring styles of their providers.

The majority of these recent family care studies have focused on identifying resident, care provider and environmental variables associated with positive resident adaptive behavior change. However, Intagliata and Willer (1980) also examined how these factors relate to resident maladaptive behavior. Their results indicated that the family care residents most likely to be seen as exhibiting a wide range of maladaptive behaviors tended to be those who were younger and higher functioning. However, regardless of their individual characteristics, residents were perceived as exhibiting more maladaptive behavior in family care homes in which providers were overprotective and dominating and less maladaptive behavior in homes where family cohesion and mutual support were stressed and where residents were encouraged to act openly and express their feelings directly.

Together, these studies of resident adjustment in family care begin to provide an understanding of the variety of factors that account for observed variation in the quality and effectiveness of family care home placements. Clearly, residents' own characteristics are powerful determinants of their degree of adjustment in the community. However, the characteristics of family care home environments, especially care provider style, also have important effects. Nevertheless, though evidence regarding the importance of community environments for resident development is accumulating, "much more work needs to be done for a complete understanding on the extent to which retarded behavior can be modified and how environments interact to produce desired behavior" (Eyman & Begab, 1979, p. 12). In the meantime the research results to date should prove useful in guiding the selection, training and monitoring of family care providers.

Discussion

For nearly fifty years, foster family care has been used in this country as a placement alternative enabling mentally retarded persons to leave institutions and return to more normal community living. In addition, it has also been used extensively to avoid the institutionalization of mentally retarded persons whose families are no longer willing or able to maintain them at home. Foster family care presently provides an important component in the continuum of residential alternatives developed in response to the current public policy of deinstitutionalization. However, its use preceded the current push toward deinstitutionalization and is likely to outlive it as well.

As a placement model with a substantial history the specific ideologies guiding its use at different points in time have changed along with the broader ideologies that have characterized the general system of services and care for mentally retarded persons. At present, with the principles of normalization, least restrictive environment and the developmental model being emphasized, there are indications that foster family care programs have begun to shift away from their prior custodial orientation toward a more active, habilitation-oriented emphasis. However, given that this residential model was well established prior to the emergence of current ideological positions this transition toward newer service ideologies within family care programs has been neither rapid nor complete.

There are quite a number of indications, however, that a transition is taking place. Perhaps the most significant change within the foster care model is the trend toward greater expertise and professionalism among care providers. This trend was identified by Adams (1975) and there is a variety of evidence that suggests it is growing. One indication is the movement to offer family care providers the specialized training programs that they need in order to facilitate effectively the growth and development of their residents (Baker et al., 1974; Mamula, 1970; Meyers et al., 1979; Willer & Intagliata, 1979). Another indication is the trend toward altering reimbursement practices so that family care providers are paid a salary that recognizes the skills in the tasks they are now expected to perform to meet program expectations (Adams, 1975; Baker et al., 1974; Lei et al., 1979; Willer & Intagliata, 1979). This salary is remuneration above and beyond the mere reimbursement for resident room and board that had been customary when these homes were seen as primarily custodial. Third, the number and strength of family care provider associations is growing. These associations are a crucial development that can facilitate care providers' competence and growing sense of professionalism. Finally, evidence of their growing professional identity is provided by studies of certain family care programs in which providers have begun to be viewed as equal colleagues with other agency staff in making plans for the placement and care of residents (Baker et al., 1974; Willer & Intagliata, 1979).

However, as a residential care model in transition, the diversity in the character and quality of individual family care homes at present is great. While there is consistent evidence that many of these homes are successfully meeting habilitative and normalization goals for their residents, there are numerous examples of homes that fall far short of these objectives. The lack of quality and effectiveness in such homes may be due to a variety of factors. These include a custodial orientation of the agency administering the homes, the lack of programs to train providers in the skills and attitudes necessary for taking a more habilitative role, the lack of adequate training for agency workers who are expected to monitor the quality of care in the homes, and the lack of general support services needed by both residents and care providers.

In spite of such inadequacies, it is reasonable to assume that foster family care will continue to be a widely used placement for mentally retarded individuals. At least two recent trends seem especially important to maintaining this momentum. The first of these is the trend toward professionalization of foster care providers. Perhaps the most important component of this trend is the proliferation of training programs designed to increase the skills of providers and give them a more active role in the habilitation of residents. This development clearly has the potential to improve considerably the quality of care provided to foster care residents. Thus, it is essential that these training programs be implemented more widely and that they continue to be refined and adapted to better meet the changing needs of both family care providers and their mentally retarded residents.

The second trend which needs to be maintained is that of family care research being directed toward identifying factors associated with residents' community adjustment rather than mere community tenure. Since the goal of deinstitutionalization is not merely to change or relocate people into the community, but to also improve the quality of their lives, this change in research orientation is crucial. As indicated previously, such research has already highlighted the significant impact of particular care provider styles on resident development and behavior. It needs to be emphasized, however, that the ultimate value of this type of research depends on the extent to which it is used to guide the selection and training of care providers as well as the overall orientation of agencies administering foster family care programs.

Foster family care as a community residential alternative for mentally retarded persons has a number of important strengths. If properly managed it can provide a cost-effective, normalizing living environment for mentally retarded persons of varying ages and levels of disability. However, its continued valuable contribution as a placement alternative depends on the strength of the commitment that is made to monitoring and improving the quality and consistency of the care offered by individual providers.

References

Adams, M. Foster care for mentally retarded children: How does child welfare meet this challenge? *Child Welfare*, 1970, *49*, 260-269.

Adams, M. *Mental retardation and its social dimensions*. New York: Columbia University Press, 1971.

Adams, M. Foster family care for the intellectually disadvantaged child: The current state of practice and some research perspectives. In M. Begab & S. A. Richardson (Eds.), *The mentally retarded and society: A social perspective*. Baltimore: University Park Press, 1975.

Babcock, C. G. Some psychodynamic factors in foster parenthood. *Child Welfare*, 1965, *44*, 485-493, 570-577.

Baker, B. L., Seltzer, G. B. & Seltzer, M. M. *As close as possible*. Cambridge, MA.: Behavioral Education Projects, 1974.

Birch, H. G. & Belmont, L. The problem of comparing home rearing versus foster-home rearing in defective children. *Pediatrics*, 1961, *28*, 956-961.

Bishop, E. B. Family care: The patients. *American Journal of Mental Deficiency*, 1957, *61*, 583-591.

Bjaanes, A. T. & Butler, E. W. Environmental variation in community care facilities for mentally retarded persons. *American Journal of Mental Deficiency*, 1974, *78*, 429-439.

Browder, J., Ellis, L. & Neal, J. Foster homes: Alternatives to institutions? *Mental Retardation*, 1974, *12*, 33-36.

Brown, S. J., Windle, C. & Stewart, E. Statistics on a family care program. *American Journal of Mental Deficiency*, 1959, *64*, 535-542.

Bruininks, R., Hill, B. & Thorsheim, M. J. *A profile of specially licensed foster homes for mentally retarded people in 1977*. Minneapolis: University of Minnesota, Department of Psychoeducational Studies, 1980.

Butler, E. W. & Bjaanes, A. T. A typology of community care facilities and differential normalization outcomes. In P. Mittler (Ed.), *Research to practice in mental retardation: Care and intervention*. Baltimore: University Park Press, 1977.

Caplan, R. *Psychiatry and the community in nineteenth century America*. New York: Basic Books, 1969.

Caplan, G. *Support systems and community mental health*. New York: Behavioral Publications, 1974.

Conroy, J. Trends in deinstitutionalization of the mentally retarded. *Mental Retardation*, 1977, *15*, 44-46.

Culley, J. D., Settles, B. H. & VanName, J. B. Foster parents and social workers' attitudes on foster care issues. In *Understanding and measuring the cost of foster family care*. Newark, DE: University of Delaware, Bureau of Economic & Business Research, 1975.

Dick, K. What people think about foster care. *Children*, 1961, *8*, 48-52.

Doll, E. A historical survey of research and management of mental retardation in the U.S. In E. P. Trapp & P. Himelstein (Eds.), *Readings on the exceptional child*. New York: Appleton Century Crofts, Inc., 1962.

Eagle, E. Prognosis and outcome of community placement of institutionalized retardates. *American Journal of Mental Deficiency*, 1967, *72*, 232-243.

Edgerton, R. B. *The cloak of competence: Stigma in the lives of the mentally retarded*. Berkeley: University of California Press, 1967.

Eyman, R. K., Silverstein, A. B., McLain, R. & Miller, C. Effects of residential settings on development. In P. Mittler (Ed.), *Research to practice in mental retardation: Care and intervention*: Baltimore, MD: University Park Press, 1977.

Eyman, R. K. & Begab, M. Relationship between foster home environments and resident changes in adaptive behavior. *Proceedings of the Fifth International Congress of the International Association for the Scientific Study of Mental Deficiency*, 1979.

Eyman, R. K., DeMaine, G. C. & Lei, T. Relationship between community environments and resident changes in adaptive behavior: A path model. *American Journal of Mental Deficiency*, 1979, *83*, 330-338.

Fanshel, D. *Toward more understanding of foster parents*. Unpublished doctoral dissertation, New York School of Social Work, Columbia University, 1960.

Fanshel, D. Specializations within the foster care role: A research report. Part II. Foster parents care for the "acting out" and the handicapped child. *Child Welfare*, 1961, *40*, 19-23.

Fanshel, D. *Foster parenthood: A role analysis*. Minneapolis: University of Minnesota Press, 1966.

Fanshel, D. Status changes of children in foster care: Final results of the Columbia University longitudinal study. *Child Welfare*, 1976, *55*, 143-169.

Freeman, H. Foster home care for mentally retarded children: Can it work? *Child Welfare*, 1978, *57*, 113-121.

Gardner, J. M. Community residential alternatives for the developmentally disabled. *Mental Retardation*, 1977, *15*, 3-8.

Garrett, B. L. Meeting the crisis in foster family care. *Children*, 1966, *13*, 3-8.

Garrett, B. Foster family services for mentally retarded children. *Children*, 1970, *17*, 228-233.

Gollay, E., Freedman, R., Wyngaarden, M. & Kurtz, N. R. *Coming back*. Cambridge, MA.: Abt Books, 1978.

Gray, P. A. & Parr, E. A. *Children in care and the recruitment of foster parents*. S. S. 249, London, 1957.

Guerny, L. A description and evaluation of a skills training program for foster parents. *American Journal of Community Psychology*, 1977, *5*, 361-371.

Heal, L. W. & Daniels, B. S. *A cost-effectiveness analysis of residential alternatives for selected developmentally disabled citizens of three Northern Wisconsin counties*. Paper presented at the 102nd Annual Meeting of the American Association of Mental Deficiency, Denver, Colorado, May 1978.

Heal, L., Sigelman, C. & Switzky, H. Research on community residential alternatives for the mentally retarded. In N. R. Ellis (Ed.), *International review of research in mental retardation* (Vol. 9). New York: Academic Press, 1978.

Intagliata, J. *Post-institutional adjustment of retarded persons placed in family care homes*. Paper presented at the Annual Convention of the American Association on Mental Deficiency. Denver, Colorado, May 19, 1978.

Intagliata, J. & Willer, B. *Factors associated with success in family care homes and community residential facilities*. Paper presented at the annual meeting of the American Academy on Mental Retardation, San Francisco, California, May 12, 1980.

Intagliata, J., Willer, B. & Cooley, F. Cost comparison of institutional and community based alternatives for mentally retarded persons. *Mental Retardation*, 1979, *17*, 154-156.

Jaffee, B. A comparative study of the Case Family Program for Youth and the Older Children's Department of the Children's Home Society of Washington. In B. Jaffee & D. Kline (Eds.), *New payment patterns and the foster parent role*. New York: Child Welfare League of America, 1970, 25-96.

Justice, R. S., Bradley, J. & O'Connor, G. Foster family care for the retarded: Management concerns of the caretaker. *Mental Retardation*, 1971, *9*, 12-15.

Kaplan, B. H., Cassel, J. C. & Gove, J. Social support and health. *Medical Care*, 1977, *15*, 47-50.

Kay, N. A systematic approach to selecting foster parents. *Case Conference*, 1966, *3*, 49-51.

Kraus, S. *Community based alternatives to institutionalization: An historical perspective*. Paper presented at the annual meeting of the American Psychological Association, Toronto, Canada, August, 1978.

Lei, T. *Foster family care for mentally retarded children: What are the dimensions*? Paper presented at the annual conference of the American Association on Mental Deficiency, Miami, Florida, May 1979.

Lei, T., Sheehy, N. & Wilson, S. *Who provides small family care for mentally retarded children*. Paper presented at the Annual Conference of the Pacific Sociological Association, San Francisco, California, April 1980.

Maas, H. S. & Engler, R. *Children in need of parents*. New York: Columbia University Press, 1959.

Madison, B. & Schapiro, M. Permanent and long-term foster family care as a planned service. *Child Welfare*, 1970, *49*, 131-136.

Mamula, R. Developing a training program for family caretakers. *Mental Retardation*, 1970, *8*, 30-35.

Mamula, R. A. & Newman, N. *Community placement of the mentally retarded: A handbook for community agencies and social work practitioners*. Springfield, IL: Charles C Thomas, 1973.

McCarver, R. B. & Craig, E. M. Placement of the retarded in the community: Prognosis and outcome. In N. R. Ellis (Ed.), *International review of research in mental retardation* (Vol. 7). New York: Academic Press, 1974.

Meyers, C. E., Lei, T., Nihira, L. & Eyman, R. *How much room at the inn? Are there limits on small family placement*? Paper presented at XIII Annual Gatlinburg Conference on Research in Mental Retardation, Gulf Shore, Alabama, 1979.

Moos, R. H. *Family Environment Scale (FES). Family work and group environment scales*. Palo Alto, CA: Consulting Psychologists Press, Inc., 1974.

Morrissey, J. R. Status of family care programs. *Mental Retardation*, 1966, *4*, 8-11.

Murphy, H., Rennee, B. & Luchins, D. Foster homes: The new back wards? *Canada's Mental Health*, 1972, Monograph Supplement No. 71.

Newman, E. & Sherman, S. Foster family care for the elderly: Surrogate family or mini-institution. *International Journal of Aging and Human Development*. 1979-1980, *10*, 165-176.

New York State Department of Mental Hygiene. *Summary of plans of compliance for meeting ICFMR requirements*. Albany, NY: NYSDMH, 1975.

New York State Department of Mental Hygiene. Office of Social Rehabilitation. *Manual for family care providers*. Albany, NY: NYSDMH, 1976.

Nihira, L. & Nihira, K. Normalized behavior in community placement. *Mental Retardation*, 1975, *13*, 9-13.

Nirje, B. The normalization principle and its human management implications. In T. Kugel & W. Wolfensberger (Eds.), *Changing patterns in residential services for the retarded*. Washington: President's Committee on Mental Retardation, 1969.

O'Connor, G. *Home is a good place: A national perspective of community residential facilities for developmentally disabled persons* (Monograph No. 2). Washington, DC: American Association on Mental Deficiency, 1976.

Parks, J. M. *Characteristics of foster care sponsors*. Unpublished master's thesis, University of Utah, 1959.

Penniman, T. L. *Initial screening and identification of predictors for possible use in selecting foster mothers for the mentally retarded*. Dissertation Abstracts International, 1974, *35* (6-A), 3879.

Pollock, H. M. Organization of a family care colony for mental defectives. *American Journal of Mental Deficiency*, 1940, *45*, 73-77.

Pollock, H. M. Family care of mental defectives in Scotland. *American Journal of Mental Deficiency*, 1947, *52*, 89-90.

Reistroffer, M. E. Participation of foster parents in decision-making: The concept of collegiality. *Child Welfare*, 1972, *51*, 25-28.

Rich, M. Foster homes for retarded children. *Child Welfare*, 1965, *44*, 392-395.

Scheerenberger, R. C. *Deinstitutionalization and institutional reform*. Springfield, IL: Charles C Thomas, 1976.

Scheerenberger, R. C. & Felsenthal, D. *A study of alternative community placements*. Madison, WI: Research Institute of the Wisconsin Association for Retarded Citizens, 1976.

Sigelmen, C., Bell, N., Schoenrock, C., Elias, S. & Danker-Brown, P. *Alternative community placements and outcomes*. Paper presented at the annual meeting of the American Association on Mental Deficiency, Denver, May 1978.

Smitson, W. S. Foster mothers and mental patients. An exploratory study of interpersonal relationships. *Mental Hygiene*, 1970, *54*, 251-255.

Stedman D. J. & Eichorn, D. H. A comparison of the growth and development of institutionalized and home-reared mongoloids during infancy and early childhood. *American Journal of Mental Deficiency*, 1964, *69*, 391-401.

Sternlicht, M. Variables affecting foster care placement of institutionalized retarded residents. *Mental Retardation*, 1978, *16*, 25-28.

Vaux, C. L. Family care of mental defectives. *American Association on Mental Deficiency Proceedings*, 1935, *40*, 168-189.

Willer, B. & Intagliata, J. *Columbia County personal care pilot program: Final evaluation report*. Buffalo, NY: TEFCO Services, 1979.

Willer, B. & Intagliata, J. *Evaluation of the impact of deinstitutionalization of mentally retarded persons in New York State*: Final project report, 1980.

Willer, B., Intagliata, J. & Atkkinson, A. C. Crisis for families of mentally retarded persons including the crisis of deinstitutionalization. *British Journal of Subnormality*, 1979.

Willer, B., Scheerenberger, R. C. & Intagliata, J. Deinstitutionalization and mentally retarded persons. *Community Mental Health Review*, 1978, *3*, 3-12.

Windle, C. Prognosis of mental subnormals. *American Journal of Mental Deficiency*, 1962, *66* (Monograph Supplement), 8-25.

Windle, C. D. Sabagh, G., Brown, S. J. & Dingman, H. F. Caretaker characteristics and placement, success. *American Journal of Mental Deficiency*, 1961, *65*, 739-743.

Windle, C. D., Stewart, E. & Brown, S. J. Reasons for community failure of released patients. *American Journal of Mental Deficiency*, 1961, *66*, 213-217.

Wolfensberger, W. & Glenn, L. *PASS 3: A method for qualitative evaluation of human services*. Toronto: National Institute on Mental Retardation, 1975.

Zigler, E. & Balla, D. Impact of institutional experience on the behavior and development of retarded persons. *American Journnal of Mental Deficiency*, 1977, *82*, 1-11.

Matching Developmentally Disabled Client Characteristics to Careprovider and Employer Preferences

Patricia Sutter
Tadashi Mayeda

University of California, Los Angeles
Neuropsychiatric Institute Research Group
at Lanterman State Hospital and Development Center
Pomona, California

Frequently decisions must be made which involve changing the placement settings in which developmentally disabled persons live, work and learn. The current focus on deinstitutionalization is resulting in decisions to move increasing numbers of developmentally disabled clients from institutions to community residential settings. Likewise, sheltered workshops across the country are adopting objectives and goals which result in the placement of the developmentally disabled in competitive employment.

Regardless of the care with which placement changes are made, a substantial number of placements are unsuccessful, and many clients are being returned to the original placement settings. Placement failure rates for developmentally disabled persons were presented by Eagle (1967) for community residential placements and by the United State Department of Labor (1977) for vocational placements. These reports give reason for concern.

It seems apparent that the better suited the placement is to the needs and abilities of the client the greater the probability of placement success. Recently the authors have examined the extent to which placements were suitable in terms of the compatibility of match between careproviders and clients (Sutter, Mayeda, Yee, & Yanagi, 1980) and between employers and developmentally disabled employees (Farber, Kaplan, Mayeda, & Sutter, 1980).

Both studies were based on the hypothesis that variability exists in the criteria of both employers and careproviders in terms of those client characteristics with which they feel they are able to deal. The authors believed that they would find a relationship between the success of the placement and the extent to which individual careprovider or employer criteria were matched with the actual characteristics of the clients placed under their supervision.

In the Sutter et al. (1980) study the number of mismatches between careproviders and successfully placed clients were compared with the number of mismatches found between careproviders and unsuccessfully placed clients. Clients were labeled as unsuccessful by virture of having been reinstitutionalized within the 12 months immediately preceding the study. A mismatch was defined as a client exhibiting a characteristic which his or her careprovider had indicated was undesirable.

Unsuccessful careprovider/client pairs were found to be significantly more often mismatched in terms of client maladaptive behavior than successful

This research was supported by ODH-DHEW Developmental Disabilities Grant Number 54-P-71117/9.

careprovider/client pairs. This relationship remained statistically significant even for cases where clients manifested a large number of maladaptive behaviors (5 or more per client). Clients manifesting a large number of maladaptive behaviors who had been placed with careproviders who indicated a tolerance for those behaviors tended to remain in community care while clients who had not been so well matched to the criteria of the careprovider did not.

Likewise in the Farber et al. (1980) study successful employer/employee pairs were compared with unsuccessful employer/employee pairs for number of mismatches. Unsuccessful developmentally disabled employees were found to have been significantly more often mismatched with their employers than were successful developmentally disabled employees.

The results of these studies led to the conclusion that the probability of placement success might be increased if placement settings were selected on the basis of a point by point match between the criteria of client acceptability of the supervising adult with whom the client potentially is to be placed and the characteristics of the client. Since appreciable variability was noted in the criteria of the different careproviders and employers participating in the studies, it appeared that a wide variety of placement settings were potentially available to accommodate clients with varying characteristics.

Basically the same methodology was used in the two studies. A description is presented here since it is not given in detail elsewhere and since the simplicity of the procedure suggests that this technique may prove to be a viable and practical tool for assessing the suitability of placement settings.

A separate form was designed for use in each study to collect data on the criteria of client acceptability. Each form consists of objective items (26 for employers, 21 for careproviders) which depict client characteristics that previous research and clinical experience indicate are potentially problematic in the placement setting. Items such as "Wanders off or runs away" and "Has frequent toileting accidents" are representative of the careprovider form. Items such as "Is often late or absent" and "Must be closely supervised" are representative of the form designed for employers. These forms are shown in Figures 1 and 2.

The instruments were self-administered. The authors attempted, therefore, to minimize any element of implied judgement or criticism that might be associated with negative responses by giving special consideration to the nature of the instructions for completing the forms and to the wording of item alternatives.

Both instruments were described to respondents as preference surveys. Respondents were told that the purpose of the survey was to provide placement staff with more accurate information regarding the respondents' preferences in client characteristics in order that more suitable placements might be made. No mention was made of either success or failure in terms of clients associated with that placement setting. It was believed that this was a fair representation of the purpose of the studies since the ultimate goal was to develop procedures that would aid in making successful placements.

Items were completed by checking the alternatives of choice. The wording of item alternatives was intended to be neutral and not such as to elicit reluctance in respondents who might prefer to select a negative response to an item. Careproviders were asked to indicate for each item on the careprovider preference form whether they considered the characteristic depicted by the item to be "not serious," "somewhat serious," or "very serious" if exhibited by a client in their home and, independently of seriousness, whether they "would handle" or "preferred not to handle" a client with that characteristic. Employers were asked to indicate for each item on the employer preference form whether they "will hire" or "cannot hire" a client with the characteristic described by the item.

Employer Preference Survey

Company Name ______________________________ Individual Completeing Form ______________________ Date ________________	Will hire	Cannot hire
Has trouble seeing	1	2
Has trouble hearing	1	2
Has seizures	1	2
Must take medication regularly for physical problems	1	2
Is poorly groomed	1	2
Leaves work early, comes late, or is often absent	1	2
Dresses sloppily	1	2
Gets lost within facility	1	2
Has difficulty making change or working with numbers	1	2
Is unable to run errands outside place of employment	1	2
Has trouble initiating own tasks	1	2
Takes poor care of own or company's belongings	1	2
Must be closely supervised	1	2
Is unlikely to initiate helping others	1	2
Is negligent in using phrases such as "please" and "thank you"	1	2
Lets simple injuries (e.g., cuts, burns) go unattended	1	2
Has difficulty remembering names of items	1	2
Has trouble mixing well with co-workers	1	2
Reacts poorly to criticism or frustration	1	2
Demands excessive attention or praise	1	2
Is unable to read signs or simple instructions	1	2
Is poorly coordinated	1	2
Requires additional job training	1	2
Doesn't tell you when he doesn't understand	1	2
Works well but slowly	1	2
Is unable to fill out an application	1	2

Figure 1. UCLA-NPI-LSH Research Group/EMPLOYER PREFERENCE SURVEY (7/80).

Careprovider Preference Survey

Facility Name ______________________________

Name of Individual Completing Form ______________________________

State __ __ County __ __ __ Type __ __ ID # __ __ __ __ __ __ __ __ __ Date __ __/__ __/__ __	Not serious	Somewhat serious	Very serious	Can handle	Prefer not to handle
When a client: It is:					
Is hyperactive and cannot settle down	1	2	3	1	2
Has trouble seeing and gets hurt	1	2	3	1	2
Has trouble hearing	1	2	3	1	2
Can hear but does not listen	1	2	3	1	2
Has seizures and gets hurt	1	2	3	1	2
Drools and/or has mouth odor	1	2	3	1	2
Must take medication regularly	1	2	3	1	2
Refuses to take medication	1	2	3	1	2
Has tantrums and becomes uncontrollable	1	2	3	1	2
Is a messy eater and is sloppy	1	2	3	1	2
Has frequent toilet accidents	1	2	3	1	2
Cannot wash self and has body odor	1	2	3	1	2
Wanders off or runs away	1	2	3	1	2
Cannot tell you what he wants and causes problems	1	2	3	1	2
Does not understand instructions and seems stubborn	1	2	3	1	2
Does not pay attention and gets into trouble	1	2	3	1	2
Gets into fights, threatens or hurts others	1	2	3	1	2
Damages or takes things	1	2	3	1	2
Shows unacceptable sexual behavior	1	2	3	1	2
Hurts self on purpose	1	2	3	1	2
Does odd things or makes odd noises	1	2	3	1	2

Figure 2. UCLA-NPI-LSH Research Group/CAREPROVIDER PREFERENCE SURVEY (7/80)

The source of the client data was different in the two studies. In the careprovider study, information on client characteristics was obtained from the Behavior Development Survey (BDS) item scores. The BDS is a modified version of the AAMD Adaptive Behavior Scale (Nihira, Foster, Shellhaas, & Leland, 1974).[1] For the employer study, data for each client were collected on forms which duplicated the items on the employer preference form. Information was obtained from workshop files and through interviews with workshop staff familiar with the client.

The responses of individual careproviders and employers were then matched on an item by item basis to the characteristics of the clients who were or who had been under their supervision. The number of mismatches for each careprovider/client pair and for each employer/employee pair were determined by tallying those characteristics that were exhibited by clients and that corresponded to negative careprovider or employer responses.

These investigations have not been comprehensive enough to indicate the probability of success or failure that might be associated with varying degrees of mismatch. The results of these studies seem to indicate, however, that a relationship does exist and that the more compatible the match between the client and the supervising adult with whom he is to be placed the higher the probability of placement success. The implementation of a procedure similar to the one described in this paper when assessing the suitability of a potential placement setting might be expected to increase the probability of placement success.

References

Eagle, E. Prognosis and outcome and community placement of institutionalized retardates. *American Journal of Mental Deficiency*, 1967, *72*, 232-243.

Farber, F., Kaplan, D., Mayeda, T., & Sutter, P. *Relationship of employer performance criteria to client failure in competitive employment*. Manuscript submitted for publication, 1980.

Nihira, K., Foster, R., Shellhaas, M., & Leland, H. *AAMD Adaptive Behavior Scale*. Washington, DC: American Association on Mental Deficiency, 1974.

Sutter, P., Mayeda, T., Yee, S., & Yanagi, G. *Community placement success based on client behavior preferences of careproviders*. Manuscript submitted for publication, 1980.

United States Department of Labor. Sheltered workshop study: A nationwide report on sheltered workshops and their employment of handicapped individuals (Volume 1). Washington, DC: Employment Standards Administration: Employment and Training Administration, 1977.

[1]Copies of the BDS as well as copies of the two preference forms may be obtained from the UCLA/NPI Research Group at Lanterman State Hospital and Developmental Center, P.O. Box 100-R, Pomona, CA 91769.

A Study of Small Family Care for Mentally Retarded People

Tzuen-jen Lei
Lyly Nihira
Nancy Sheehy
C. Edward Meyers

School of Medicine
University of California, Los Angeles
The Neuropsychiatric Institute
Lanterman State Hospital Research Group

In 1935, an experimental placement of 32 mentally retarded children in 14 community families established the foster care model for paid care of retarded clients in homes other than their own (Heal, Sigelman & Switzky, 1978). With the thrust for normalization through deinstitutionalization and for retention of the mentally retarded population in the community, a number of alternative residential placements have been used. Among these alternatives, foster family care is regarded as the closest substitute to the care provided by the natural family. This surrogate care presumably offers the most intimate surroundings and maximal personal interaction for mentally retarded persons along socially normal lines within the community settings. It has been assumed that a well-planned foster family care placement system will help the retarded person achieve specific developmental goals and maximize individual potential.

With expanded use of community placement, there is growing interest among researchers in the evaluation of various types of community residential care for retarded persons. Although a fair amount of literature exists on the subject of foster family care (Adams, 1970, 1975; Adams & Calvin, 1969; Ambinder, Fireman, & Sargent, 1963; Fanshel, 1961, 1966; Mamula, 1971; Murphy, 1964; Parker, 1966; Peterson, 1974; Taylor & Starr, 1967; Williston, 1963), the majority of the work evaluates the general foster family care system. Only a small amount of research has centered around foster family care provided to mentally retarded persons. Thus, information on foster family care for mentally retarded people is still limited. (A review of available literature is provided in this volume by Intagliata, Crosby, and Neider.)

The purpose of this study is to describe the various components (i.e., clients, careproviders, and home environments) of a foster family care system for mentally retarded persons. In California "foster care" is provided to mentally retarded individuals by community facilities licensed as "small family homes," serving from one to six developmentally disabled residents through contact with regional centers. The data reported here were collected on a sample of 245 mentally retarded clients (21 years of age or younger) who lived in 112 small family homes at the time of the survey in 1978. These homes were located in a four-county area

This study was supported by contract No. HD-7-2847 from the National Institute of Child Health and Human Development, U.S. Department of Health, Education, and Welfare, Richard K. Eyman, Principal Investigator; Public Health Service General Research Grant No. FR-05632, National Institute of Health; and Grant No. HD-04612, Mental Retardation Research Center, UCLA, George Tarjan, Principal Investigator.

of southern California having a total population of over one million people. The area is served by one of the 21 regional centers which provide services for developmentally disabled individuals, including the mentally retarded.

Characteristics of the Clients

Among the 245 sampled clients, approximately 60% were children under 18 years of age at the time of initial sample selection. The remaining 40% were between ages 18 and 21. This proportion should not be taken as representative. The main focus of the study was to be upon homes serving children and young adults, so only those homes in the area having clients under 22 years were included. This constituted approximately 40% of all small family homes of the area. The data reported here are based solely on the clients aged 21 or under residing in the selected homes.

For mentally retarded children, especially the younger ones, out-of-home placement is considered only upon exhaustion of all other available resources designed to aid the parents to take care of their retarded child at home (e.g., daytime programs, respite care, specialized equipment). The regional center generally considers placement in a small family home preferable to placement in a larger facility or an institution since the small family home presumably provides a more natural and normalized environment for its residents. To be placed in a licensed small family home, a child must be ambulatory, have no medical problems which require close medical supervision, and be without symptoms of any major emotional disturbance. In addition, previous research has indicated that foster family care is usually provided for the retarded persons who do not have serious functional impairment (Eyman & Borthwick, 1980; Eyman & Call, 1977; Lei & Eyman, 1979).

The total client sample contained 58% male and 42% female clients. Sixty-five percent of the sample were in the mild-moderate range of mental retardation, 34% were in the severe-profound range, while the remaining 1% was unknown. Thirty-nine percent of the clients were placed in the current facility within the last 2 years, 27% had been in current placement for 3 to 5 years, and the remaining 34% had been there for more than 5 years, up to the longest period of 14 years. As indicated in Table 1, a higher proportion of the severely/profoundly retarded children were placed outside their natural home as infants, while mildly/moderately retarded children tended to be placed at older ages.

Table 1

Age of Initial Out-of-Home Placement by MR Level

	MR Level	
Age Category	**Mild/Moderate (N = 153)**	**Severe/Profound (N = 81)**
0-1	13.7%	22.2%
2-4	32.7%	28.4%
5-9	30.1%	39.5%
10-20	23.5%	9.5%
Median age	5.11	4.43

$X^2 = 9.27$, d.f. $= 3$, $p < .05$.

Most of these clients (89%) were in good health. In fact, nearly half of the clients did not have any medical problems at the time of the survey. About 40% of the clients previously had chronic diseases. However, their health problems were under control with easily administered medications. Only 11% of clients in these homes still had uncontrolled medical problems. If the health of the 11% would continue to require close medical care, these clients very possibly would be relocated into a different residential setting where intensive medical supervision is available.

Clients' Education and Training

Nearly 90% of the 245 clients were enrolled in special education classes or other training programs during the regular school hours. The school-aged children were distributed in the following programs: classes for educable mentally retarded students (2%), classes for trainable mentally retarded students (52%), developmental centers for handicapped children (24%), programs for the multiply handicapped (4%), and programs for autistic children (3%). Other programs including workshops, work activity centers, and adult education were specially geared to the needs of mentally retarded adults who comprised a total of 14% of clients enrolled in special training programs. Teachers or program directors were requested to complete a School Behavior Development Survey form (School BDS) for the clients in their class or program. The school BDS is a modified version of the Behavior Development Survey (BDS) which is a short form of the AAMD Adaptive Behavior Scale (Nihira, Foster, Shellhaas, & Leland, 1974). The purpose of this survey was to assess the competence and behavior of the mentally retarded clients outside the home settings. The regular BDS form has been completed annually by the careproviders since 1973 to evaluate the overall behavioral adaptation and development of each client residing in the home. Item by item comparison between careproviders' responses to the regular BDS and teachers' responses to the School BDS on 190 clients (78% of the total sample) showed a high degree of consistency (approximately 90% of agreement) between the two ratings. These results have suggested there was little or no variation between clients' behavioral performance at home and their behavior in school.

For the clients aged 13 or older, vocational readiness and level of occupational competence were also evaluated by the teacher or program director. The instrument used for this evaluation was the modified San Francisco Vocational Competency Scale, which, in its original form, was designed to provide an assessment of the personal-social development and vocational competence of mentally retarded adults based on observation of their characteristic performance in varied work situations (Levine & Elzey, 1968). The scale contains 30 items. Each item provides either four or five descriptive statements that represent varying degrees of competence for a particular task. The descriptive statements within each item are ordered by ability level and are numbered from 1 through 4 or 5, with a score 1 representing the lowest degree of vocational competence and a score 4 or 5 representing the highest degree of competence. The total vocational competency score is the sum of all individual item scores. It should be noted that for the experimental use of the prevocational evaluation of younger and lower functioning clients in this project, some items have been revised and response formats have been slightly changed to make the items appropriate to the clients in the sample. However, the basic scoring procedure has remained the same as that of the original scale.

The results of complete evaluation on the 150 retarded adolescents by sex and level of retardation are presented in Table 2. No significant differences were found between vocational competency scores for males and females. This finding was in contrast to the study reported by Levine and Elsey (1968) on a normative sample consisting of 562 mentally retarded individuals (ages 18+ and IQs between 20-75) in which significant sex differences were observed. However, as Table 2 indicates, significant differences were found between the mildly/moderately retarded group and the severely/profoundly retarded group.

Table 2

Scores on the Modified San Francisco Vocational Competency Scale by Sex and MR Level

	Median	Mean	S.D.	N
Sex				
Male	66.0	72.3	24.4	88
Female	61.5	68.8	24.4	62
MR Level[a]				
Mild-moderate	75.2	76.5	24.6	89
Severe-profound	59.5	61.9	21.4	60
Unknown	—	—	—	1

[a] $t = 3.81$, $p < .01$

Since the scale has been modified for the younger and lower functioning clients in this project, the results were not compared with percentile norms of the original scale (Levine & Elsey, 1968). However, the distribution of the scores seemed to indicate the vocational readiness and occupational potential of mentally retarded persons can be measured at an earlier age by using appropriate evaluation instruments.

Placement Background

Among the 245 sampled clients, 27% (N = 67) were in their initial out-of-home placement, but one-third (N = 80) were deinstitutionalized cases, and 40% (N = 98) were transferred from other community residential facilities, the majority of which were other small family homes. Generally, the clients who had their first out-of-home placement were considerably younger (median age = 14 years) than the clients who were previously institutionalized or had other experiences in out-of-home placement (median age = 17 years).

Table 3 shows the relationship between the clients' prior living arrangements and reasons for their current placement. The results indicated that a majority of the deinstitutionalized cases were placed in the small family homes to conform to the principle of normalization. Placements of most clients who were in their initial residential placement were judged to be the result of failing home environments in which their parents were no longer able to cope with their problems. Relocation from other community residential facilities was usually the consequence of previous unsuccessful placements, closure of the facilities, residential mobility of client's own family, and similar reasons.

Although foster care is designed to provide "substitute" family care for a "planned period," in many cases the placement becomes permanent. Examination was made of the relationship between the reason for parents' requesting out-

Table 3
Prior Living Arrangement by Reason of Current Placement

Reasons for Current Placement	Prior Living Arrangement		
	Other Community Facilities (N=98)	Homes of Parents, Relatives or Friends (N=67)	Institutions or Convalescent Hospitals (N=80)
Parent's inability to cope	16.0%	82.1%	16.3%
To achieve a normalized environment	13.8%	6.0%	76.3%
Other (conflict in previous placement, closure of prior facility, residential mobility, etc.)	70.2%	11.9%	7.5%

$X^2 = 165.26$, d.f. = 4, $p < .001$

of-home placement and various individual and family characteristics at the time of initial placement (cf. Table 4). The level of retardation of the clients apparently bears no relationship to any reported reason for out-of-home placement. Most retarded children placed at infancy were among those who were placed immediately after birth (69%), had never lived with their natural family (60%), and were more likely to have been abandoned by their younger mother (16% among mothers aged under 30 vs. 9% of mothers in the 30-59 age category). Many of these children (approximately 25 cases) have had court appointed guardians. Significantly more older mothers (age 30 or over) with other children at home reported the need for a more suitable environment for their retarded offspring than younger mothers (age below 30) with no other children.

Natural Parent Evaluation of Placement

Among the 245 sampled clients, 180 natural parents (73%) were located and gave consent to an interview. Nearly 90% of the parents who were interviewed expressed satisfaction with their child's placement. A majority (over 80%) of them had never considered trying to bring their child back home permanently and did not think there would be a possibility for them to do so, even if they were to receive financial reimbursement at the current level of payment for the out-of-home care (Nihira & Lei, 1979). It is our judgment that the above findings would be altered very little if contact had been made with the remaining 27% of parents. If anything, the satisfaction with the foster placement and the intention not to take the client back home would be increased. Most of the 27% could not be reached or refused to be involved. The findings suggested that foster care placement for most mentally retarded persons is permanent. Therefore, the qualities and characteristics of foster home environments and careproviders are of vital importance to the growth of the retarded clients placed in these small family homes.

Characteristics of Careproviders

Both group surveys and individual interviews were carried out with the primary careproviders of each sampled foster home to collect data regarding their socio-demographic characteristics, attitudes, experiences, and preferences in

Table 4

Reasons for Initial Out-of-Home Placement by Individual and Family Characteristics

Characteristics	Total N[a]	Reasons for Initial Out-of-home Placement: Family Problems	Placement Immediately After Birth	Supervised Environment and Training	Others	X^2
		%	%	%	%	
MR Level						
Mild/Moderate	153	51.0	10.5	30.0	8.5	1.0
Severe/Profound	84	46.4	14.3	32.2	7.1	
Age of Client						
0-1	39	20.5	69.2	5.1	5.1	149.6***
2-4	74	63.5	0.0	28.4	8.1	
5-9	77	51.9	0.0	40.3	7.8	
10-20	43	51.2	0.0	39.5	9.3	
Mother's Age						
19-29	70	52.9	15.7	18.5	12.9	12.4**
30-59	151	49.0	8.6	37.7	4.9	
Family Composition						
Both Bio. Parents	131	56.5	5.3	31.3	6.9	93.0***
One Bio. Parent	74	47.3	1.4	40.5	10.8	
Other	35	25.7	60.0	8.6	5.7	
No. of Siblings						
None	29	48.3	27.6	20.7	3.4	13.6*
1-2	119	50.4	10.1	32.8	6.7	
3-8	56	51.3	3.9	36.9	7.9	

[a]Total N varies in the different characteristics because of the missing data
*$p<.05$
**$p<.01$
***$p<.001$

handling the behavior and care of mentally retarded children. Of the 112 homes, approximately 50% were licensed to serve only developmentally disabled children (under 18 years of age), 13% of the homes were licensed to serve both children and adults, and the remainder of the homes (37%) were licensed to provide services only for adults (18 years or older). The homes that provided services to both children and adults were in a transitional period of changing their license from serving mentally retarded children to caring for adult clients. Often when clients reach the age of adulthood (18 years old), instead of relocating the clients to an adult home, many careproviders prefer to change their license to care for adult clients because of their attachment to the clients. The residents of this type of home are most likely to be older adolescents and young adults. About 37% of the homes provide services only to male clients, nearly 29% only to female clients, and 33% serve both male and female clients. The majority of the careproviders (approximately 90%) served only ambulatory residents. The remaining 10% might consider serving non-ambulatory clients. However, as the personnel of the regional center serving the catchment area in which this study was conducted is very reluctant to place any non-ambulatory clients in small family care, the mentally retarded persons in this sample were all ambulatory.

Socio-demographic Characteristics of Careproviders

The distributions of sex, age, ethnicity, marital status, and education were examined among the primary careproviders of the 112 small family homes (Lei, Sheehy, & Wiilson, 1980). All but 5% of the primary careproviders responding to our survey were females. Apparently the foster mother had the primary responsibility of providing care for the residents. The distribution of marital status showed that about 80% of the homes were two-parent families. Thus, most of the foster homes had a male figure as a secondary careprovider and supplied a home environment similar to the traditional family. At the time of the survey, nearly 40% of the careproviders had their own children living at home. Most homes provided care to two or more residents, up to the legal maximum of six. More than half of the careproviders had at least 8 years of experience in serving developmentally disabled clients.

There was a substantial difference between the ethnic composition of careproviders and the clients whom they served. The majority of the careproviders were non-white (53%), whereas the majority of the clients were white (87%). Among the non-white careproviders, the majority (approximately 75%) was black. Other non-white careproviders (a total of 16) included Spanish-speaking Americans, Asian-Americans, and other ethnic minorities.

About two-thirds of the careproviders were at least 50 years old. Ethnic differences were revealed in the age distribution of careproviders. Half of the white careproviders were at least 50 years old whereas over 80% of the non-white careproviders were in the same age category. Since there was no ethnic difference in length of service in providing residential care to mentally retarded clients, the data may suggest that non-white careproviders are more likely to become involved in foster care as they approach the time they will be forced to retire from other jobs or in the years after their own families have been raised. More white careproviders may undertake their role as a job held within the home while raising their own children.

Approximately 60% of the primary careproviders had completed a minimum of 12 years of formal education, and 90% responded that they had taken one or more special training classes designed to assist them in caring for the retarded client. There was a difference in educational level between the white and non-white groups but not in the number of training sessions in which they had participated. Nearly three-fourths of the white careproviders had completed at least 12 years of school, compared with less than half of the non-white careproviders. However, no significant ethnic difference in education was found after controlling for age, since age and level of education were inversely related and non-white careproviders tended to be older than the white careproviders.

Careproviders and Client Characteristics

Some associations were found between careproviders' characteristics and types of home classified by age and sex of the clients. The variables measuring the careproviders' characteristics were dichotomized: age (under 50 years vs. 50 years or over); ethnicity (white vs. nonwhite); education (less than 12 years vs. 12 years or more); presence of own children at home (no vs. yes); number of clients in residence (one to three clients vs. four to six clients); and years of experience in providing residential services to mentally retarded clients (five years or fewer vs. more than 5 years).

Table 5 shows that a significantly higher proportion of the careproviders who served only the adult clients were non-white, less educated (less than 12 years of education), without any of their own children living at home, and having four or more residents. On the other hand, the careproviders of the homes providing services to children and young adults were more likely to be white, more educated (at least completion of high school), to have their own children living in the same residence, and to provide services to fewer than four clients. Age and experience of the careproviders were not associated with the age of clients served.

Table 5

Careprovider Characteristics and Homes Classified by Age of Residents Served

Dichotomized Careprovider Characteristics	Residents Served: Adults Only (N=42)	Residents Served: Children Under Age 18[a] (N=70)	X^2
Age			
Under 50	33.3%	43.5%	1.1
50 or over	66.7%	56.5%	
Ethnicity			
White	23.8%	60.0%	13.8**
Non-white	76.2%	40.0%	
Education			
Less than 12 years	52.4%	32.9%	4.2*
12+ years	47.6%	67.1%	
Own children at home			
No	73.8%	54.3%	4.2*
Yes	26.2%	45.7%	
No. of clients			
1-3	26.2%	48.6%	5.5*
4-6	73.8%	51.4%	
Experience			
5 years or less	38.1%	34.3%	.2
More than 5 years	61.9%	65.7%	

[a]Including 15 homes in the transitional period of license change for providing the services to young adult clients
*$p<.05$
**$p<.001$

Whether the home provided services only to male clients or female clients was not associated with any characteristics of careproviders. However, significant differences were found between the homes providing services to the clients of same sex (either male or female) and those homes having residents of both sexes (cf. Table 6). It appeared that careproviders of the homes having same sex clients were older (at least 50 years of age), non-white with more than 5 years of experience in foster care business, and without any of their own children living at home. In contrast, careproviders of the homes serving both male and female clients were younger (under 50 years of age), white, less experienced (5 years or less), and with their own children living at home. Education of the careproviders and the number of residents were not related to whether clients of the same sex or both sexes were served.

Table 6

Careprovider Characteristics and Homes Classified by Sex of Residents Served

Dichotomized Careprovider Characteristics	Residents Served: Single Sex (N=74)	Residents Served: Both Sexes (N=38)	X^2
Age			
Under 50	30.1%	61.1%	9.6**
50 or over	69.9%	38.9%	
Ethnicity			
White	39.7%	62.2%	4.9*
Non-white	60.3%	37.8%	
Education			
Less than 12 years	42.5%	37.8%	.2
12+ years	57.5%	62.2%	
Own children at home			
No	69.9%	45.9%	6.0*
Yes	30.1%	54.1%	
No. of clients			
1-3	39.7%	43.2%	.1
4-6	60.3%	56.8%	
Experience			
5 years or less	28.8%	51.4%	5.4*
More than 5 years	71.2%	48.6%	

*$p<.05$
**$p<.01$

Careprovider Preferences

One of the primary concerns of the study was to investigate whether different demographic characteristics of the careproviders were related to their attitudes and preferences in providing foster care to mentally retarded clients with various behavior problems. The careproviders were given a questionnaire, the Careprovider Preference Survey, listing 50 behavioral problems which residents might present. The purpose of the survey was to assess the experiences and preferences of careproviders regarding physical and behavioral problems or deficits, excluding medical problems (except seizures), commonly displayed by developmentally disabled or mentally retarded clients in community residential care. Each of the items in the survey elicited responses pertaining to: (1) the preference for or willingness to handle the problem and the perception of the degree of seriousness of the problem; and (2) the personal experience in handling the problem.

The responses to preference in handling each of the 50 listed behavioral problems were coded in an ordinal scale from 1 to 4. A score of 1 represents the attitude of a careprovider who considers the problem very serious and prefers not to handle it; and a score of 4 represents the attitude of a careprovider who is willing to handle the problem regardless how serious it is. A principal component factor analysis on these coded responses given by the 112 careproviders who participated in this study (Nihira, Meyers, & Lei, 1979) yielded seven oblique factors:

(1) anti-social behavior (e.g., disrupting others' activities, verbal threats to others, damaging property); (2) potentially jeopardizing behavior (e.g., self-abuse, running away); (3) chronically dependent behavior (e.g., need of daily help with bathing or dressing); (4) inadequate self-care behavior (e.g., spilling, lack of toilet training); (5) socially dependent behavior (e.g., incapable of handling money, inactive in group activities); (6) low functioning behavior (e.g., trouble with drinking, making strange noises); and (7) physical handicap (e.g., difficulty in using hands, trouble seeing). The factor scores were constructed by summing the coded preference scores of each factor's individual items. The total number of items that the careprovider reported having had experience in handling was also summed on each factor.

Items that careproviders were most likely to consider as very serious and to prefer not to handle are clustered under Factor 2, potentially jeopardizing behavior, i.e., running away, homosexual behavior, stereotyped behavior, self-abuse, public masturbation, and removal of clothing at an inappropriate time. Items clustered under Factor 7 also showed that careproviders tended to be seriously concerned about clients' physical condition, i.e., being deaf, blind or epileptic, or any act that involved jeopardy, and that they were reluctant to handle such behavior. Their responses further suggested they were least concerned about clients' need for help in more advanced self-care behaviors, such as handling of money or meal preparation.

Careprovider Characteristics and Preferences

The five variables measuring the careprovider characteristics, age, ethnicity, education, number of clients served, and years in foster care service, were related to the seven factor scores of careproviders' preferences and experiences in handling client's problem behaviors. Relationships between each factor score and careprovider characteristics were evaluated by multiple regression analysis, with simultaneous control of the effects of other characteristics in the same equation. The results showed that different careprovider characteristics were significantly associated with their preferences for handling different behavioral problems of clients. The older careproviders were more likely than the younger ones to report willingness to handle clients' anti-social behavior (Factor 1). White careproviders were more likely than non-white careproviders to be willing to handle low functioning clients (Factor 6). The less educated careproviders were more likely than the better educated ones to express willingness to handle potentially jeopardizing behavior (Factor 2). The careproviders who served more clients were more likely than those careproviders of smaller homes to report their willingness to handle inadequate self-care behavior (Factor 4). Finally, the more experienced careproviders (having provided services for more than 5 years) were more likely than the less experienced careproviders to be willing to handle clients who might display socially dependent behavior (Factor 7). None of the careprovider characteristics was associated with willingness to care for clients with chronically dependent behavior (Factor 3) and problems relevant to physical disabilities.

All the careprovider characteristics were significantly associated with experience in handling clients' behavioral problems clustered in Factors 4, 6, and 7: inadequate self-care behavior, low functioning behavior, and physical disabilities. Careproviders characterized as younger, white, more educated, serving more clients, and having provided foster care services for longer periods, were more likely than their counterparts to have had experience in handling clients behavioral problems pertaining to these factors. Most care-provider characteristics, except

Table 7

Careprovider Preferences and Experience Related to Careprovider Characteristics: Multiple Regression Analyses[a]

Preferences and Experience Factors	Careproviders' Characteristics					
	Age	Ethnicity	Education	No. of Clients	Years in Foster Care Service	Multiple R
Preferences						
1 Anti-social behavior	.148	—	—	—	—	.274
2 Potentially jeopardizing behavior	—	—	−.163	—	—	.269
3 Chronically dependent behavior	—	—	—	—	—	.127
4 Inadequate self-care behavior	—	—	—	.201	—	.220
5 Socially dependent behavior	—	—	—	—	.163	.206
6 Low functioning behavior	—	−.263	—	—	—	.271
7 Physical disabilities	—	—	—	—	—	.183
Experience						
1 Anti-social behavior	−.171	—	.174	.185	.233	.354
2 Potentially jeopardizing behavior	−.168	—	.217	.379	.295	.516
3 Chronically dependent behavior	—	—	—	.145	.182	.245
4 Inadequate self-care behavior	−.197	−.134	−.155	.320	.298	.515
5 Socially dependent behavior	—	—	.158	—	.309	.334
6 Low functioning behavior	−.141	−.189	.136	.207	.284	.450
7 Physical disabilities	−.187	−.138	.137	.295	.290	.488

[a]Non-significant standardized multiple regression coefficients (ß) are not presented. Ethnicity is coded as 0 = white and 1 = non-white

ethnicity, were significantly associated with experience handling clients' anti-social behavior (Factor 1) and potentially jeopardizing behavior (Factor 2). Similarly, the younger, better educated careproviders, operating larger homes, and having more years of service experience were more likely than the older, less educated careproviders, operating smaller homes, and having provided foster care service for shorter lengths of time, to have had experience in handling these behaviors. Generally, the careproviders who had been in foster care business for years were more likely than those who started providing foster care for mentally retarded clients in recent years to have experience in handling all types of behavioral problems that clients might display. In addition, a careprovider of a larger home was more likely than a careprovider of a small home to have experience in handling chronically dependent behavior (Factor 3). The better educated careproviders were more likely than those less educated to have reported experience in handling clients' socially dependent behavior.

Characteristics of the Home Environment

In assessing the foster home environment for mentally retarded residents, in addition to the physical environment, the social and psychological dimensions of the foster parent-client relationship must be measured. The importance of both of these dimensions has been demonstrated in the literature examining parent-child relationships in natural homes. Three survey instruments were used to evaluate the physical, social and psychological environments of the 112 small family homes in the study: the Program Analysis of Services Systems (*PASS 3*, Wolfensberger & Glenn, 1975); the Home Inventory Form, an adapted version of Home Observation for Measurement of Environment (Caldwell, Heider, & Kaplan, 1966; Caldwell, 1968), and the Home Quality Rating Scale, a subjective rating completed by a trained rater immediately following home observation and an interview with the careprovider. Among these three instruments, the Home Quality Rating Scale appeared to be the most appropriate for measuring foster home environment and showed most promising results in this study when related to careproviders' characteristics.

The Home Quality Rating Scale consists of items that were designed to measure the socio-psychological atmosphere and physical environment of a small family home. All items are scored from 1 to 5, with a score of 1 representing the lowest rating and a score of 5 representing the highest rating of the home environment. A principal component factor analysis on the data collected for this study (Meyers, Sheehy, & Lei, 1979), with squared multiple correlations on the diagonal and varimax rotation, yielded six interpretable factors: (1) parenting quality and harmony in home (e.g., growth promotion in client care, acceptance of client); (2) additional support in providing care (e.g., secondary care providers, burden of care shared by others); (3) quality and safety of dwelling and physical surroundings (e.g., cleanliness of the home, house structure and appearance); (4) size of home and sibling influence (e.g., presence of siblings, number of bedrooms); (5) residential environment (e.g., residential quality of neighborhood, quiet home atmosphere); and (6) protective tolerance (e.g., absence of overprotection of clients, lack of hazards in home). The factor scores were the sum of individual item scores of each factor.

Careprovider Characteristics and Home Environment

As the home environment directly influences clients' behavior and growth (Eyman & Begab, 1979), it is necessary to examine the relationship between careproviders' socio-demographic characteristics and quality of the home environment. Among the careprovider characteristics examined, five variables, age, ethnicity, education, presence of own children at home, and number of clients served, were associated with one or more of the six factors of the Home Quality Rating Scale (cf. Table 8). Under the multiple regression procedure with simultaneous control of the five selected careprovider characteristics, three variables were significantly associated with the factor of parenting quality and openness (Factor 1). The careproviders characterized as white, better educated, and having at least one of their own children living at home were more likely than the non-white, less educated careproviders who had none of their own children at home to have received a higher rating on the factor pertaining to parenting quality and openness. Higher scores on additional support in providing care (Factor 2) were found among homes whose careproviders had received higher levels of education and provided services to more clients than those homes whose careproviders were less educated and served fewer clients. While a higher score on quality and safety of home surroundings (Factor 3) was associated with ethnicity (white) and education (better educated) of careproviders and number of clients served at home (fewer clients), a higher rating of the size of home and sibling influence (Factor 4) was related with the careproviders who were younger, having at least one of their own children living at home, and serving more clients. Number of clients served at home (fewer clients) was the only characteristic associated with the higher rating of the residential quality of the home environment (Factor 5). The last factor, protective tolerance, was moderately associated with better educated careproviders.

Table 8

Home Quality Rating Scale and Careprovider Characteristics: Multiple Regression Analyses[a]

Home Quality Factors	Careproviders' Characteristics: Age	Ethnicity	Education	Own Children At Home	No. of Clients	Multiple R
1 Parenting quality and openness	—	−.182	.195	.185	—	.374
2 Additional support in providing care	—	—	.253	—	.226	.348
3 Quality and safety of home surroundings	—	−.171	.164	—	−.166	.295
4 Size of home and sibling influence	−.123	—	—	.693	.235	.745
5 Residential environment of home	—	—	—	—	−.162	.194
6 Protective tolerance	—	—	.137	—	—	.264

[a]Non-significant standardized multiple regression coefficients (ß) are not presented. Ethnicity is coded as 0 = white and 1 = non-white; own children at home is coded as 0 = no and 1 = yes.

Discussion and Summary

This paper has examined the characteristics of 245 mentally retarded children and young adults who have received residential care in 112 foster family homes located in southern California. Data reported in this study have suggested that foster family care can provide effective services for certain categories of mentally retarded persons, i.e., children without a serious functional impairment, medical problems, or maladaptive behavior. The majority of mentally retarded clients in foster family care have participated in special education or other training programs. Most of clients who were not in any training program were of preschool age. Programs for the school-aged children emphasized cognitive development, while programs for mentally retarded adults were specially geared to vocational training.

The authors compared careproviders' and teachers' evaluations of clients' adaptive behavior and found a high degree of agreement for those clients who attended school. A measure of vocational competence for clients 13 years of age and older demonstrated that the moderate-mild group was superior to the severe-profound group on that measure. The scale employed for the purpose (a modification of the San Francisco Vocational Competency Scale) was found to discriminate at low ability levels and with subjects at a prevocational age. Hence, it has been demonstrated that it is possible to make an early evaluation of vocational readiness to permit early training of mentally retarded adolescents.

Data collected on this sample have indicated that reasons for seeking out-of-home placement by the natural parents were unrelated with clients' level of retardation, but were rather significantly related with some characteristics of the client's family. Out-of-home placement seemed to be sought most frequently as a relief from socially induced problems as a consequence of having a retarded person at home, rather than a search for therapy for a client's condition. Parents of the retarded clients generally expressed satisfaction with their children's placements and felt unable to take permanent responsibility of raising their retarded children at home.

Most primary careproviders who offer small family care for the mentally retarded clients in this sample were female householders in their 50's and were adequately educated. The majority of these homes were operated by a husband-wife team, and if the husband was also providing care, it was in a secondary role. Our data have shown that most careproviders had years of experience in caring for retarded clients and had attended at least one training session since they were licensed to operate a family care home for mentally retarded clients. Thus, despite a wide range in all characteristics, most careproviders were mature and experienced. More than one-third of the careproviders in the sample were black. This proportion may be compared with the two percent of clients who were black and the four percent of the total population of the entire catchment area.

A number of careprovider characteristics were related to clients' behavior problems. Greater willingness to accept clients with antisocial behavior was found in older careproviders. Greater willingness to accept clients with jeopardizing behavior was found in careproviders who were less educated. Greater willingness to accept clients with inadequate self-care behavior was found in careproviders who served more clients at home. Greater willingness to handle clients' socially dependent behavior was found in careproviders who have more years of experience. Greater willingness to accept low functioning clients was found in careproviders who were white. More experience in handling clients with behavior problems, on the other hand, was reported by younger and better educated careproviders who operated larger homes and had provided foster care for more years. Better home qualities (as operationalized by the Home Quality Rating Scale) were generally found in the homes of careproviders who were younger, better educated, and who had their own children at home. Larger homes with more clients were positively associated with higher ratings of additional support in care and sibling influence, but negatively related to the quality and safety of home surroundings, as well as to the residential environment of home.

These relationships should be regarded only as tentative results because of the crude measurement and basic statistics used in the present study. A separate study (Lei & Sheehy, 1980), using a more sophisticated multivariate technique to analyze the relationship between careproviders' characteristics and the quality of home environment, found most relationships were not of a simple strict linear nature. Complex, curvilinear relationships were observed between careprovider characteristics similar to the variables investigated in this paper, and the six factors of the home quality rating scale.

Some earlier studies have found moderate but significant association between changes in clients' adaptive behavior scores and factors of home environment measured by *PASS 3* environmental ratings (Eyman, Demaine, & Lei, 1979), by Caldwell's Home Inventory (Eyman, Kawakami, Litchfield, & Moss, 1978), or by Home Quality Rating Scale (Eyman & Begab, 1979). All these studies were carried out under the assumption of strict linear relationships. For future research, possible curvilinear relationships should be considered for studying the complex associations among careproviders' characteristics, home environment, and clients' behavioral development. In addition, it must be noted that certain variables in this study, particularly "ethnicity," are strongly affected by economic and social conditions. For example, on Factor 3 (quality and safety of dwelling and physical surroundings) the differences between whites and non-whites are clearly more a function of a deep-rooted social problem than they are reflective of real differences among members of the two groups.

Data reported in this paper have provided a fairly optimistic picture of small family care for the mentally retarded people. Although there may be a practical limit to the types and number of mentally retarded people that can be placed into foster care homes, this model of residential care provides an opportunity for its clients to live in a home environment with a careprovider who is presumably more experienced and trained, and potentially not as emotionally involved as the natural parent with the problems that the mentally retarded person may display.

This paper also suggested some tentative associations between socio-demographic characteristics of careproviders and the types of clients they choose to serve, their attitudes toward foster care practice and clients' behavioral problems, and the quality of foster home environments. It is hard to characterize a general profile of foster care homes that are most conducive to clients' development. It is possible that the combination of certain careprovider characteristics and certain environmental factors may meet the needs of one type of client, while other combinations are effective in providing services to other clients with different needs. As was shown, careproviders have their own individual preferences for the kind of clients they are most willing to serve or the type of clients' problems they are willing and capable of handling. Therefore, when careproviders' preference meets the characteristics and needs of the clients, there should be a good chance of successful placement. As more clients are placed in foster homes under the general policy of promoting community placement, careproviders may end up having to provide services to more seriously handicapped clients, thus increasing the risk of failure in placement (Meyers, Lei, Nihira, & Eyman, 1979).

A well-planned foster family care system can provide specific services to help a mentally retarded individual grow to his/her developmental potential with proper treatment and professional training in a normalized environment. As California continues its policy of deinstitutionalization, the need for residential facilities in the community continuously grows. Particularly, the number of small family homes has been steadily increasing. However, as the deinstitutionalized population stabilizes, the number of small family homes targeted for the mentally retarded population is also likely to stabilize. In addition, a new trend in deinstitutionalization encourages natural parents to take care of their retarded children at home, with the continuous expansion of respite care services and daytime training programs in the community. Thus, it is likely that the number of homes for adults may continue to increase in order better to accommodate the needs of the mentally retarded adults who no longer can live with the natural family, while the number of small family homes for developmentally disabled children may grow very slowly or may even decrease somewhat.

References

Adams, M. E. Foster family care for the intellectually disadvantaged child: The current state of practice and some research perspectives. In M. J. Begab & A. Richardson (Eds.), *The mentally retarded and society: A social science perspective*. Baltimore: University Park Press, 1975.

Adams, M. E. Foster care for mentally retarded children: How does child welfare meet this challenge? *Child Welfare*, 1970, *49*, 260-269.

Adams, M. E., & Calvin, R. W. The deprivation hypothesis: Its application to mentally retarded children and their needs. *Child Welfare*, 1969, *46*, 136-141.

Ambinder, W., Fireman, L., & Sargent, D. Verbal abilities and literacy levels required of foster parents. *Child Welfare*, 1963, *42*, 501-53.

Caldwell, B. *Instruction manual: Home observation for measurement of the environment*. Unpublished manuscript, 1968.

Caldwell, B., Heider, J. & Kaplan, B. The inventory of home stimulation. Paper presented at the annual meeting of the American Psychiatric Association, September, 1966.

Eyman, R. K., & Begab, M. J. Relationship between foster home environments and residential changes in adaptive behavior. *Proceedings of the Fifth International Congress of the International Association for the Scientific Study of Mental Deficiency*, 1979.

Eyman, R. K., & Borthwick, S. A. Patterns of care for the mentally retarded. *Mental Retardation*, 1980, *18*, 63-66.

Eyman, R. K., & Call, T. Maladaptive behavior and community placement of mentally retarded persons. *American Journal of Mental Deficiency*, 1977, *82*, 137-144.

Eyman, R. K., Demaine, G. C., & Lei, T. Relationship between community environments and resident changes in adaptive behavior: A path model. *American Journal of Mental Deficiency*, 1979, *82*, 330-338.

Eyman, R. K., Kawakami, K., Litchfield, R., & Moss. W. Environmental stimulation and adaptive behavior of mentally retarded residents. *Pacific State Archives*, 1978, *3*.

Fanshel, D. *Foster parenthood: A role analysis*. Minneapolis: University of Minnesota Press, 1966.

Fanshel, D. Studying the role performance of foster parents. *Social Work*, 1961, *6*, 74-81.

Heal, L., Sigelman, C. K., & Switzky, H. N. Research on community residential alternatives for the mentally retarded. In N. R. Ellis (Ed.), *International review of research in mental retardation* (Vol. 9). New York: Academic Press, 1978.

Lei, T., & Eyman, R. K. Characteristics of individuals referred to services for the developmentally disabled. *Mental Retardation*, 1979, *17*, 196-199.

Lei, T., & Sheehy, N. Physical and parenting characteristics of foster homes for retarded children. Paper presented at the annual meeting of the American Academy on Mental Retardation, San Francisco, California, May, 1980.

Lei, T., Sheehy, N., & Wilson, S. Who provides small family care for mentally retarded children? Paper presented at the annual meeting of the Pacific Sociological Association, San Francisco, California, April, 1980.

Levin, S., & Elzey, F. F. *San Francisco Vocational Competency Scale*. New York: The Psychological Corporation, 1968.

Mamula, R. A. The use of developmental plans for mentally retarded children in foster family care. *Children,* 1971, *18,* 65-68.

Meyers, C. E., Lei, T., Nihira, L., & Eyman, R. K. How much room in the inn? Are there limits on small family placement? Paper presented at the 13th Annual Gatlinburg Conference on Research in Mental Retardation, Gulf Shore, Alabama, 1979.

Meyers, C. E., Sheehy, N., & Lei, T. Post interview home evaluation of foster family care environments. Paper presented at the 103rd Annual Conference on the American Association of Mental Deficiency, Miami, Florida, May, 1979.

Murphy, H. B. M. Foster home variables and adult outcomes. *Mental Hygiene,* 1964, *48,* 587-599.

Nihira, K., Foster, R., Shellhaas, M., & Leland, H. *AAMD Adaptive Behavior Scale, 1974 revision*. Washington, DC: American Association of Mental Deficiency, 1974.

Nihira, L., & Lei, T. Parental response to foster care of their mentally retarded offspring. Paper presented at the 13th Annual Gatlinburg Conference on Research in Mental Retardation, Gulf Shore, Alabama, April, 1979.

Nihira, L., Meyers, C. E., & Lei, T. Careprovider preference and mentally retarded client behavior. Paper presented at the 103rd Annual Conference of the American Association of Mental Deficiency, Miami, Florida, May, 1979.

Parker, R. A. *Decision in child care: A study of prediction in fostering*. London: Allen & Union, 1966.

Peterson, J. C., & Pierce, A. D. Socioeconomic characteristics of foster parents. *Child Welfare,* 1974, *53,* 295-304.

Taylor, D. A., & Starr, P. Foster parenting: An integrative review of the literature. *Child Welfare,* 1967, *46,* 371-385.

Williston, G. C. The foster parent role. *Journal of Psychology,* 1963, *60,* 263-272.

Wolfensberger, W., & Glenn, K. *PASS 3, A method for the quantitative evaluation of human services*. Toronto: National Institute on Mental Retardation, 1975.

A Review of Training Programs for Providers of Foster Family Care to Mentally Retarded Persons

James Intagliata
Barry Willer

Division of Community Psychiatry
State University of New York at Buffalo

The use of foster family care homes for mentally disabled persons has been traced as far back as sixth century in Belgium (Camplan, 1969; Smitson, 1970). However, such homes were not used for mentally retarded persons in this country until 1931 in New York State (Heal, Sigelman & Switsky, 1978). They were begun as an alternative to institutions because it was felt that they provided a more natural and congenial life, gave altruistic employment to community families, and lessened the need for institutions, thereby reducing costs (Pollock, 1936, 1947). Though the interest in and use of this placement option waned somewhat in the late 1940s and 1950s, by 1966 foster care homes were serving more than 5,700 mentally retarded persons in 26 states (Morissey, 1966).

As a result of the widespread deinstitutionalization of mentally retarded persons since that time, the use of foster family care has greatly expanded. The results of a recent national survey (Bruininks, Hill & Thorsheim, 1980) indicated that in 1977 there were more than 8,600 mentally retarded persons living in specially certified family care homes in 21 states. Further, the authors reported that the number of states making use of such homes reached 32 in 1978.

The current rationale for utilizing family care homes is not unlike that offered by Pollock (1947) more than 30 years ago. In keeping with the principle of normalization, family care is seen as the placement of choice for an individual who is capable of living in a home-like setting but whose own family cannot provide it (Adams, 1970; Nirje, 1969). Further, family care homes provide a much less expensive placement when compared to most other community-based alternatives (Gardner, 1977; Heal & Daniels, 1978; Intagliata, Willer & Cooley, 1979).

As the use of family care homes for the mentally retarded has increased, so has the recognition that the care provider's role is a difficult one. To begin with, the demands of caring for disabled persons requires specialized skills beyond those required for normal parenting (Dorgan, 1974; Shah, 1971). Indeed, the stress experienced by foster care providers who serve the mentally retarded has been well documented (Intagliata, Willer & Wicks, 1979; Justice, Bradley & O'Connor, 1971; Maluccio, 1966; Rich, 1965; Wilkes, 1974). What is more, recent studies (Gollay, Friedman, Wyngaarden & Kurtz, 1978; Willer, Intagliata & Wicks, 1979) have reported that the retarded persons placed in family care homes tend to be more severely handicapped than individuals placed in community residences.

Along with recognition of the significant demands placed on foster care providers serving the mentally retarded has come the realization that providers must be carefully prepared if they are to function effectively in their role. The need to develop specialized training for these providers has been repeatedly acknowledged in the professional literature (Dick, 1961; Garrett, 1966; Guerny, 1977; Mamula, 1970; Mamula & Newman, 1973). Further, foster parent associations have grown rapidly since the 1960s and have strongly supported the development of training programs designed to increase the professional competence of their members (Goldstein, 1967; Stone & Hunzeker, 1975). Demanding that homes meet certain physical standards and that care providers have good health and character references are simply no longer sufficient criteria for assuring the quality of foster family care programs, especially those intended to serve handicapped individuals (Mamula, 1970).

In response to the evident need, a number of training programs have been developed specifically for foster family care providers serving mentally retarded/developmentally disabled residents. However, while these training programs are available, their wide scale implementation with care providers has lagged. Further, no systematic critical review of existing training packages has appeared in the professional literature. The present paper will present such a review of training programs for family care providers serving mentally retarded persons.

The reader should be aware that there has been a corresponding development of training packages for those caring for mentally retarded persons in a variety of settings other than family care homes. Specifically, training packages have been developed for staff of small community residential facilities (e.g., ENCOR, 1977), the natural parents of mentally retarded persons (Porter, 1978) and those who provide respite care for the mentally retarded (e.g., Murstein, 1978). Also generic training packages have been developed to be used with almost any group of individuals providing community based care to mentally retarded/developmentally disabled individuals (cf. Appendix for Way-to-Go Program). Though these training programs will not be reviewed in the present paper, they are mentioned here because much of what will be said about foster care training can be readily applied to them.

This review will begin with a discussion of the basic types of foster care provider training programs which can be developed. Following this, six selected programs will be described and compared. They will be discussed in terms of their objectives, content, educational methods and intended use. The lack of evaluation data on these programs will be noted and a model for designing training evaluations will be presented. Finally, the authors will present a series of suggested steps for those readers interested in developing their own training programs. For those interested in obtaining specific training materials mentioned in this review, the authors have prepared an appendix that identifies where one can write to obtain further information on each program.

Types of Training Programs

Several different types of training have been suggested and developed for foster care providers. The National Foster Parent Association stated in 1973 that there should be a continuum of development opportunities having three mandatory components: preservice training, ongoing inservice training, and agency supervision of foster homes (Stone & Hunzeker, 1975). The supervision component generally refers to supervision of care providers by professionals of a government funded agency. It has generally been less structured than preservice or inservice education and has been oriented to monitoring rather than training. However, a good foster care program will have all components of provider training and will probably include training of supervisory personnel as well.

Preservice Training

Preservice training is generally designed to serve as a mandatory prerequisite for persons who are seeking certification as foster care providers. In most cases, applicants are not eligible to enter such training until they have passed through an initial screening phase in which they and their home must meet certain agency standards (Mamula, 1970; Stone & Hunzeker, 1975). Preservice training varies in length but generally involves six to ten separate sessions scheduled over a one-to-three-month period. The content is chosen to provide prospective care providers with a general orientation to such topics as the philosophy and specific operating regulations of the foster care agency, the administrative responsibilities of care providers, the nature of developmental disabilities, the concepts of normalization and deinstitutionalization and principles of basic care procedures for residents (Dickerson, 1977; Mamula, 1970; Murphy, 1975; Provencal & Evans, 1977).

Inservice Training

Inservice training is generally viewed as an ongoing educational process which supplements the preservice training program. It is provided to individuals who have successfully passed through preservice training and who are working as certified foster care providers. Unlike the more intensive preservice phase, inservice training sessions are typically offered no more than once a month. Frequently they take the form of advanced workshops focusing on topic areas which were addressed only briefly during preservice training (Goldstein, 1967; Provencal & Evans, 1977). An extensive inservice training program is currently available at Eastern Michigan University (Ryan, Warren & McFadden, 1977). Once care providers have completed the 20-hour introductory course for foster parenting, they may select from eighteen separate, advanced courses dealing with special topics such as guiding sexual development or dealing with emotional disturbance.

Inservice training is offered to, and in some cases mandated for, foster care providers in order to provide them with ongoing opportunities to develop and refine their caring skills. The demands placed on foster care providers are great, especially when the resident placed in the home is mentally retarded. Most preservice training programs can only provide caretakers with a basic introduction to the important aspects of their role. Thus, if providers are to be able to deal more independently and effectively with the wide range of problems which will confront them, ongoing inservice training may be a necessity.

Agency Supervision

The success of structured educational programs, preservice and inservice, will depend in part on the extent to which professional supervisory staff of agencies reinforce concepts taught during the training sessions. Much of what is taught in training programs revolves around the use of some form of individual program planning. The development of individual plans clearly requires the assistance of professional staff, especially in determining the most effective methodology for reaching individual goals. The professional staff will also be expected to provide information to the care provider about each resident's activities and programs in other life areas such as vocational and recreational.

An effective way to link the inservice and preservice programs with ongoing supervision is to involve the agency professionals in providing or receiving the training. In addition, it is probably a good idea to design a supplementary series of special training sessions for supervisory personnel on such topics as leadership, case management, individual program planning, and effective supervisory styles.

In summary, comprehensive training programs should include preservice training, inservice training and supervision. Preservice training is designed to prepare new care providers through a basic understanding of their role, agency regulations, and the needs of the developmentally disabled. Inservice training is generally oriented to teaching basic behavior management skills, individual programming, crisis management and a host of other content areas. Supervision should include monitoring of standards and reinforcement of concepts taught during training sessions.

Selection of Training Programs for Review

Identifying the foster care training programs for this review was a difficult process. The authors began with a thorough review of the mental retardation and foster care literature. However, while there was frequent mention of the need for such programs, descriptions of programs which had actually been implemented simply did not appear (with the exception of Mamula, 1970). As an alternative strategy the authors contacted a few individuals who were generally knowledgeable about training-related endeavors in the mental retardation field. These persons were able to identify one or two groups who they knew had developed training programs for foster care providers. The authors then contacted these individuals, requested information about their training programs and asked them to identify any other persons whom they knew to be directly involved in developing training programs. If they could not identify anyone else who had developed a similar training program, the authors asked them to name anyone who they thought might be of assistance in searching out other foster care provider training packages. Thus, the authors were able to contact an ever expanding network of persons involved in foster care training.

The process of identifying existing foster care training programs took almost one year and involved phone calls and correspondence to individuals throughout the country. Eventually, the same training programs continued to be identified and there were no new leads. At this point a number of different types of training programs had been identified. These included programs for training foster care providers, community residence staff, parents, and respite care providers. The authors, however, had decided to focus the review on just those programs developed for or used with foster care providers. Further, a decision was made to review only those programs that were relatively comprehensive in coverage. Of the eight programs which met these criteria, three had been developed exclusively for training foster parents working with mentally retarded children (Dickerson, 1977; Marr, 1976; Nowak & Reistroffer, 1970), while the other five were designed to train care providers working with mentally retarded persons of various ages. The five more generic programs along with the most generically oriented program for training foster parents working with children (Dickerson, 1977) were selected for the present review. The reason for this is that while the authors thought that it was useful to include at least one program designed for a specialized resident population (Dickerson, 1977) it was felt that this review would be more widely useful if it focused on programs designed to train foster care providers in general.

The six training programs selected for review are: (1) Caretakers Training Program (Mamula, 1970), (2) Foster Care of the Developmentally Disabled (Murphy, 1975), (3) Resident Manager Education (Provencal & Evans, 1977), (4) Fostering Children with Mental Retardation (Dickerson, 1977), (5) Living in a

Family Environment (LIFE) training program (Waisman Center on Mental Retardation and Human Development, 1976) and (6) New Directions in Community Care (California Instructional Television Consortium, 1975). All six programs have been used in training foster care providers, although some were developed for a broader range of community care providers, including staff in group homes, hotels and other community residential facilities.

Comparison of Selected Programs

Brief descriptions of each program are presented on the next few pages. These summary sketches are offered so that the reader can refer back to program descriptions as this review proceeds to compare and contrast the programs on a number of their component aspects. The particular aspects on which programs will be compared include objectives, content, educational methods and intended use.

Title: **Training Program for Family Caretakers**

Author: Mamula (1970)

Objectives:

(1) To provide participants with a basic knowledge base regarding mental retardation and specific problems related to family care.

(2) To help participants view their role not as custodial, but rather as demanding active involvement with residents.

(3) To give participants a sense of ego identification with the family care program.

Content:

(1) Introduction to Family Care—I

(2) Mental Retardation and Mental Illness

(3) Field Visits to State Institutions

(4) Introduction to Family Care—II

(5) Field Visits to Family Care Homes

(6) Caretakers Discuss Family Care

(7) Special Problems in Family Care (e.g., health, behavior)

(8) General Aspects of Certification

Educational Methods: Lecture, discussion, field trips, role playing

Intended Use: Preservice training of family care providers for mentally ill and mentally retarded persons.

Title: **Foster Care of the Developmentally Disabled: A Basic Course for Foster Parents and Foster Care Workers**

Author: Murphy (1975)

Objectives:

(1) To provide participants with a basic understanding of developmental disabilities and the foster care system.

(2) To increase participants' awareness of how they respond emotionally to developmentally disabled persons.

(3) To help participants develop the skills necessary for providing basic care and dealing with behavior problems.

Content:

(1) An Overview of Care of the Developmentally Disabled
(2) Foster Care System
(3) Clarification of Role of Foster Parents
(4) Developmental Disabilities
Part I: Mental Retardation
(5) Developmental Disabilities
Part II: Cerebral Palsy, Epilepsy
(6) Emotional Response to Developmentally Disabled Persons
(7) Understanding the Developmentally Disabled Child
(8) Developmental Disabilities: A Family Problem
(9) Foster Care of the Developmentally Disabled
Part I: Placement Considerations
(10) Foster Care of the Developmentally Disabled
Part II: Basic Care Considerations
(11) Special Problems: Separation, Discipline, Mental Health
(12) Summary, Evaluation, Termination of Course

Educational Methods: Lecture, discussion, field visits, films, guest speakers

Intended Use: Preservice and inservice training of family care providers and family care staff.

Title: **Resident Manager Education (Macomb-Oakland)**

Authors: Provencal and Evans (1977)

Objectives:

(1) To provide participants with a knowledge base of mental retardation and the responsibilities of care providers.
(2) To give participants the skills for responding effectively to problems and crises.
(3) To prepare participants to maintain a safe, healthy living environment.
(4) To introduce participants to individual program planning for clients.

Content:

Preparational Education

(1) An Orientation to Mental Retardation
(2) Maintaining Healthy Environments, Providing Emergency Care
(3) Fire and Safety Considerations
(4) Administrative Responsibilities
(5) Elements in Programming
(6) Normalization

Continuing Education

(1) Managing Behavior
(2) Leisure Time/Recreational Considerations
(3) Educational Considerations
(4) Community Placement
(5) Relationships with Natural Families
(6) Thoughts on Sexuality

Educational Methods: Lecture, group discussion, guest speakers.

Intended Use: Preservice and inservice education of family care providers and group home personnel.

Title: **Fostering Children with Mental Retardation**

Author: Dickerson (1977)

Objectives:

(1) To give participants insight into personal attitudes and values and how these affect care.

(2) To assist participants in understanding normal child development.

(3) To develop participants' skills in assessment and planning for special needs of developmentally disabled children.

(4) To assist participants in understanding effective management techniques for behavior problems.

Content:

Part I: Providing Postive Parenting for the Child with Mental Retardation

(1) Introduction

(2) Facts About Mental Retardation

(3) Home Safety and Routines

(4) Positive Parenting

(5) Getting to Know Your Foster Child

(6) Learning the Specifics of Behavior

(7) Introduction to Positive Behavior Management

(8) Who Will Help the Foster Parent?

Part II: Assessing and Planning for the Child with Mental Retardation

(9) Focusing on Your Foster Child

(10-11) Assessing Adaptive Behavior

(12) Recognizing and Setting Priorities

(13-15) Focus on Particular Developmental Needs

(16) Keeping Records

Educational Methods: Lecture, group discussion, homework assignments.

Intended Use: Preservice and inservice education of family care providers.

Title: **The Life Project**

Authors: Waisman Center on Mental Retardation and Human Development (1976)

Objectives:

(1) To provide participants with a basic understanding of mental retardation.

(2) To prepare participants to maintain a safe, well-organized, healthy living environment.

(3) To develop participants' skills for teaching clients self-help skills, community living skills and constructive use of leisure time.
(4) To attune participants to the need to integrate their residence into the community.

Content:
(1) Introduction to mental retardation and community living
(2) Home Management
(3) Health and Hygiene
(4) Behavior Management
(5) Teaching Social Competency Skills
(6) Sexuality
(7) Use of Leisure Time
(8) Community Resources and Relations

Educational Methods: Self-teaching manuals, audio-cassettes and film strips.

Intended Use: Preservice or continuing education for group home parents and foster parents.

Title: **New Directions in Community Care**

Producer: California Instructional Television Consortium (1975)

Objectives:
(1) To provide a basic understanding of developmental disabilities and the system of services in the state of California.
(2) To prepare participants to maintain a safe, healthy, residence.
(3) To prepare participants to respond effectively to routine behavior problems as well as emergency situations.
(4) To develop participants' skills for teaching clients basic self-care skills and increasing their social competence.
(5) To increase participants' awareness and sensitivity to the human and legal rights of their residents.

Content:
Part I
(1) Introduction (one module)
(2) Medications (three modules)
(3) Health (two modules)
(4) Emergencies (one module)
(5) Nutrition (three modules)
(6) Activities (three modules)
(7) Human Needs (two modules)
(8) Preplacement (one module)

Part II (Each topic covered in one module)
(1) Developmental Disabilities
(2) Self-help Skills
(3) Safety
(4) Behavior Problems

(5) Sexuality
(6) Recreation and Leisure
(7) Transition: Encouraging Resident Independence
(8) Community
(9) Team Planning
(10) Agencies

Educational Methods: Series of videotape modules (1/2 hour each), accompanying written materials, study questions, discussion, guest speakers.

Intended Use: Inservice education of administrators and staff of community care facilities and family care providers for mentally ill and developmentally disabled persons, as well as elective use with students in the health sciences.

Objectives

Although the content of the objectives for each program is substantially similar, the specificity with which each is conceptualized varies a great deal. Mamula (1970) provides general objectives for the entire training package but does not provide specific learning objectives for the individual training sessions. Provencal and Evans (1977) and the California Instructional Television Consortium (ITV) (1975) state no overall program objectives but present specific learning objectives for each training module. This latter approach is desirable since it provides a basis on which the content of specific modules can be evaluated separately.

Whether objectives are presented for modules or for the entire training program, objectives should be clearly stated. Murphy (1975) states that the single objective of her training program is to help participants to work more effectively and collaboratively to provide community-based residential services to developmentally disabled persons. This objective is stated in most general terms and does not make clear what type of behavior might be required for a participant to be able to work more effectively as a care provider. As a contrast to Murphy's (1975) singular program objective, the Waisman Center (1976) listed ten program objectives for the LIFE training program. These, however, vary greatly in their specificity, from very general "to help participants guide residents," to specific "to help participants assist residents in developing personal care skills."

Given the wide variation in the form (level, number, specificity) in which they have been stated, it was impossible to compare the content of each program's objectives without devising a standard approach for redefining them. In order to do this, the overall content of each program was surveyed, and in each case general training objectives consistent with the program's content were inferred.

Taking this approach, it appears that all six programs reviewed share three basic objectives for participants. These are to provide them with (1) fundamental knowledge about mental retardation, (2) an understanding of their responsibilities as care providers, and (3) the basic skills needed to care for residents in their homes. The depth and breadth of the knowledge and skills taught, however, vary greatly from one program to another and will be discussed in more detail in the section of this paper which compares program content.

In addition to these basic objectives which are shared by all programs reviewed, two other objectives relating to care providers' attitudes are included in some programs. First, four of the programs (Mamula, 1970; Murphy, 1975; Provencal & Evans, 1977; California ITV Consortium, 1975) encourage participants to assume the attitude that they are part of a "foster care team" which also includes agency caseworkers, natural family, and other skilled professionals. Consistent with the team concept, the importance of coordinating the responsibilities and skills of all these persons is stressed.

While this first attitudinal objective deals with the way in which care providers relate to professionals and significant others, the second deals with care providers' attitudes toward the residents placed in their care. In her training program, Murphy (1975) attempts to help participants "come to grips" with personal feelings and reactions toward a disabled resident in order to help them get beyond the handicap and respond directly to the person. This is, however, the only program reviewed that confronts this important issue directly. The reasons why it is neglected in the other five programs are not clear. It is possible that the authors have assumed either (1) that participants have already faced and resolved this issue prior to entering training, or (2) that those persons who use their training curriculum will present this issue to participants on their own initiative. However, these are unfortunate assumptions if they lead to this important issue of care providers' emotional response to handicapped persons being ignored in training.

In general, most of the training programs did not appear to deal directly with affective or attitudinal topics. Most programs, especially the most structured ones, are focused primarily on teaching knowledge and skills. While these are clearly important aspects of providing quality care, it must not be overlooked that care providers are likely to be highly influenced by attitudes and beliefs as well.

Whether objectives relate to knowledge, skills or attitudes, clearly stated objectives are a definite asset to any training program. Objectives provide the program with a fundamental rationale which can help to integrate subsequent decisions regarding the specific content and methods of training. Further, clearly stated objectives provide the framework for evaluation of the training program. Unless a training program has a clear purpose, it is difficult to devise a fair and useful evaluation of its impact.

Content

Table 1 presents a scheme for categorizing the content covered in the training programs and indicates which programs deal with which particular content areas. Clearly, no single program includes all topic areas and perhaps no program should. The programs all represent the particular bias of their authors and presumably reflect the needs of the particular audience for whom the program was designed.

A thorough review of the specific topic areas of each training program reveals that there is no unanimous content overlap between programs with the exception of one topic, facts of mental retardation. The specific facts about mental retardation presented in each program are relatively consistent and typically include information on definition, cause and diagnostic categories. In addition, Murphy (1975) includes a discussion of the psychological and social impact of labeling. Dickerson (1977) presents information on the additional physical handicaps that frequently accompany mental retardation.

1. *Caretakers Training Program*

The variation in content covered by each training program calls for review and comment on each program individually. Of all the individual programs reviewed,

Table 1
Content of Training Programs

Topics	Programs					
	Mamula	Murphy	Provencal-Evans	Dickerson	Waisman Center	California ITV*
Orientation to Mental Retardation						
Facts about mental retardation	X	X	X	X	X	X
Ideologies and services		X	X			X
Orientation to Care Provider Role						
History and role of foster care	X	X				
Care provider responsibilities	X	X	X			X
Relationship with natural family		X	X		X	
Community relations					X	X
Utilizing support services				X	X	X
Emotional response to mental retardation		X				
Basic Home Management						
Maintaining a safe home			X	X	X	X
Dealing with general emergencies			X		X	XX
Establishing routines		X		X	X	XX
Establishing limits/rules				X		XX
Basic Resident Care						
Teaching self-care skills		X			X	X
Routine health care	X		X		X	XX
Medical emergencies			X		X	XX
Medications/administration			X		X	XX
Nutrition					X	XX
Positive parenting				X		
Behavior management			X	X	X	X
Individual Program Planning						
General principles			X	X	X	X
Behavior assessment				X	X	XX
Setting goals/contracting				X	X	XX
Behavioral sequences/ task analysis				X	X	
Keeping records				X	X	X
Effective team work						X

*Note: XX indicates that this topic is covered only in Part I of the training and is excluded from Part II which was designed specifically for those working with developmentally disabled persons.

Table 1 *(Continued)*
Content of Training Programs

Topics	Mamula	Murphy	Provencal-Evans	Dickerson	Waisman Center	California ITV*
Advanced Resident Training						
Teaching social competence					X	X
Use of leisure time			X		X	X
Human sexuality			X		X	X
Special Problems						
Discipline	X	X				
Mental health		X				
Separation		X				X
Individual rights					X	XX

*Note: XX indicates that this topic is covered only in Part I of the training and is excluded from Part II which was designed specifically for those working with developmentally disabled persons.

the one described by Mamula (1970) is the most limited in content. In all it is comprised of eight sessions and is intended to provide basic training to family care providers serving either mentally ill or mentally retarded residents. The first session provides participants with orientation to the training program and to their prospective role as care providers. As part of this session they are given presentations on the history of family care and some general information about mental illness and mental retardation. The second session of the program is designed to provide a more extensive orientation to mental illness and mental retardation. Specifically, diagnostic categories and their implications for family caretakers are discussed.

This orientation is continued in a more experiential fashion with field visits to state institutions serving the mentally ill and mentally retarded. During these visits participants meet and speak with hospital staff as well as prospective family care residents. Following these visits, participants attend their fourth training session in which they are acquainted with the various types of community placement options available to patients and the role played by family care homes in the deinstitutionalization effort. They are also introduced to various basic regulations regarding the operation of family care homes.

Once again, field visits are used to provide an experiential supplement to participants' orientation. Specifically, the fifth training session involves field visits to selected family care homes where participants are given an opportunity to interact with both caretakers and residents. The sixth session involves a panel discussion by experienced family caretakers. These caretakers share their experiences and perceptions and respond to any questions raised by participants.

The seventh session focuses on introducing participants to a variety of practical problems which they will face as family caretakers. In particular, health problems are discussed by nursing staff. Further, this session involves the role playing of selected resident behavior problems and suggested techniques for handling them. The eighth and final session focuses on various aspects of home certification and prepares participants for their future contacts with residents' social workers.

The strength of this program lies in the thoughtful attention given to orienting potential family caretakers to their role. Unlike any of the other programs reviewed, this one supplements didactic orientation material with experiential input. During the course of training, participants are given several opportunities to meet and interact with experienced caretakers and potential residents. Such an approach seems an excellent way to bring naive trainees into real contact with the role they intend to assume.

The weakness of the program is its failure to address such important training topics as basic home management, basic resident care, individual program planning and advanced resident training. Thus, in its present state the authors would recommend that it be used only as a guide in developing the orientation stage of a more comprehensive training program. If one intends to prepare participants to take a treatment rather than custodial-oriented role, far more attention must be given to training residents in self-care skills and social competence. Further, basic principles of individual program planning need to be included. These content areas could be the focus of a supplemental continuing education training package.

2. *Foster Care of the Developmentally Disabled: A Basic Course for Foster Parents and Foster Care Workers*

The program developed by Murphy (1975) is more extensive in its content than that of Mamula. Three of the twelve content units in the program are devoted to providing participants with a thorough orientation to developmental disabilities. One entire unit is devoted to mental retardation and includes discussion of definition, diagnosis, causes, and levels of subnormality. The unit on other developmental disabilities focuses on cerebral palsy and epilepsy and includes information on the types, causes, medical and psychosocial effects, attitudes toward and management of these disabilities. The third unit compares the developmental stages for normal and developmentally disabled children and explains the social and psychological impacts of labeling. The special impairment problems and behavioral characteristics of developmentally disabled persons are also presented.

A fourth unit of this program provides participants with further orientation by providing an overview of care for the developmentally disabled. Deinstitutionalization is discussed in the context of a historical presentation on service ideology. Three additional units are devoted to orienting participants to their care provider role. Specifically, participants are familiarized with the foster care system in which they will work and their roles and responsibilities in relation to natural families and other professionals in this system. Participants are also given information regarding the practical realities and problems which will accompany the placement of a developmentally disabled child into their home.

In addition to these units which provide participants with primarily cognitive input, Murphy (1975) supplements the orientation to the care provider role by including two sessions which focus on care providers' affect. One of these is devoted to giving participants an appreciation of the emotional impact that having a developmentally disabled child has on his/her family. The purpose of this is to facilitate better relationships between foster care providers and the residents' natural family by giving the former greater empathy for the latter. Another unit in Murphy's program has participants identify and confront their own emotional reactions to disabled persons. As noted previously, this is the only program reviewed which includes any attention to the emotional aspects of providing foster care to the mentally retarded.

In the unit devoted to basic care considerations, participants are encouraged to set realistic expectations for the resident placed in their home. Brief coverage is given to the need to teach residents to become as independent as possible with respect to selected self-care skills (e.g., grooming, eating, dressing, toileting). While no elaboration is included, participants are also encouraged to train residents in household skills, money management, community travel and other areas required for independent living.

In a final content unit, Murphy's program addresses three special topics not dealt with in most other programs reviewed. These include fair and effective approaches to discipline for residents, dealing with resident mental health problems, and coping with residents' reactions to separation from a familiar environment.

The major strength of this program, like that of Mamula (1970), is in providing participants with a sound orientation to the role of care provider. In addition, it also provides participants with knowledge and insight into the way that one's attitudes can affect response to developmentally disabled persons. The major deficit of the program, however, is that it neglects to train participants in specific caring skills. Too little attention is given to training participants in basic home management and resident care while no attention is given to teaching participants individual program planning or advanced social skills training. Thus, the effectiveness of this program could be greatly enhanced by supplemental inservice workshops devoted to addressing these serious deficits.

3. Resident Manager Education

This program developed by Provencal and Evans (1977) is organized to serve as a model for both preservice and inservice training. Both the preservice and inservice segments include six content units which are intended to be covered in five to eight sessions, each lasting two to three hours.

Readers should be aware that the training manual for this program is unlike that of any other program reviewed here. Instead of including specific content for each of the topics addressed, Provencal and Evans simply present a curriculum model. For each content area the authors specify (1) the learning objectives for the area, (2) discussion stimulants related to these objectives, (3) a list of resources which suggests where users might seek out expert presenters for the content area, and (4) a list of readings from which users might draw the specific content needed to meet the suggested learning objectives. Thus, while the manual provides the structure for each session, the specific content to be communicated must be developed by individual users.

The preservice component includes two units which focus on providing participants with a thorough orientation to mental retardation and current service ideology. The unit on mental retardation suggests coverage of causative factors of mental retardation, behavioral characteristics of mentally retarded persons, and similarities and differences in the growth and development of mentally retarded and intellectually normal persons. The unit on service ideology focuses on the principle of normalization and its application in human service settings. The corollary principle of "dignity of risk," the concept of deinstitutionalization, and the direction of future service design also receive attention.

With respect to orienting participants to the care provider role, however, the only content suggested for the preservice component is included in a unit devoted to describing the administrative responsibilities of care providers in relation to other actors in the foster care system.

The area of basic home management is touched on in a content unit focusing on fire and safety considerations. Specific safety issues which are listed include identifying fire hazards, developing a home evacuation plan, basic rules for extinguishing fires and how to maintain a hazard-free home.

The area of basic resident care is dealt with in one unit which focuses on routine personal health needs as well as the emergency medical needs of residents. Health issues suggested for coverage include basic personal hygiene, storage and administration of residents' medication and dealing with epileptic seizures. Users are also encouraged to provide participants with demonstrations of cardiopulmonary resuscitation and the Heimlich maneuver.

A final content unit of the preservice segment touches on the area of individual program planning. Specifically, this unit is intended to prepare participants for assessing residents' strengths and weaknesses in adaptive behavior and establishing intermediate and long-range goals. As part of this unit, users are encouraged to orient participants to the AAMD Adaptive Behavior Scale.

The topics which comprise the inservice training segment build upon the preservice sessions. The six units which comprise this segment are devoted to specialty areas which Provencal and Evans feel users might wish to include as part of continuing care provider education. One of these units is devoted to strengthening participants' orientation to the care provider role by dealing with relationships to natural families. Issues to be addressed include establishing procedures for residents' visiting and vacationing with their families, reinforcing the interest families give their relative, and developing increased sensitivity to the feelings of natural families.

Another unit is intended to strengthen participants' orientation to mental retardation by focusing on issues related to trends toward community placement of former institutional residents. Users are encouraged to provide participants with an historical frame of reference for current deinstitutionalization ideology, the rationale for current roles played by foster care and group homes, and explanations of how the normalization principle and developmental model should be applied in establishing quality community placements.

Enhancing the participants' knowledge in the area of basic resident care is the intent of a unit devoted to behavior management. Users are encouraged to instruct participants in understanding the causes of behavior, the importance of defining behavior in specific terms and the advantages of using reinforcement rather than punishment to shape behavior. In general, this unit is intended simply to present the basic principles which underlie learning theory and to lay the groundwork for future sessions dealing with individual program planning.

The final three units are devoted to considerations regarding residents' sexuality, leisure time/recreational needs, and educational development. The intent of the unit on sexuality is to assist program participants in developing a healthy attitude toward the sexuality of residents. The suggested content is also intended to aid mentally retarded residents to become more knowledgeable about themselves as sexual beings. The unit on residents' leisure time is structured to help participants learn how to stimulate new leisure time interests in their residents and how to introduce recreational opportunities which encourage residents' self-actualization. The suggested content of the final unit on educational considerations is intended to help participants understand educational service structures, procedures for obtaining services, and the value of continuing education for adult residents.

Of those programs discussed thus far, this one is clearly the most comprehensive in its content. However, since this program only offers users an outline for each training session, the adequacy and quality with which specific content is addressed will vary widely from one user to another. In spite of the fact that Provencal and Evans' manual does not provide specific content, its usefulness can be assessed based upon the adequacy of curriculum outlines and the selection of content areas. In general, the suggested structure for each session has been well-developed. The learning objectives are very specific and clearly indicate to users not only what content should be covered but also how to cover it. The suggested discussion stimulants, resources, and reading lists are both detailed and comprehensive.

However, users should be attuned to certain deficits in the content areas outlined in the manual. In orienting participants to the care provider role, this program fails to address the issues of relating to and obtaining support services from the community. It also neglects to include material intended to help care providers confront their emotional responses to handicapped persons. Further, too little attention is given to the specifics of individual program planning and no attention is given to training participants in the skills necessary for teaching residents self-care and social competency. Admittedly, the authors did not intend this curriculum model to fill all the educational needs of care providers. However, those who utilize Provencal and Evans' curriculum model ought to give first consideration to the deficits that have been identified when designing any supplemental inservice educational sessions for care providers.

4. *Fostering Children with Mental Retardation*

This training developed by Dickerson (1977) is similar to that of Provencal and Evans in that it is a two-part program including both basic and advanced training components. Both parts of the program are comprised of eight sessions. The entire program is designed to be presented in 16 weekly meetings, each of 2½ hours duration.

Part I of the program is intended as preservice training for both new foster parents who need an introduction to their role and for other persons who need information before deciding whether they should take children into their care.

The first of the eight sessions is spent on helping participants get to know each other and acquainting them with the outline and objectives of the training sessions. After this introduction the second session is devoted to factual information on mental retardation, including discussion of definitions, etiology, incidence, prevalence, accompanying physical handicaps, and severity classification schemes.

The third session is devoted to basic home management. Specifically, participants are presented with the characteristics of a healthy, growth stimulating home. Common safety hazards, as well as the importance of structure, order, and routine in a well managed home, are discussed. Session four deals with material related to basic resident care. Specifically, participants are taught principles of positive parenting. The main concern here is to attune participants to helping a child to develop feelings of self worth. The important role played by reasonable, enforceable rules is highlighted.

The next three sessions are intended to provide participants with an introduction to basic resident care and individual program planning. Participants are expected to prepare a detailed behavioral profile of their foster child, learn that simple behaviors like dressing are composed of many particular minute tasks, and become familiar with how to proceed with reinforcing or extinguishing behaviors. The eighth and final session of Part I is devoted to orienting participants to the care provider role by helping them become aware of and prepared to utilize important resources and support services available to them in their community. Unfortunately, this is the only attention given to orienting participants to the care provider role.

Part II of this program also consists of eight sessions and is designed as advanced inservice training to help foster parents facilitate the child's growth and development by focusing almost exclusively on the area of individual program planning.

After an introductory session to allow participants to become acquainted with each other and the objectives of Part II, the second and third sessions are devoted to teaching participants to use the AAMD Adaptive Behavior Scale. The participants learn the purpose and structure of the scale and must complete the entire instrument on the child in their home.

The next session is devoted to interpreting the results of the scale and using it to identify and prioritize the needs of their child. This work sets the stage for sessions five, six, and seven in which participants learn specific problem-solving techniques for dealing with high priority needs of their child. In these sessions, participants have an opportunity to learn how to actually apply the concepts of behavior assessment and goal setting, as well as to learn how to plan and implement specific behavioral interventions. The final session of Part II is devoted to teaching participants how to use a simple individualized monthly chart for recording the behavioral goals and achievement of the foster child in their care.

The major strength of the Dickerson program is its comprehensive treatment of the topic of individual program planning. At the completion of this program one would expect that participants would be intimately familiar with the strengths and capabilities of their residents and have had substantial practice in designing and carrying out individual program plans which meet resident needs.

The major limitations of this program include its inadequate orientation of participants to the care provider role and the lack of attention given to teaching them the specific skills required for training residents in basic self care or advanced social behavior. The inadequate treatment given to care provider orientation may be due to the possibility that participants are required to complete an introductory course in foster parenting (also offered at Eastern Michigan University) before being admitted to this specialty course in mental retardation. However, if this is the case, it is not made clear by Dickerson.

The lack of attention given to the details involved in teaching specific behavior skills to residents is consistent with this program's particular approach to individual program planning. Rather than focusing on specific skill areas (e.g., personal hygiene, money management), Dickerson teaches participants a general approach to training residents which can be applied to many different areas of need. While such a process-oriented approach may be useful, it might be helpful to supplement it with more specific information regarding the common problems and sticky issues which may arise when training residents in particular areas (e.g., human sexuality).

5. *Living in a Family Environment: A Training Program for Group Home Parents*

The fifth program reviewed is the LIFE Project developed at the Waisman Center (1976). The reason it was included in the present review is that it was oriented for small group homes run by live-in, parental model staff. Such homes are, in many cases, not significantly different from foster care homes. This program consists of eight separate content units with no particular indication of whether it is intended for preservice or inservice training.

The first unit provides a good orientation to mental retardation. Specifically, it includes information on mental retardation and other developmental disabilities, as well as on the principles of normalization and dignity of risk. It also includes a brief history of care for the developmentally disabled and a discussion of the rights of mentally retarded persons. A second unit provides participants with information useful in orienting them to their care provider role. Specifically, it focuses on how participants should proceed to obtain the support services they need and to establish good community relations. Information is provided on how to identify formal and informal helping resources, as well as how to advocate effectively for needed services. Also, participants are sensitized to the importance of developing and maintaining good community relations since a supportive community will more readily provide needed cooperation.

A third unit focuses on basic home management. It contains a wealth of information on a variety of important topics, including: getting to know new residents and easing their transition into the home, relating to residents' natural families, individual program planning, management of the household budget, meal planning and preparation, cleaning and laundry. Strategies for assigning selected household tasks to residents are also discussed. To aid participants in individual program planning, a comprehensive resident skill evaluation form is included. This form is designed for assessing residents' level of skill with respect to basic self-care, routine household responsibilities, and more advanced social competencies (e.g., use of public transportation, shopping in community). This assessment is intended to be the basis from which individual program plans are developed. Supplemental information is also included to aid participants in menu planning and meal preparation (e.g., number of food servings per weight of various foods, selected food recipes).

A fourth unit deals with the area of basic resident care and focuses on health, hygiene and home safety. With respect to health, information on the management of common health problems as well as seizures is included. First aid is also covered. Further, participants are encouraged to ensure that residents receive routine health and dental check-ups. The final health-related information in this unit focuses on the proper administration of medications and on selected prescribed drugs and their side effects. Personal hygiene of residents is also covered in this unit with specific attention being given to menstrual hygiene. Finally, common household hazards are discussed along with the precautions which need to be taken to keep a home a safe place.

A fifth unit builds participants' skills for individual program planning by providing comprehensive coverage of principles and techniques of behavior management. Participants are instructed in how to observe and monitor behavior, how to break complex behavior into smaller discrete tasks, how to use general learning principles to teach new skills, and how to make use of a formal contract to involve residents in their own behavior change.

Unlike most of the other programs which focused on teaching residents only basic self-care skills, this program includes three additional units devoted to advanced resident training. One of these deals with teaching residents social competency skills. In addition to the skills necessary for basic self care and appropriate behavior in the home, this unit focuses on methods of teaching residents socially appropriate behavior necessary for attending school, holding a job, and using such community resources as public transportation, restaurants, libraries, movies, and bars.

Another unit is devoted to teaching residents about sexuality. Specifically, this unit includes information regarding: facts of sexuality, how to talk about sex, socially appropriate expressions of sexuality, and methods of birth control. The unit on recreation and leisure time provides a great deal of information on suggested age-appropriate activities for children, adolescents, and adults, both within and outside of the home. Further, it includes specific suggestions on how to use such activities to develop individual resident's behavioral skills.

In summary, this program offers comprehensive coverage of a wide range of topics important for providing quality care to residents. A major strength throughout the program is the wealth of specific practical information included in the self-teaching manuals. Further, this is the first program discussed thus far to focus attention on teaching residents useful community living skills. Moreover, it provides participants with a more comprehensive treatment of how to utilize community resources and support services than any other program reviewed. The only important area not sufficiently covered regards orienting participants to their particular care provider responsibilities. Thus, anyone using this program ought to supplement it with several sessions providing information of this type.

6. *New Directions in Community Care*

This program was developed by an interdisciplinary design team and was produced as a cooperative effort by the California Department of Health and the Instructional Television Consortium. It is substantially different from all others reviewed because it was intended for use with administrators and staff of community care facilities and nursing homes, and because the first of its two parts was intended for those working with the mentally ill as well as those working with the mentally retarded. It qualifies for this review, however, because it has been used for training family care providers and because it provides a unique example of how such a program can be implemented on a state-wide basis using public television.

As mentioned, the program is divided into two parts. Part I is intended for those working with any mentally handicapped persons. It covers seven content areas with 16 one-half hour videotape modules, each accompanied by written materials. Following an introductory session to acquaint participants with the overall aim and method of the course, the first four major content areas presented are devoted to various aspects of basic resident care. These aspects include medications, health, medical and behavioral emergencies, and nutrition.

The first content area presented is medications and it is covered in three one-half hour modules. Specific issues addressed include the role of medications in the deinstitutionalization movement, the use and side effects of psychotropic medications, knowing your own residents' medications, secure storage of drugs, keeping medication records and teaching clients self-medication. This is the only program reviewed which dealt with the subject of medications in a comprehensive manner. Given that the mentally retarded residents served in foster family care are frequently prescribed a variety of drugs, including this component in a provider training program is recommended.

The second content area addressing basic resident care is health. It is covered in two modules. The first deals with the relationship between basic resident health and well-being. The importance of good personal hygiene and grooming in developing resident self-esteem and pride is emphasized. However, participants are not given any specific guidance in how to teach self-care skills to residents. The second module is devoted to a presentation of basic medical facts relating to skin problems, dental disease and water retention. Participants are also given general guidelines for assessing medical problems and for deciding when to seek out help.

The third content area dealing with basic resident care focuses on the handling of medical and behavioral emergencies. Participants are provided with basic information regarding how to deal with fires and first aid emergencies. In addition, legal responsibilities in managing emergencies are discussed.

The fourth content area devoted to basic resident care issues is nutrition. It is covered in three modules. The first gives participants a basic orientation to major nutrient groups and basic food groups. It also gives suggestions for doing daily menu planning and meeting individual resident food preferences. The second module focuses on more administrative concerns such as food cost records, cost-control methods and food storage hints. The final module covers food preparation and gives specific attention to diets to meet specialized resident needs (e.g., weight control, diabetes, low-sodium and low-fat diets). As with the topic of medications, this program provides a more comprehensive treatment of nutrition than any other program reviewed.

The fifth content area deals with a topic in the category of advanced resident training. Specifically, three separate modules are devoted to training participants to meet the activity needs of residents. The first describes the important place of activities in creating a healthy home atmosphere. It also discusses different categories of activities and the various possible levels of resident involvement. The last two modules deal with how to develop ongoing activity programs and how to motivate residents to participate.

The sixth content area falls into the special problems topic category and is labeled "human needs." It is comprised of two modules dealing with such specific issues as the human rights of administrators and residents, residents' need for privacy, and the importance of involving residents in discussions and decisions regarding house policies and rules. The Waisman Center program is the only other program reviewed that deals with the issue of resident rights. This is an important topic and ought to be a standard component of any comprehensive provider training program.

The final content area in Part I deals with the importance of participants getting ready to serve the clients who will be placed in their facilities. In fact, it is the only session in Part I which is directed to provide participants with a general orientation to their care provider role. Specifically, it presents care providers with a picture of how they fit into the team of individuals responsible for developing residents' placement plans. This final session also lays out some of the basic issues involved in individual program planning. Specifically, it provides the outline of a comprehensive behavioral assessment which participants are recommended to use in order to get to know their clients and to provide a basis for developing behavioral objectives for their residents' program plans.

New Directions in Community Care, Part II, was developed specifically for community care administrators and staff who have developmentally disabled residents in their facilities. It includes ten content areas, each covered by a single one-half hour videotape program.

The first module provides participants with an orientation to developmental disabilities. Specifically, it defines such conditions as mental retardation, autism, cerebral palsy and epilepsy and discusses the causes of each. The second module addresses the area of basic resident care and is devoted to teaching participants how to teach self-help skills to their residents. Specific skill areas covered include dressing, eating, grooming, oral hygiene and toileting.

The third module deals with basic home management and is devoted to home safety. It provides participants with information regarding common household accidents and how to prevent them. Fire safety issues are also discussed, including common fire hazards, proper use of extinguishers and evacuating the residence in case of fire. The fourth module once again addresses the area of basic resident care and focuses on resident behavior problems. Participants are given a framework for understanding and dealing with behavior problems in a systematic fashion. Basic principles of behavior modification are also presented. While this session's focus on managing problem behaviors has practical utility, the principles of behavior modification are not placed in a broader perspective which would allow participants to see how they apply to individual program planning in general. Giving trainees the broader picture is recommended since it would facilitate their use of these principles in a proactive rather than a reactive manner.

The fifth module deals with sexuality, a topic in the advanced resident training category. It emphasizes the importance of open communication between staff and residents regarding human sexuality. Privacy is presented as a central factor in sexual expression and guidelines for appropriate expression of intimacy by residents are included. The sixth module is devoted to recreation/leisure, another topic in the advanced resident training category. Specific issues discussed include how to get residents involved and how to match activities to clients' functional level and individual preferences. Examples of specific recreational activities are also presented.

The seventh and eighth modules are also devoted to issues of advanced resident training. Module seven deals with how to move residents to their highest level of independence. Specific topics discussed include improving residents' work and personal care habits as well as ability to manage money. Module eight deals with residents' relationship with their community. Specific skills which residents need in order to make effective use of community resources (e.g., restaurants, stores, bus) are discussed. These include self-control, good manners, respect for property, and good grooming habits. In addition, participants are given guidelines for training residents to use public transportation and prepare for job interviews. This program and that of the Waisman Center (1976) are the only ones reviewed which focused attention on teaching residents how to make more effective, independent and normalized use of community resources. While the specific treatment given to this area of social competence may need to be adjusted depending on the functioning level of residents served, it should be addressed in some fashion in all foster care provider training programs.

The ninth module deals with the topic of individual program planning and describes the importance of taking the team approach. It presents information on the roles of community residence staff, other professionals, as well as the resident in establishing plans of action and setting behavioral objectives. However, while basic principles of program planning are presented, the attention given to this topic in Part II is far too cursory. More extensive materials were provided in the final module of Part I and should be considered essential for an adequate treatment of this topic.

The tenth and final module deals with the system of services in California, the effect of current legislation and the roles of regional centers in meeting the needs of administrators and residents. As such, it is the least applicable in its present form if used in other states. However, if properly adapted, a similar presentation could provide an important component in the orientation of participants to the service system in other states.

Together, Parts I and II of this California ITV program provide the most comprehensive training of all programs reviewed. However, while promotion materials suggest that Part II is sufficient training for providers serving the developmentally disabled, the authors of this review disagree. In their view, the topics of medication, health care, emergencies and nutrition, which are covered only in Part I, are an essential supplement to Part II and should not be viewed as optional. Part II should also include the materials from Part I that deal with care provider and resident rights (modules 14,15) as well as the development of individualized resident program plans (module 16).

The only noticeable deficit in content in the overall program is the failure to include materials dealing with affective issues in caring for residents. As mentioned previously, only one of the six programs reviewed (Murphy, 1975) has dealt with this important issue as part of preparing providers to work more effectively with their residents.

An additional problem with the program is that it was not designed specifically for family care providers serving the mentally retarded and, therefore, contains a great deal of information which may be of secondary importance when providing training to this group. On the other hand, because training programs are costly to produce, a program developed for wider audiences such as this one must be considered an attractive option. In addition, this program's segments are all on half hour videotapes and include supplemental written material. This makes this program the most transportable of any training program developed to date. More will be said on this issue in the discussion of educational methods.

Educational Methods

An overall comparison of the educational methods used by the programs reviewed is presented in Table 2. This table demonstrates that the most commonly utilized methods are lecture and group discussion. With respect to group discussion, it should be noted that several authors offer some excellent suggestions for those intending to use discussions in teaching. Dickerson (1977) for example, presents a number of techniques which session leaders can use to encourage participants to involve themselves actively and to keep their discussion focused. Provencal and Evans (1977) include an extensive list of specific discussion stimulating questions with each of their program sessions. These questions are extremely useful because they push participants to take the concepts and skills being taught and discuss how they might actually be applied in a variety of real-life problem situations. The selection of problems posed in these discussion questions is comprehensive and demonstrates that the authors are well attuned to the daily difficulties that confront care providers.

Several programs (California ITV Consortium, 1975; Murphy, 1975; and Provencal & Evans, 1977) also suggest the use of guest speakers. Such individuals might be recognized local experts in particular content areas or experienced care providers who can share their first-hand knowledge with trainees. These guest speakers are typically asked to present either lectures or demonstrations as well as lead group discussion.

Table 2

Educational Methods of Training Programs

Methods	Mamula	Murphy	Provencal-Evans	Dickerson	Waisman Center	California ITV
Lecture	X	X	X	X		
Discussion	X	X	X	X		X
Guest speakers		X	X			X
Role playing	X					
Field trips	X	X				
Films		X				
Homework/Quizzes				X	X	X
Self-teaching manual					X	
Audio-cassette and filmstrip					X	
Videotape						X

In addition to lecture and discussion, there are a variety of other teaching methods used in the programs reviewed. Both Mamula (1970) and Murphy (1975) include field visits to give participants a firsthand look at foster care homes. Role playing is used by Mamula (1970) to give participants an opportunity to practice responding to problem situations, and though Dickerson (1977) does not include it in any of the session outlines in her manual, she notes how role-playing can help participants gain a new perspective of a problem situation.

Films or filmstrips are used as a teaching modality by both the Waisman Center (1976) and Murphy (1975) programs. Further, though Dickerson (1977) does not include any in session outlines, she suggests that films can be a useful supplement to stimulate good discussion. For those who wish to consider using films in their training programs, an excellent resource is the foster parent training program developed by Nowak and Reistroffer (1970). Since this program was designed for teaching generic foster care providers, it was not reviewed in detail in this paper. However, it includes an extensive list of films on topics relevant to all care providers, whether for normal or disabled persons.

Another teaching method used in several programs is to give participants periodic quizzes on training content and/or regular homework assignments. The California ITV program (1975) includes a set of study questions for participants to complete as they watch each separate videotape module. These questions, however, are intended more to keep participants attuned to the videotape presentations than to serve as an assessment of learning. The Waisman Center (1976) program includes a pre-test and post-test with all eight of its program units. This approach is intended to help participants monitor their own learning progress on an ongoing basis. Such feedback is especially important in this program since it is basically a self-teaching approach.

The Dickerson (1977) program is the only one to give participants regular written homework assignments. Giving such assignments appears to be an excellent way to encourage participants to begin to apply concepts and skills in their own homes. It would seem that giving participants an opportunity to practice their learning and discuss difficulties in applying it increases the likelihood that training will have long-range behavioral impact on care providers. Guerny (1977) strongly agrees with this perspective and includes such assignments as an integral part of her skills-training program for generic foster parents.

While the majority of programs reviewed require groups of participants to gather together and be trained in person by lecturers, discussion leaders, or expert panels, two programs offer alternative approaches. The Waisman Center (1976) program is designed so that trainees can teach themselves. Program materials include self-teaching training manuals, filmstrips and audio cassettes. Such a program offers greater flexibility in terms of implementation, especially if trainees are located at great distance from one another. Nevertheless, to get the most out of this program it would seem advisable to suggest that trainees periodically gather into small groups to discuss training content and that they have ongoing contact with a training supervisor who could answer questions and provide personal feedback.

The other alternative approach involves the use of videotapes. The California ITV Consortium (1975) has prepared half hour tapes for each segment of their training program. The use of this medium has a number of distinct advantages. Although initial production of training materials would be expensive, for a large state-wide program it would probably be less expensive in the long run especially if specific videotape segments could be broadcast to individual care providers' homes. The use of pre-recorded programs also increases the consistency with which content is presented. In addition, with videotapes important ideas can be demonstrated graphically without field trips and other aids. The videotapes also increase the general use of programs in other locations although there are several cautions to be noted. First, the program developed for California included some comments on history, agencies, and legislation that is specific to California. Second, the use of videotapes especially through public television is a somewhat untested approach. Although the idea of pre-recorded training tapes is attractive, no one to date has carefully evaluated the effectiveness of this technique.

Intended Use

The variation in comprehensiveness in the content of the programs reviewed can be attributed, in part, to variation in the intended use of these programs. For example, Mamula's (1970) program was intended as general orientation for naive care providers and was thus very introductory in nature. Murphy's (1975) program was designed for experienced and inexperienced care providers and thus included some content on more advanced training issues as well as basic introductory information.

The Dickerson (1977) training program for family care providers and the Provencal and Evans (1977) program for managers of group homes both divide their programs into preservice, for inexperienced providers, and inservice for experienced providers. This distinction is important because it recognizes the advantages of participants having had actual care providing experience before being exposed to educational material on individual program planning, teaching basic life skills, behavior management and other aspects of training the mentally retarded. However, establishing a separate preservice training program may not be justified unless there is a sizeable new population of care providers or if there has been a dearth of training provided to current care providers.

The programs developed by Provencal and Evans (1977), the Waisman Center (1976) and the California ITV Consortium (1975) provide further opportunities to offer training to mixed audiences. Potentially, any of these programs could be used to train both family care providers and staff of community residential facilities. Of the three, the California ITV program is intended to serve the broadest audience. According to its developers, it is intended for use with administrators and staff of community care facilities as well as for students in the health sciences. It has also been used to train family care providers. Moreover, it is intended as training both for those who work with the mentally ill as well as the mentally retarded.

Such broadly focused programs offer some advantages. In states where there is a small population of individual provider groups, it may prove cost efficient to use such programs to train groups of family care providers and community residence staff at the same time. Those who choose to train such a mixed audience should be aware that certain portions of both the Provencal and Evans (1977) and California ITV (1975) programs are clearly intended primarily for the community residence staff. On the other hand, the Waisman Center (1976) program is oriented more to the generic needs of any care provider and is probably the best example of a good mix between the training needs of various individual audiences. While there are many similarities in the skills and knowledge required for providing care in any type of community residence, there may be major and important differences between the groups of trainees for given residence types.

Examples of the kinds of potentially important differences can be drawn from the authors' experience in New York State. When the characteristics of family care providers and the staff of group homes in New York are compared, the following differences emerge: (1) family care providers tend to be older (average age 51) than the group home staff, many of whom are young people either attending or just completing college, (2) family care providers tend to vary greatly with respect to educational background (ranging from individuals with little formal education to those with college or graduate degrees) but, in general, are a less educated group than group home staff, and (3) many family care providers have had years of experience in working with mentally retarded persons while many group home staff are relatively new to the human services field and are relatively inexperienced due to their young age. Further, the training needs of the two groups differ because of differences in the population of residents served. In New York State, family care providers generally serve a more disabled, lower functioning population of mentally retarded residents than are served in group homes. Hence, while family care providers are oriented to providing residents with a stable organized home life, group home staff are more likely to expect their residents to move to a less supervised living arrangement. The orientation of group home staff is thus more toward providing residents with structured learning experiences and teaching self-sufficiency.

Clearly, the nature and degree of differences between the individual characteristics and training needs of family care providers and group home staff will vary from one state to another. However, anyone considering implementing a generic training program for a mixed audience should thoroughly assess such differences before proceeding. If major differences exist, it may, in fact, not be possible to adopt a single generic training program.

Evaluation of Foster Care Training Programs

A great deal of effort and time has been devoted to the development of each of the programs reviewed. However, with only one exception, insufficient attention has been paid to evaluation. The only program for which any formal evaluation efforts have been reported is that developed by Mamula. In his published report (1970), he stated that his training program had (1) provided an additional screening mechanism which helped the agency to identify potentially poor care providers and (2) given participants greater confidence as they began their care-providing jobs. While the first of these may be a useful outcome, it does not really relate to the impact of training on the participants themselves. Moreover, although the second outcome is related to participants, it was based on the subjective reports of social workers and is of undetermined reliability or validity.

The only other program reporting evaluation information of any type was the Waisman Center (1976) LIFE program. However, this evaluative information consisted entirely of the testimony of one user of the program which was incorporated into an advertisement promoting sales of the training manuals. The testimony stated that participants in the program had undergone attitude changes. However, what kind of attitude change was being reported or how it had been assessed was not made clear.

The importance of evaluating training seems to be recognized in each of the other four programs reviewed. For example, Murphy (1975) and Dickerson (1977) include short evaluative questionnaires which can be distributed to participants when they have completed the programs, and the California ITV (1975) program provides evaluative questions for each videotape module. Further, though Provencal and Evans (1977) do not include any examples of evaluation in questions, they do provide program users with a good discussion of what issues must be considered in designing evaluation materials. Nevertheless, while evaluation is acknowledged as useful, no results of actual evaluations have been reported by either program authors or users.

Clearly, there is a need for foster care training programs to be evaluated in a thorough and systematic fashion. While there are various types of evaluations that could be conducted (e.g., process, adequacy, efficiency), it is outcome evaluation that is most seriously needed.

Outcome evaluation involves measuring the various effects of a given program or intervention. With respect to evaluating the outcome of training programs, the main focus could be determined by the objectives established for each program. Such an approach would be feasible to the extent that programs have developed objectives which are clearly stated, specific, and well operationalized. However, as noted in this paper, statements of program goals are too frequently vague, general, or nonexistent. In such cases, evaluators must set out with less structure and look for a broad range of program effects, including those which were intended, unintended, positive, and negative. Taking such an approach, in fact, has some advantages over an evaluation which is focused entirely on predetermined program goals. The less an evaluator is guided by specific program objectives, the less tunnel vision will develop, and the more attention will be devoted to looking for actual rather than merely intended effects.

However, while there may be some advantage to taking a broad ranging approach to evaluating a training program, there is a need for evaluators to approach their task with some guiding paradigm. One such useful paradigm suggests that the kinds of effects which ought to be assessed for training programs occur at four basic levels: (1) participants' perception and opinions of the training program; (2) participants' knowledge and attitudes following training; (3) participants' behaviors in their actual work settings; and (4) impact of changed behaviors and attitudes on the home organization and clients (Brethower & Rummler, 1976; Dixon, 1977).

The first level focuses on the participants' reactions to the training program. Typically questionnaires are designed to solicit participants' perceptions and opinions of such program aspects as adequacy and relevance of content selected for training sessions, the helpfulness of instruction materials, the competence of the individual instructors, and the overall program quality. Such an evaluation is usually conducted immediately after completion of the entire program. However, if it were conducted on a periodic basis during training, the information could be used to modify the program so that it would be more effective for the particular group of participants providing the feedback. On the other hand, if it were conducted six months or a year after training, participants' feedback might prove even more valuable since their perspective would be broadened by their on-the-job experience. The choice of when or how often to administer such a questionnaire should be made with these various consequences in mind. The questionnaire developed by Dickerson (1977) for rating instructor effectiveness is just one example of an evaluation instrument designed to assess such first level effects.

The second level of effects to be measured related to the impact of training on participants' knowledge, attitudes, or skills. This type of impact can be assessed in a variety of ways. Provencal and Evans (1977) discuss the possible use of frequent short quizzes, a written in-class final examination, or a rigorous take-home exam. Exams can also be given before and after training to allow participants and the instructors to see the kinds of progress made. In the Waisman Center (1976) program, for example, participants are provided with pre- and post-tests for each training unit.

While impact on knowledge may be readily measured by written examinations, impact on attitudes and skills is not as easily assessed. Accurate measures of attitudes are not easily constructed. Furthermore, a change in a participant's attitude may not be reflected likewise in behavior. With respect to measuring acquired skills, the creative use of simulation or structured role-playing provides a far more useful and reliable assessment of learning than does a written exam. However, no such in-vivo assessments were constructed or conducted for the participants of any of the training programs reviewed in this paper.

The third level of training effects to be measured relates to the participant's use of learned concepts and skills. Such effects can be measured in a variety of ways. One indirect method suggested by Murphy (1975) is simply to ask training graduates such questions as (1) What content have you actually used?, (2) What content did you find most useful?, (3) What content was most effective when you put it to use?, and (4) What content did you feel was irrelevant? Another possible indirect method would be to look for various signs that would demonstrate that participants had used training concepts. For example, one might compare the quality of individualized program plans written by care providers who had been trained with those of providers who were not trained.

Clearly, the more direct the measure of a participant's use of training concepts, the more reliably one can evaluate the impact of training. Ideally then, measurement of concept or skill use would be based on direct observation of care providers' behavior with mentally retarded residents. Understandably, such an evaluation approach may not always be feasible and a more indirect measurement must be utilized.

The final level of training effects to be measured relates to the impact of training on the administrative agency and on the clients served by care providers.

With respect to the first of these impacts, administrative agencies may reasonably anticipate that training care providers for their job will ease a variety of administrative burdens since trained providers can be expected to be more confident and independent (Mamula, 1970, 1971). Evaluative indices which could be utilized to assess such impact might include number of supervision hours requested by providers or care-provider turnover rates.

A training impact far more fundamental than administrative burden, however, is the impact that trained care providers have on their mentally retarded residents. After all, the fundamental rationale for the development of care-provider training programs is to assure better quality care for the clients being served. To be judged effective, then, a program ought to be able to demonstrate that training providers creates direct benefits for clients. Indices to evaluate such benefits could include such positive measures as amount or rate of progress in clients developing self-care or social competency skills and reported satisfaction of clients or their natural families.

The four-level model described here is presented as merely one way to stimulate and organize systematic evaluative research on care-provider training programs. Many important questions need to be explored in a variety of topic areas including the selection and sequencing of training content, the choice of teaching methods, and the integration of preservice and inservice training components. However, evaluators are cautioned to be careful in how research questions are posed. Attempting to identify which training program is the ''best,'' for example, may be a futile if not meaningless task. The authors of this paper, for example, have not attempted to identify the ''best'' program reviewed. This is because the decision as to which program is ''best'' depends so heavily on the particular needs of potential users. Thus, in evaluating programs it may prove far more useful to ask more complex but precise questions such as what programs, taught with which methods are most effective in achieving which particular objectives with what types of trainees? It is this strategy that will produce the kind of information that potential users of these programs need in order to make intelligent decisions about how best to meet their particular training needs.

Developing a Training Program

As suggested by Mamula (1970), a logical first step in developing a training program is to establish evidence for its need. Rarely, however, is this need established in a formal manner. More typically, a few concerned foster care providers, case workers, or other agency staff who are already convinced of the need for training simply begin the process of developing a program by forming a training committee. A common strategy in forming a committee is to include persons who represent the interests of both the agency administering the foster care program and the foster care providers. Other persons who are frequently invited to join such a committee include Association of Retarded Citizens members, educational specialists, and any other local experts with relevant experience (Dorgan, 1974; Provencal & Evans, 1977; Stone & Hunzeker, 1975). The rationale is that such a representative membership provides greater assurance that the committee's final training program will not only be effectively organized but will also receive the political support necessary for its smooth and successful implementation.

One way for a training committee to begin is to develop the general philosophy and objectives from which the particular educational programs will evolve

(Provencal & Evans, 1977). Once the framework for the programs is set, the decisions regarding the specific content and methods of training can follow more smoothly. Numerous program developers have also stressed that as the training committee proceeds with its work, it should maintain a regular interchange with the foster care providers for whom the training is being designed (Dorgan, 1974; Goldstein, 1967; Mamula & Newman, 1973; Nowak & Reistroffer, 1970). It is felt that actively involving prospective participants helps to produce a training package which is not only tailored to their needs but to which they are also more likely to be committed.

There are a variety of methods which training committees have utilized to obtain valuable input from foster care providers. They include distributing a questionnaire (Levine & Zubrack, 1975), holding a series of meetings with small groups of foster care providers (Dorgan, 1974, 1975), or merely relying upon the opinions of those few care providers who are already on the training committee. The type of input sought typically relates to the selection of specific content areas on which the care providers would like the training to focus.

Those designing training programs for care providers who have previously received no training should carefully consider the type of program they choose to develop. The usual beginning point for the development of a training program is to establish an effective inservice training program. This is practical because it addresses the training needs of the many care providers already providing care to the developmentally disabled. It is also practical because it can draw on the extensive experience base of the care providers. Preservice training programs are practical when there is a large number of new providers entering the system. This program should be a condensed version of the inservice training program and should emphasize attitude formation. Inservice training which emphasizes skill development should then be provided to new providers once they have had some experience.

While the exact approach a particular committee takes in developing a training program will vary, it seems important that the overall process be systematic. One excellent model to guide the overall flow of developing a program has been offered by LeVine and Zubrack (1975). In addition to the steps which have already been discussed here, they suggest that the committee conduct a thorough review of existing training programs. While the present paper offers one such general review, individual training committees should obtain copies of those programs which seem relevant and review them to see how they can be used to meet their own particular training needs. While the committee may decide that some new materials need to be developed, some combination of the various components of programs reviewed in this paper can probably be used to meet most foster family care provider training needs.

LeVine and Zubrack (1975) also suggest that the training committee address such issues as how to staff their program, where to provide training, and the size of the training budget they can afford. A further suggestion offered by Dorgan (1974) is that the training committee should plan to pilot test their program as part of its refinement process.

A final aspect of developing training programs which is generally overlooked is designing a method for evaluating the training. This review of training programs indicated that few of them had looked at evaluation, and when they did, it involved participant feedback on training sessions. Good training programs should be developed to improve on the quality of care being provided to residents. However, whether or not the training has this desired impact can only be determined through a careful evaluation effort. Guidelines for designing such an evaluation were presented earlier. While the level of evaluation conducted may depend on available resources and expertise, no training program should be implemented without plans for collecting at least basic evaluative data.

In general, the process of developing a training program should include the following steps: (1) form a representative training committee, (2) conduct a systematic assessment of providers' training needs, (3) determine what resources (e.g., budget, manpower) will be available for developing and implementing the training program, (4) develop the general philosophy and broad objectives for the training, (5) decide on the type (preservice, inservice) of training to be developed, (6) review existing training materials to determine how they can be utilized or adapted to meet program objectives, (7) develop new training materials to meet those objectives not adequately addressed by existing materials, (8) select and train those individuals who will conduct the training, (9) plan to pilot the training program to determine what further refinements are needed, and (10) design a method for evaluating the training program before it is implemented.

Summary

The training needs of foster care providers serving mentally retarded persons have been acknowledged for some time. This review of specific training programs demonstrates that a variety of excellent materials and strategies for meeting these needs are now available. A number of important tasks remain. First, existing training programs need to be implemented more widely. Second, new programs and training materials need to be developed to address needs not adequately met by existing programs. Finally, there is a need to conduct systematic evaluations of care provider training on a more regular basis. The results of these evaluations must then be used to guide refinements in future training efforts. This is an essential step if these programs are to be effective in meeting their goal of improving the quality of care offered to mentally retarded persons by foster family care providers.

References

Adams, M. Foster care for mentally retarded children: How does child welfare meet this challenge? *Child Welfare*, 1970, *49*, 260-269.

Brethrower, K. S., & Rummler, G. A. *Evaluating training*. Unpublished manuscript, 1976.

Bruininks, R. H., Hill, B. K., & Thorsheim, M. J. *A profile of foster home services for mentally retarded persons in 1977*. Minneapolis: University of Minnesota, Department of Psychoeducational Studies, 1980.

California Instructional Television Consortium. *New directions in community care, Parts I and II*. Rohnert Park, CA: Sonoma State University, 1975.

Caplan, R. *Psychiatry and the community in nineteenth century America*. New York: Basic Books, 1969.

Dick, K. What people think about foster care. *Children*, 1961, *8*, 48-52.

Dickerson, M. W. *Fostering children with mental retardation*. Ypsilanti, MI: Eastern Michigan University, Foster Parent Training Project, 1977.

Dixon, J. K. *Methodological considerations in evaluation of continuing education in the health professions: Utilization of chain of events models in determining evaluation criteria*. Paper presented at the Annual Convention of the American Educational Research Association, New York, April 1977.

Dorgan, M. Initiating a program of foster parent education. *Child Welfare*, 1974, *9*, 588-593.

Dorgan, M. Three models of preservice programs. In H. Stone & J. Hunzeker (Eds.), *Education for foster family care: Models and methods for foster parents and social workers*. New York: Child Welfare League of America, Inc., 1975.

ENCOR (Eastern Nebraska Community Office of Retardation). *Residential specific training*. Omaha, NE: ENCOR, 1977.

Gardner, J. M. Community residential alternatives for the developmentally disabled. *Mental Retardation*, 1977, *15*, 3-8.

Garrett, B. L. Meeting the crisis in foster family care. *Children*, 1966, *13*, 3-8.

Goldstein, H. Group learning for foster parents in a voluntary agency. *Children*, 1967, *14*, 180-184.

Gollay, E., Freedman, R., Wyngaarden, M., & Kurtz, N. R. *Coming back*. Cambridge, MA: Abt Books, 1978.

Guerny, L. A description and evaluation of a skills training program for foster parents. *American Journal of Community Psychology*, 1977, *5*, 361-371.

Heal, L. W., & Daniels, B. S. *A cost-effectiveness analysis of residential alternatives for selected developmentally disabled citizens of three Northern Wisconsin counties*. Paper presented at the 102nd Annual Meeting of the American Association of Mental Deficiency, Denver, Colorado, May 1978.

Heal, L., Sigelman, C., & Switzsky, H. Research on community residential alternatives for the mentally retarded. In N. Ellis (Ed.), *International Review of Research in Mental Retardation* (Vol. 9). New York: Academic Press, 1978.

Hill, B., Sather, L., Kudla, M., & Bruininks, R. *A survey of types of residential programs available for mentally retarded people in the United States in 1978*. Unpublished paper from the Developmental Disabilities Project on Residential Services and Community Adjustment, University of Minnesota, Minneapolis, 1978.

Intagliata, J., Willer, B., & Cooley, F. Cost comparison of institutional and community based alternatives for mentally retarded persons. *Mental Retardation*, 1979, *17*, 154-156.

Intagliata, J., Willer, B., & Wicks, N. *Factors related to the quality of communtiy adjustment in family care homes*. Paper presented at the Conference on Community Adjustment, Minneapolis, Minnesota, March 16, 1979.

Justice, R. S., Bradley, J., & O'Connor, G. Foster family care for the retarded: Management concerns of the caretaker. *Mental Retardation*, 1971, *4*, 12-15.

LeVine, S., & Zubrack, F. Five models of inservice programs. In H. Stone & J. Hunzeker (Eds.), *Education for foster family care: Models and methods for foster parents and social workers*. New York: Child Welfare League of America, Inc., 1975.

Maluccio, A. N. Selecting foster parents for disturbed children. *Children*, 1966, *13*, 69-74.

Mamula, R. A. Developing a training program for family caretakers. *Mental Retardation*, 1970, *8*, 30-35.

Mamula, R. A. The use of developmental plans for mentally retarded children in foster family care. *Children*, 1971, *18*, 65-68.

Mamula, R. A., & Newman, N. Training programs for care providers. In *Community placement of the mentally retarded: A handbook for community agencies and social work practitioners*. Springfield, IL: Charles C Thomas, 1973.

Marr, P. *Introduction to foster parenting* (Volumes 1 and 2). Manhattan, KS: Kansas State University, 1976.

Meyers, C. E., Lei, T., Nihira, L., & Eyman, R. *How much room at the inn? Are there limits on small family placement?* Paper presented at XIII Annual Gatlinbury Conference on Research in Mental Retardation, Gulf Shore, Alabama, 1979.

Morissey, J. R. Status of family care programs. *Mental Retardation*, 1966, *5*, 8-11.

Murphy, G. *Foster care of the developmentally disabled: A basic course for foster parents and foster care workers*. Boston, MA: Boston University School of Social Work, 1975.

Murstein, A. *Respite aides for parents of the handicapped*. St. Louis, MO: St. Louis Metropolitan Council on Developmental Disabilities, 1978.

Nirje, B. The normalization principle and its human management implications. In T. Kugel & W. Wolfensberger (Eds.), *Changing patterns in residential services for the retarded*. Washington, DC: President's Committee on Mental Retardation, 1969.

Nowak, M. J., & Reistroffer, M. *Foster family parent education*. Milwaukee: University of Wisconsin Extension, 1970.

Pollock, H. M. Family care of mental defectives in Scotland. *American Journal of Mental Deficiency*, 1936, *20*, 414-423.

Pollack, H. M. Family care of mental defectives in Scotland. *American Journal of Mental Deficiency*, 1947, *52*, 89-90.

Porter, F. *Pilot parents program: A design for developing a program for parents of handicapped children*. Omaha, NE: Greater Omaha A.R.C., 1978.

Provencal, G., & Evans, D. *Resident manager education: A curriculum model for educating foster parents and group home personnel*. Mt. Clemens, MI: Macomb-Oakland Regional Center, 1977.

Rich, M. Foster homes for retarded children. *Child Welfare*, 1965, *45*, 392-395.

Ryan, P., Warren, B. L., & McFadden, E. J. *Course outlines for foster parent training project*. Ypsilanti, MI: Eastern Michigan University, Center for the Study of Metropolitan Problems, 1977.

Shah, C. P. Assessing needs and board rates for handicapped children in foster family care. *Child Welfare*, 1971, *50*, 588-592.

Smitson, W. S. Foster mothers and mental patients. An exploration study of interpersonal relationships. *Mental Hygiene*, 1970, *54*, 251-255.

Stone, H., & Hunzeker, J. (Eds.), *Education for foster family care: Models and methods for foster parents and social workers*. New York: Child Welfare League of America, Inc., 1975.

Waisman Center on Mental Retardation and Human Development, University of Wisconsin. *Living in a family environment (LIFE): A training program for group home parents*. Los Angeles: Stanfield House, 1976.

Wilkes, J. R. The impact of fostering on the foster family. *Child Welfare*, 1974, *53*, 373-379.

Willer, B., Intagliata, J., & Wicks, N. *Return of retarded adults to natural families: Issues and results*. Paper presented at the Conference on Community Adjustment, Minneapolis, Minnesota, March 16, 1979.

Appendix 1

Training Programs

Generic Family Care Provider Training Title/Author(s)	*For Further Information*
Training Program for Family Caretakers Richard Mamula, M.S.W.	Vallejo Community Services Division Office 1000 Marin Street Vallejo, California 94590
Foster Care of the Developmentally Disabled: A Basic Course for Foster Parents and	Boston University School of Social Work

Foster Care Workers Gwendolyn Murphy	Division of Continuing Education 264 Bay State Road Boston, Massachusetts 02215
Resident Manager Education: A Curriculum Model for Educating Foster Parents and Group Home Personnel Gerald Provencal David Evans	Macomb-Oakland Regional Center 16200 Nineteen Mile Road Mt. Clemens, Michigan
Living in a Family Environment: A Training Program for Group Home Parents Waisman Center	Stanfield House 12381 Wilshire Boulevard Suite 203 Los Angeles, Cal. 90025
New Directions in Community Care California ITV Consortium	California ITV Consortium c/o Office of Extended Education Sonoma State University Rohnert Park, Cal. 94928

Training Family Care Providers of Children Title/Author(s)	*For Further Information*
Fostering Children with Mental Retardation Martha Dickerson, M.S.W.	Foster Parent Training Project Eastern Michigan University Ypslanti, Michigan 48197
Introduction to Foster Parenting (Parts I and II) Pam Marr, M.S.	Pam Marr Dept. of Family and Child Development College of Home Economics Kansas State University Manhattan, Kansas 66506
Foster Family Parent Education Mary Jane Nowak Mary Reistroffer	Publications and Courses Dept. of Social Work University Extension University of Wisconsin 3255 N. Maryland Ave. Milwaukee, Wisconsin 53211
Foster Parenting a Retarded Child Child Welfare League of America	Foster Parent Curriculum Project Child Welfare League of America 67 Irving Place New York, New York 10003

Other Training Programs

Natural Parents	
Pilot Parents Program Fran Porter	Glenda Davis, Program Coordinator Greater Omaha A.R.C. 3212 Dodge Street Omaha, Nebraska 58131

Group Residence Staff

Residential Specific Training
Eastern Nebraska Community Office of Retardation (ENCOR)

Residential Training Specialist
ENCOR
885 South 72nd St.
Omaha, Nebraska 68114

Respite Care Providers

Respite Aides for Parents of the Handicapped
Alberta Murstein, M.Ed.

St. Louis Metropolitan Council of Developmental Disabilities
1240 Dautel Lane
P.O. Box 27480
St. Louis, Missouri 63141

Parents, Care Providers, and Professionals

Way-to-Go
William Bronston, Edward Roberts, Edward Goldman, Richard Byrne and others.

University Park Press
233 East Redwood Street
Baltimore, Maryland 21202

A Systems Approach to Community Living Skills Training

Robert L. Schalock
Roger S. Harper

Mid-Nebraska Mental Retardation Services
Hastings, Nebraska

The influx of the developmentally disabled into community-based programs has been well summarized (Bassuk & Gerson, 1978; Comptroller General, 1977; Conroy, 1977; Heal, Sigelman & Switzky, 1978; McDevitt, Smith, Schmidt & Rosen, 1978; O'Connor, 1979; Scheerenberger & Felsenthal, 1977; Willer, Scheerenberger & Intagliata, 1979). According to data presented in these reports, this influx will require the development, expansion and better integration of community-based residential and programmatic services for the developmentally disabled. One major component of those needed services is a systematic approach to developing community living skills. This chapter outlines the evolution of the Mid-Nebraska Independent Living Training Program, initiated six years ago when three realities became apparent: (1) to integrate deinstitutionlized persons into a community-based program adequate space must be available in the community residences; (2) exit from residential facilities is an important factor in providing places for persons entering the community residential service system, i.e. unless there are exits from the residences, a waiting list soon develops; and (3) the majority of clients who fail their job and independent and semi-independent apartment placements do so primarily because of skill deficits.

This chapter describes where we were, where we are, and the changes we are making in our attempt to serve well the high percentage (40%) of clients in our program who are clinically diagnosed as severely retarded. Our intent is to share our successes and failures so that others may benefit from them in seeking solutions to similar problems in their programs. The focus of the paper is on the systematic training of community living skills. Readers wanting more detail on the Mid-Nebraska program may find discussions of the historical aspects of the program in Schalock and Harper (1977), program evaluation approaches in Schalock and Harper (1978; 1979), the assessment-remediation model in Schalock and Karan (1979), and an analysis of cost effectiveness in Schalock (1980).

Phase I: The Past
Developing the Original Program

Deinstitutionalization was taking place successfully in Nebraska even before judicial involvement because of the farsightedness of a small group of consumers, mental retardation professionals, and state employees. The Nebraska strategy for developing community-based mental retardation programs was set into action through the creation of six mental retardation regions. Nebraska, like much of the Midwest, has a heavy concentration of its population in one part of the state. Regionalization and vesting the control of the regions in the hands of a multi-county board solved the problems of small town rivalry, equitable program distribution and service provision in remote parts of the state, uniformity of management, and quality control. The task facing Mid-Nebraska Mental Retardation Services (Region III) was to establish within the Region a viable service delivery system based upon the principles of normalization and community integration. Initially, a Regional Director was appointed who, with consumer and county direction, established seven area programs with an Area Director in charge of each.

The Area Director is responsible for the identification of facilities, fiscal management, local public relations, staff hiring and firing, physical plant and program supervision. The Regional Director provides general program direction and development, state-local relations, state agency interactions, and relates officially to funding and legislative sources and bodies. The regional system of service delivery is in many ways comparable to the franchise system in the private sector: an assigned area alleviates competition and duplication of services; a standardized system of management and service delivery provides the integration of a continuum of necessary services; program/cost responsibility centers can be established; achievement and failure can be objectively measured; long range and short-term goals can be established in an efficient manner; and successful treatment programs can be shared through communication.

Originally, the Mid-Nebraska programmatic services were divided into adult and children's components. Public schools now provide children's services. Each of the seven areas had an adult component that followed a sheltered workshop model in which the workshop and its contract activities were used to teach academics, competitive employment, independent living, recreation, and socialization skills. In addition, as is true of most sheltered workshops, each had its share of birthday parties, bowling trips, ceramics, and coveting of clients. Group living homes were also a part of the adult component. These were large leased houses converted into living facilities for 10 to 12 clients. The facilities were not used for any systematic training, and the programming that did take place in the evenings in many instances amounted to over-programming of the clients.

Early Problems. Despite the laudable purposes and initial successes (namely finding facilities, clients, staff and funding) in establishing Phase I of a community based mental retardation program (CBMR), the program began to experience numerous problems. First, we were beginning to develop a waiting list. Initially the waiting list was interpreted as meaning one of two things: either we were so good that everybody wanted our services; or more reasonably, there were no exits from our programs. Upon close examination, however, we discovered that the *real* reason for the lack of movement and consequently the waiting list was that staff feared that their clients would not make it in the real world. One of the most critical issues with which we had to struggle was that of the waiting list versus the "numbers game" (defined as placement at the expense of the actual needs of the client). It took us a while to realize that the argument that "we didn't want to get into the numbers game" was in reality a "cop-out" that represented both the staff's trepidation in taking chances in placing clients and the potential influx of lower functioning clients waiting in the wings. Staff feared that because of either inadequate preparation or lack of previous experience, "their" clients might fail. This was reinforced from the administration's point of view because large numbers of clients and lengthy waiting lists appeared to have good face validity. At this point, we did not realize that society's "return on investment" had to be in movement through the system, rather than being maintained in the system. In our early history, however, the emphasis was on filling the centers; if we could do that, we felt we were fulfilling our task.

A second problem, and one of our biggest, was related to the fact that the workshop was the single center in our attempt to teach academics, competitive employment, community living skills, recreation, and socialization skills. This not only confused clients, since they were receiving mixed messages, but also the staff who frequently wondered, "Where do we start with each client and where do we go?"

The third problem was so obvious that it eluded us for years. Becoming aware of this significant error of omission (a common one) provided the catalyst for a whole new programmatic approach. The problem was that most of the clients who were moving into the community were returning to the program because they could not adjust adequately to community living. Why? We discovered that most of the failures of clients to enter true independent living related to social and behavioral problems and, specifically, deficits in community living skills. What we had overlooked in our original competitive employment-oriented program was the most important aspect of community integration, namely the development and maintenance of behavioral skills related to independent community living. In retrospect, we can now see that these skills are much more complex to teach, acquire, and maintain than those related to competitive employment.

The fourth problem related to the client residence (group homes). Some Americans love buildings more than what transpires within them. We were initially guilty of perpetuating that phenomenon for we stressed the "sidewalk appeal" of the residences and were pleased about how "normalizing" and "integrative" they looked on the outside. Critical examination of the residences indicated, however, that they were too large and had too many problems of management and funding to be beneficial to client growth. In addition, because of the confusion related to the lack of clearly stated goal-oriented objectives, they were rapidly becoming community-based institutions (Moen & Aanes, 1979; Sternlicht, Schalock & Harper, 1979).

"Try Another Way." The four problems discussed above led us to seek answers regarding what skills our clients had, what problems developed regarding independent living when staff were removed from the residences, and once the problems were identified, what ideas and program changes needed to be formulated to effect change. In order to acquire data concerning the activities that clients engaged in while living in the residence, a descriptive study was conducted on 17 clients (9 males and 8 females) housed in two residential facilities. Of the 17 clients, nine had previously spent time in the large state institution and had recently entered the community program. There were separate residences for females and males. Ages ranged from 18 to 46. WAIS Full Scale IQs averaged 50.6 ($SD = 4.3$), indicating that these individuals could not be characterized as high functioning clients.

The study involved determining the time spent per day in 10 typical activities during six consecutive days (Friday evening to the following Thursday morning). The 10 activity categories rated by two staff independently (percent agreement = 96.2) and the percent of time spent in each are presented in Table 1. Since clients were away from the residences during the day Monday through Friday, residential behaviors were evaluated from 6 to 8 A.M. and 5 P.M. to midnight on those days, and 6 A.M. until 12 midnight Saturday and Sunday. Regular residential staff were not present during the study. Therefore, clients were "on their own" except for supervised medication taking, which was done by one of the observers. The study was described to the clients before it began. Clients were told that it was their responsibility to get up, fix meals (food was available), maintain personal hygiene, get to the training facility or into town, and to handle any interpersonal problems.

Programmatically, the data in Table 1 suggested that the large amount of time spent sleeping and watching TV, combined with the small percent of time away from the residence, necessitated increased training in community awareness, access, and utilization. In addition, informal observations indicated that the clients demonstrated response deficits in correct personal maintenance and the general areas of food selection and preparation.

Table 1

Average Percent of Waking Time Spent in Various Activities in the Residences[a]

BEHAVIOR	BRIEF DESCRIPTION	DAILY % OF TIME Male	Female
1. Eating	meals, snacks	7.15	9.34
2. TV	head oriented toward TV set	23.10	18.31
3. Phone	talking/directory	2.72	2.62
4. Sleep	naps, dozing	26.94	25.45
5. Absence	away from residence	13.27	9.25
6. Maintenance	personal belongings/room	2.19	7.36
7. Personal Hygiene	bathing, toileting, teeth, hair, etc.	3.67	2.60
8. Small Group	discussions, visits, games	3.72	6.19
9. Individual Activity	reading, letters, solitary games	17.52	17.05
10. Argumentation	verbal or physical argumentation	0.43	1.89

[a]This excluded working hours on week days.

So there is where we found ourselves. There was a waiting list; staff were coveting clients and were afraid to place them because of fear of failure; clients were getting mixed messages; the program was rapidly becoming a community-based institution in which clients were expected to cope with "institution-like settings" and were responding with "institution-like behaviors"; clients were failing to succeed on their own in the community; and too many competencies were expected of the staff. The collective impact of these problems resulted in sparse placement with the net effect of high cost, low yield programs.

Introspective evaluation of what we had accomplished thus far revealed that we had been busy creating environments for the clients, but we had not compared those environments to the primary goals as a service delivery system offered as a viable alternative to institutional placement. In a nutshell, we were not providing the type of an environment that would promote adaptive behavior on the part of the clients and that would allow them to move to the greatest degree of independence, productivity, and conformity with standards set by the community. Our previous efforts had been confined to the successful identification of funds, clients, manpower and facilities. The question then faced by the Board and Administration of the Region was whether to continue expanding services at an additional cost to accommodate those clients unserved in the community and underserved in the institution or to embark on a new programmatic emphasis that would be designed to serve more clients at the same cost. We chose the latter. Specifically, we set out to develop a service delivery program with the following characteristics:

1. being client centered with a lock-step progression toward defined exits;
2. providing the clients and staff with one consistent message during the program day; and
3. providing materials to and for the program staff that allowed them to assess client strengths and weaknesses, to develop remediation strategies, and to evaluate client attainments systematically.

At this point, it became clear that we had completed only the first phase of what had to be a multiphase venture. It was our feeling that the second phase would require the design of management-program technology which would remediate clients' skill deficits in the area of independent functioning, gainful productivity, and community acceptance. This technology needed to be delivered in a structure that would enhance its effect as opposed to presenting barriers to its implementation. It was felt that unless we had a comparative management-program model geared to measurable goals, we would be doomed to repeat the mistakes that had been recently discovered in our service delivery system. The following section outlines the management-program model developed and evaluates some of the results.

Phase II: The Present
Systematic Training in Community Living Skills

The management-program model chosen to implement the dual-goal of training toward independent community living and competitive employment was a systems approach. This approach to management in the private sector is well known (Anthony & Herzlinger, 1975; Borst & Montana, 1977) and therefore is not unique to Mid-Nebraska. What might be somewhat unique, however, is our application of this approach to human services with our underlying assumption being that any transaction has a consequence and the benefit of any service transaction can be assessed by the degree it diminishes the clients' future need for that service. The major variables including program management, program progressions, client services, and program monitoring involved in a systems approach are summarized in Table 2. Each is discussed in more detail below.

Program Management

In reference to the needed program changes outlined earlier, a systems approach was used to make the program changes, though at that time it was not so named. Specifically, by relating the interrogatories of a system to its management, we based decisions and program changes on objective data which improved the program and provided for accountability.

Program Progressions

The lock-step progression for the program components which eventually developed was:

ENTRY —> BASIC SKILLS —> INDEPENDENT LIVING —> COMPETITIVE EMPLOYMENT —> EXIT

Once the progressions were identified, the next step was to define and develop the procedures to move a client through the program sequence to the point of his

Table 2

Management/Program Variables Reflective Of A Systems Approach To Human Services

Variable	Input	Throughput (Process)		Output (Product)
Program Management	Program Measurability	Reportability → (Summative)	Manageability (Formative)	Program Accountability
Program Progressions	Entry (Basic Skills)	Independent Living (Community Living Skills) →	Competitive Employment	Placement
Client Services	Assessment →	Baseline data		
	→	Individual Program Plan Development		
	→	Basis for Prescriptive Programs		
	→	Skill Acquisition Data		
	→	Objectives/Goals Obtained		
	Reassessment →	Data Analysis		Client/Program Evaluation —client change —placements —cost/effective (client movement ratios')
	→	Predictive Data		
Program Monitoring	Program Function/ Dysfunction	Systems Review[a]		Program Improvement or Change in Design

[a]Systems Review (including the process and variables evaluated) is presented in Schalock (1980).

highest productivity and independence. This required divesting ourselves of both the "all encompassing" sheltered workshop model and the large group home concept. Programmatically, we divided the adult program into three separate training components that are operated in each of the seven communities throughout the Region. They include Basic Skills, Independent Community Living, and Competitive Employment. Each component has its own staff, program materials (including screening test and remediation-teaching manual), location and defined exits. Figure 1 outlines the training areas, program progressions and defined exits. Together, these reflect the operationalization of our philosophy of increasing productivity and decreasing dependency. Because of the major focus of this volume, the remainder of this paper focuses on the approach developed to train clients in community living skills.

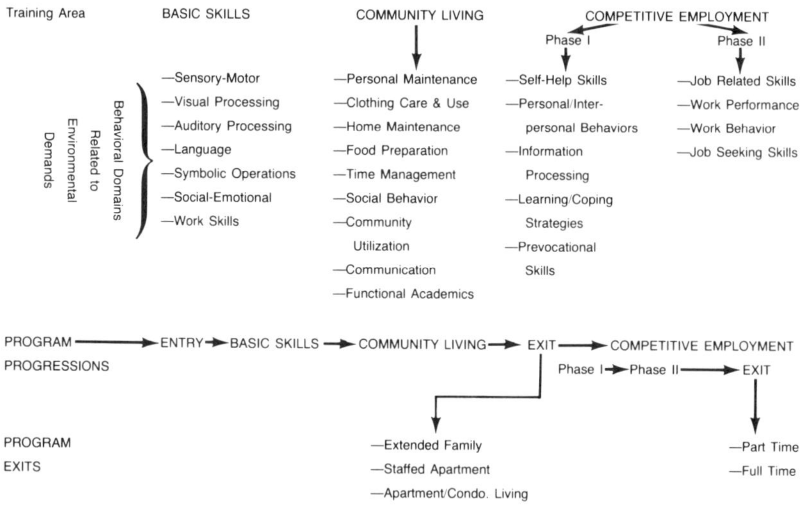

Figure 1. Training Areas and Behavioral Domains Related to Environmental Demands Program Progressions and Program Exits

Client Services

Three critical variables impact the services received by clients in a service delivery system. One is financial, a second is programmatic, and a third, case management. The relationship among these three variables as depicted in a systems approach format is presented in Figure 2. Since the programmatic flow is the most relevant to this volume, the remainder of the paper will focus primarily on that component.

	INPUT	*PROCESS*	*OUTPUT*
Financial →	Budget →	Cost Accounting → —Units of Service —Cost per Unit	Audit
Programmtic →	Assessment → (Criterion Referenced)	Remediation/ → Reassessment	Placement
Case Management →	Intake → —Demographic —Certification	Clients Monitoring → —Skills Gained —Movement/Progressions —Exits (Placement)	Follow-Along

Figure 2. Client Services Flow Analysis

Assessment

Within the Mid-Nebraska Independent Living (IL) Training Component, assessment is done by trained diagnostic programmers using the *Independent Living Screening Test* (Schalock, 1975), a criterion-referenced test yielding standard scores on each behavioral domain. Reliability, validity, normative data, and required staff competencies are presented in the *Independent Living Standardization Manual* (Schalock, 1979).

The 88 behavioral skills on which the client is assessed on entry to the IL training component and yearly thereafter were selected as a result of our experiences, environmental analyses, and from published materials. These 88 skills or adaptive behaviors are grouped into nine areas (''domains'') associated with environmental demands. These nine domains are further divided as outlined below:

Domain I: Personal Maintenance
- A. Hair Care
- B. Hygiene Aids
- C. First Aid
- D. Drugs

Domain II: Clothing Care and Use
- A. Washing/Drying
- B. Folding/Ironing/Dry Cleaning
- C. Repairs/Alterations
- D. Selecting and Wearing

Domain III: Home Maintenance
- A. Adjustment and Repairs
- B. Safety
- C. Housekeeping Skills

Domain IV: Food Preparation
- A. Meal Planning
- B. Grocery Shopping
- C. Meal Preparation
- D. Care and Safety

Domain V: Time Management
- A. Personal Schedule
- B. Leisure Time

Domain VI: Social Behavior
- A. Self-Referenced Behaviors
- B. Interpersonal Relations

Domain VII: Community Utilization
- A. Awareness and Access
- B. Community Use

Domain VIII: Communication
- A. Receptive Language
- B. Expressive Language

Domain IX: Functional Academics
- A. Money
- B. Banking
- C. Time Concepts

Prescriptive Programming (Remediation)

Following the criterion-referenced assessment, individual, prescriptive programs are developed that specify for each behavioral skill or objective the teaching strategy, accelerated-decelerated behaviors, reinforcement/correction ratios and contingencies, pass/fail criteria, programming frequency, and what data to record. The behavioral objective is either the behavioral skill itself or a component based upon a task analysis of the behavioral skill. Each program is run and graphed daily and phase changed according to standard procedures (Schalock & Gadwood, 1979). Suggested remediation activities for each behavioral skill are presented in the *Independent Living Screening Test and Remediation Manual* (Schalock, 1975). In addition, a programmatic requirement is that each client has a minimum of one prescriptive program for each of the nine domains in which assessment deficits are obtained. Each behavioral skill program then becomes an objective on the client's Individual Program Plan (IPP). This procedure results automatically in interfacing assessment, IPP, remediation strategy, reassessment, client change, and client/program evaluation.

During the duration of independent living training that occurs in the community residences, individualized remedial programming focuses on deficient independent living behavioral skills. Clients are housed in staffed apartments, eight-member group homes or family/foster homes. Placement into their own or a staffed apartment is an interdisciplinary team decision, based primarily on completing 80 to 85 percent of the 88 behavioral skills. Upon placement, clients have completed independent living training and progress programmatically to the Competitive Employment training component.

Developmental/Movement Variables (Dependent Measures)

One or more of the following dependent measures can be used to quantify client change

Development of skills. Client growth is represented by increased behavioral skills as reflected by improved scores on reassessment.

Movement within program progressions. These data reflect the client's progress from Basic Skills to Independent Living to Competitive Employment. As such, the data reflect the program's goal of increased productivity and independence. These are valid data only if the progressions are sequenced and there are clearly identified criteria for movement from one programmatic component to another.

Exits into a less restrictive environment. Most current programs for the developmentally disabled are training programs that should move clients to an environment that is more appropriate to each individual's acquired skills. Therefore, placements into less supervised living and becoming more competitively employed are major dependent variables that reflect client growth. These exists are depicted in Figure 2.

An Evaluation of Systematic Training In Community Living Skills

Given the approach to the systematic training of community living skills summarized above, one can justifiably ask, "How successful was it?" There are a number of ways to answer the question, including the four types of data presented below:

Number Placed Into Independent Housing

The number of clients placed into independent housing from 1972 to 1978 is presented in Table 3. Note the low number in 1972 which was the year before implementing systematic training in independent living skills.

Placement Success or Failure

Data summarizing a 2-year follow-up study of 60 clients placed into their own apartments following independent living training has been presented elsewhere (Schalock & Harper, 1979). As summarized in Table 4, successful placement was more frequent with younger, more intelligent individuals with better skills in personal maintenance, clothing care and use, socially appropriate behaviors, community utilization, and functional academics (money and time concepts). In general, the major reason for failure was seen as the need for additional training. Specifically, unsuccessful clients had significantly more problems in the areas of money management, home cleanliness, social behavior and meal preparation.

Table 3
Placement Into Independent Housing (1972-1978)

Year of Placement	Females # Placed	Females Mean Age	Females Mean I.Q.	Males # Placed	Males Mean Age	Males Mean I.Q.
1972	5	32	64.75	6	39.5	71.39
1973	10	36.9	69.3	15	33.27	83.6
1974	7	39.57	68.85	12	32.33	71.25
1975	15	30.53	69.33	22	34.54	70.91
1976	15	30.47	69.8	15	36.8	60.07
1977	9	31.11	67.89	12	35.25	62
1978	11	36.55	61.55	3	30.33	59.5

We recently reported (Schalock, Harper & Carver, 1980) the results of a 5-year longitudinal study of these same 47 clients—all of whom are still living in independent housing. The 12 predictor variables used in a stepwise multiple regression analysis are summarized in Table 5. Nine of these variables (comprising 88 behavioral skills) represent the behavioral domains assessed and remediated in independent living training. The other three predictor variables were chronological age, WAIS Full Scale IQ, and gender. The outcome measure (criterion variable) was successful or unsuccessful placement. Operationally, successful placement was defined as remaining in independent housing for the five years; unsuccessful was defined as returning to the group home within the first two years following placement or transfer to a more restrictive living environment.

The relationships among the predictor and criterion variables are also presented in Table 5. Statistically significant correlations ($p < .05$) were obtained between the criterion variable and personal maintenance, clothing care and use, food preparation, time management, community utilization and communication. The percent of variance explained (multiple-R squared) was 32 percent. Finally, Table 5 also indicates that, in descending order, the most significant (based on partial correlation) predictor variables were personal maintenance, communication, home maintenance, community utilization, clothing care and food preparation.

Demonstrated Effects of Training

To demonstrate that clients made greater gains on those behavioral skills programmed versus not programmed, a six month pre/post comparison study was conducted using 56 clients. These 56 had initially failed particular behavioral skills on the *Independent Living Screening Test (ILST)*. A comparison was then made on the number of these skills gained on reassessment (6 months later) for which systematic programming had been done during the six months *versus* those skills on which no systematic intervention had occurred. These data are presented in Table 6. Analysis indicated that more behaviors were gained as a function of systematic programming than no programming ($t = 2.33$, $df = 16$, $p < .05$).

Table 4
General Client Characteristics, Average Training Area Scores, and Point Biserial Correlation Coefficients

Variable	Clients' Scores		Point Biserial Correlation
	Successful (N = 47)[a]	Unsuccessful (N = 13)	
AGE:			
Mean	31.1 ± 1.4	40.7 ± 1.5*	
Females (range)	19-61	27-42	
Males (range)	21-60	32-54	
GENDER: (females/males)	(29/18)	(3/10)	
WAIS—Full Scale	65.6 ± 1.6	53.8 ± 2.2*	
REFERRAL SOURCE:			
Natural Home	19	2	
MR State Institution	16	9	
Other (Regional Center) or Private MR Facility	12	2	
IL TARGET BEHAVIORS:			
Total Number	69 ± 1.8	51.8 ± 7.3*	
Number Gained During Training	15 ± 1.2	11.5 ± 1.0*	
DURATION OF TRAINING (months)[b]	12 ± 1.1	8.7 ± 1.0*	
INDEPENDENT LIVING ASSESSMENT AREAS:			
I. Personal Maintenance (N = 47)[c]	14 ± 0.4	11 ± 0.6*	.37**
II. Clothing Care/Use (N = 14)	11 ± 0.2	8 ± 0.2*	.32**
III. Home Maintenance (N = 12)	9 ± 0.3	9 ± 2.0	.09
IV. Food Preparation (N = 9)	7 ± 0.3	6 ± 1.0	.24*
V. Time Management (N = 4)	3 ± 0.2	3 ± 0.3	.25*
VI. Social Behavior (N = 8)	6 ± 0.2	4 ± 0.4*	.37**
VII. Community Utilization (N = 7)	5 ± 0.2	3 ± 0.8*	.33**
VIII. Communication (N = 9)	8 ± 0.2	8 ± 0.8*	.26*
IX. Functional Academics (N = 8)	5 ± 0.3	1 ± 0.6*	.41**

*$p < .05$; **$p < .01$

[a]Successful was defined operationally as remaining in the community living placement for two years; unsuccessful = returning to the training component any time after placement.

[b]Correlation between training duration and number of target behaviors gained = .58 ($p < .01$).

[c]Number of behavioral skills per area; score represents average number passed per group.

Table 5
Multiple Regression Summary

Predictor Variables

Variable	Description
IQ	WAIS—Full Scale
Age	
Gender	
Independent Living Screening Test Areas[a]:	
I. Personal Maintenance (No. of items = 17)	Hair Care (2), Hygiene Aids (6), First Aid (5), Independent Drug Usage (4)
II. Clothing Care and Use (N = 14)	Washing/Drying (6), Folding/Ironing (4), Repairs/Alterations (2), Selecting/Wearing (2)
III. Home Maintenance (N = 12)	Adjustment/Repairs (3), Safety (5), Housekeeping Skills (4)
IV. Food Preparation (N = 9)	Meal Planning (2), Grocery Shopping (3), Meal Preparation (2), Care/Safety (2)
V. Time Management (N = 4)	Personal Schedule (2), Leisure Time (2)
VI. Social Behavior (N = 8)	Self Referenced Behaviors (4), Interpersonal Relations (4)
VII. Community Utilization (N = 7)	Awareness/Access (2), Community Use (5)
VIII. Communication (N = 9)	Receptive Language (5), Expressive Language (4)
IX. Functional Academics (N = 8)	Money (3), Banking (3), Time Concepts (2)

Step-Wise Multiple Regression Analysis Results

Predictor Variable	Partial-R	Multiple-R	Correlation With Outcome Measure
I. Personal Maintenance	.36	.36	.36**
VIII. Communication	.33	.42	.26*
III. Home Maintenance	.27	.46	–.10
VII. Community Utilization	.25	.51	.33**
II. Clothing Care & Use	.22	.54	.32**
IV. Food Preparation	.20	.54	.25*
IQ (WAIS Full Scale)	.11	.55	.11
IX. Functional Academics	.15	.56	–.07
VI. Social Behavior	–.10	.56	.17
V. Time Management	–.06	.56	.25*
Gender	–.05	.57	–.16
Age	–.04	.57	–.04

* $p < .05$
** $p < .01$

[a]Factor analysis indicates four orthogonal facors:
1. Domestic Skills—Areas II, III and IV
2. Community Orientation and Use—Areas V and VII
3. Social Skills—Areas I and VI

Table 6

Comparison of Behavior Skills Gained As a Function of Prescriptive Remedial Programming (N = 56)

ILST Area	Number of Behavioral Skills Programmed and Gained	Number of Behavioral Skills Gained without Programming
I	57	35
II	78	22
III	64	24
IV	48	14
V	11	8
VI	14	10
VII	23	3
VIII	27	8
IX	12	7

Cost Effective Analysis

Once behavioral and financial data are referenced to the same client and training component that component's cost effectiveness can be evaluated. One way to accomplish this is through the calculation of a Client Movement Ratio (CMR) which is operationalized as follows:

$$\left[\frac{\text{Absolute Number of Behavioral Skills Gained}}{\text{Units of Serve x Cost Per Unit}}\right] \times 100$$

Client Movement Ratios are calculated separately for each client and then aggregated for each training component and geographical area. For example, average CMRs for the seven Mid-Nebraska independent living (IL) training programs for each of the nine IL Domains for a one-year period are presented in Table 7. As presented, more progress was made in areas I through IV, with a net loss in Area VIII. Used wisely, CMR's provide an objective basis for planning, funding and program evaluation.

Thus we came to the end of Phase II of our multiphased venture. During Phase II we designed and implemented a management-program model that was geared to measurable goals of increasing a client's independence and productivity. That management-program model resulted not only in a significant increase in the number of clients who moved through the system but also generated data which permitted an evaluation of the model. Although the data summarized above suggested that our approach to independent living training was successful, we are currently having to make some significant programmatic changes. These are described in the next section.

Table 7

Average Client Movement Ratios (CMRs)

IL Domain	Average CMR	IL Domain	Average CMR
I	+.05	VI	+.02
II	+.05	VII	+.03
III	+.05	VIII	−.01
IV	+.05	IX	+.01
V	+.01		

Phase III: The Future
A Comprehensive Service Delivery System

In the multiphased venture of providing community-based services, it has been our experience that as we came to grips with one set of problems that present themselves as barriers to goal attainment, new problems inevitably surface. Three of these new problems that we currently face include interagency coordination, refinement of programmatic technology, and expanded training-placement options. Each is discussed below.

Interagency Coordination

One of the most persistent and difficult problems that a service delivery program faces is the lack of interagency coordination. For example, depending upon the program one can find individual program, habilitation, education, work, or treatment plans—with the only common elements being that they are individualized plans for some part of a client's life. Currently, the notion of what should constitute an individual plan at any part of the developmental continuum does not necessarily reflect the types of environmental demands placed on the client in his next step up the continuum. The net result is that clients currently entering community-based programs have not been oriented to the behaviors required in coping in the less structured, but more demanding community environments. Part of this problem relates to the lack of agreement as to what are the relevant developmental domains, exemplified by the four major sets of standards or regulations presented in Table 8.

It is reasonable to assume that interagency coordination will be facilitated if a continuum of needed services can be conceptualized and implemented based upon the environmental demands required to meet the standards of personal independence and social responsibility expected of one's chronological age group (Grossman, 1973). Since these expectations vary for different age groups, deficits in adaptive behavior will vary at different ages as reflected below:

During Infancy and Early Childhood

—Sensory-motor skills development
—Communication skills (including speech and language)
—Self help skills
—Socialization (development of ability to interact with others)

During Childhood and Early Adolescence

—Application of basic academic skills in daily life activities
—Application of appropriate reasoning and judgment in mastery of the environment

Table 8

Behavioral Domains as Reflected in National Standards or Regulations

EXISTING DEVELOPMENTAL DOMAINS			
ACMR/DD ACCREDITATION COUNCIL FOR SERVICES FOR MENTALLY RETARDED AND OTHER DEVELOPMENTALLY DISABLED PERSONS	ICF/MR INTERMEDIATE CARE FACILITY FOR THE MENTALLY RETARDED	PROPOSED NATIONAL DEVELOPMENTAL DISABILITIES STANDARD	PL 94-142
1. physical development & health	1. perceptual skills	1. communication	1. academic
2. sensorimotor development	2. sensorimotor skills	2. independent living skills	2. social adaptation
3. communicative development	3. self-help skills	3. learning & problem solving abilities	3. prevocational skills
4. social development	4. communication skills	4. maladaptive behaviors	4. vocational skills
5. affective development	5. social skills	5. physical development	5. self help skills
6. cognitive development, and	6. self direction	6. emotional development	
7. adaptive behaviors or independent living skills	7. emotional stability; and	7. socialization	
	8. effective use of time (including leisure time)	8. work habits & work adjustment	

—Social skills (participation in group activities and interpersonal relationships)

During Late Adolescence and Adult Life

—Vocational and social responsibilities and performances

The implementation of such a "life span continuum" will require at least the following:

1. continua of facilities and training areas geared toward the dual goal of increasing a person's independence and productivity;
2. one responsible agency to insure movement within and between steps on the continuum, necessitating the development of (and funding on the basis of) coordinated activities among public and private service providers;
3. a management-program system that will be able to evaluate both client and programmatic achievements;
4. specific behavioral criteria for movement along the continuum;
5. assessment and reassessment of specific adaptive behavioral skills associated with environmental demands;
6. computerized client-referenced monitoring systems; and
7. an operationalized systems review process.

Programmatic Refinement

One of the Phase II byproducts is that as clients move through the service delivery system, lower functioning clients take their place. For example, the average WAIS Full Scale IQ of the 50% of our current Basic Skills clientele who were testable is 34 (SD = 10.7); for Independent Living, 52 (SD = 11.2). Similarly, as one demonstrates that low functioning clients can adjust adequately to either extended families or staffed apartments (both of which are less restrictive than a large group home), it becomes apparent that the skills required are somewhat different from those involved in having or sharing one's apartment. These two byproducts have resulted in changes in our approach to developing community living skills (CLS). These changes are outlined below.

The expansion in the CLS curriculum will reflect the needs of lower functioning clients who are presently in the Mid-Nebraska Program and will allow training in a number of environments including the institution, intermediate care facilities (ICF-MRs), group homes, extended (foster) families, staffed apartments and independent housing. At this point, implementing a coordinated approach to assessment and remediation among the institution, ICF-MRs and Mid-Nebraska is being pursued. The relationship among community living program goals, living-training facilities and appropriate training areas is presented in Figure 3. The coordination of services across agencies must be developed since the lower functioning clients will require more extensive and prolonged training, but *always* with available movement up the dual continua of increased independence and productivity.

Create More Placement Options

Creating more placement options that reflect less restrictive and more independent living will require both interagency coordinated services that will maximize movement up the "independence continuum" as outlined in Figure 3 and the development of additional staffed apartments and independent housing.

GOAL: INDEPENDENCE	FACILITIES		COMMUNITY LIVING SKILLS ASSESSMENT AND TRAINING AREAS									
HIGH ↑			I Personal Maintenance	II Dressing & Clothing Care	III Eating & Food Mangement	IV Social Behavior	V Expressive Skills	VI Home Living	VII Money Management	VIII Time Awareness & Utilization	IX Recreation & Leisure Skills	X Community Awareness & Utilization
	Independent Housing Staffed Apartment	C—Level Skills	Medication Use	Wardrobe Maintenance	Independent Food Handling	Interpersonal Relations	Language Generalization	Implementation of Home Living Skills	Maintains a Money Management System	Independent Scheduling	Uses Community Recreational Facilities	Independent Community Use
	Extended (Foster) Family (Group Homes) Small, Medium, Large	B—Level Skills	Health Care	Laundry Skills	Meal Preparation	Social Integration	Interpersonal Expression	Home Safety Skills	Independent Money Usage	Follows Daily Schedule (No Prompting)	Recreation & Leisure Activities	Community Access
↓ LOW	ICFMR Institution	A—Level Skills	Grooming Skills	Dressing	Eats Independently	Self Referenced Behaviors	Expresses Self	Cleaning Skills	Understands Utility of Money	Follows Daily Routine (Staff Prompting)	Perceptual Motor Skills	Community Awareness

Figure 3. Relationship Among Goals, Facilities and Appropriate Training Areas—Community Living Skills

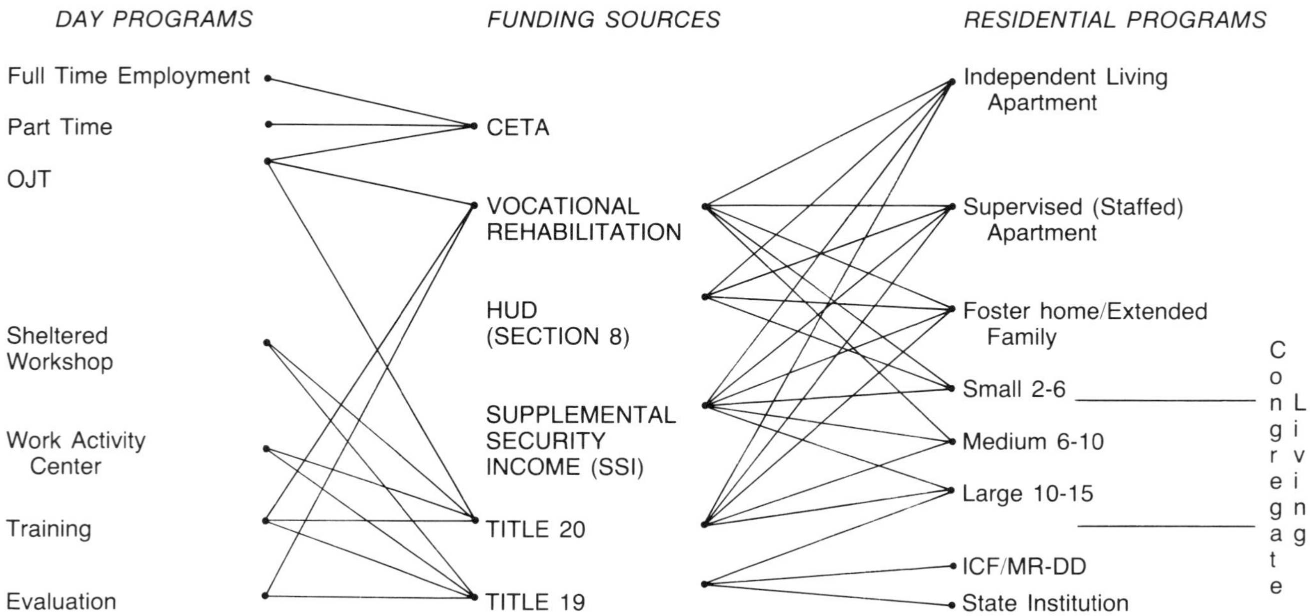

Figure 4. Relationship Among State and Federal Funding Sources and Residential or Day Programs

The relationship among various state and federal funding sources and residential programs is presented in Figure 4. Additional funding sources are discussed in more detail in Harper (1980).

Conclusion

Our experiences over the last 10 years have indicated that the development of community based programs will evolve through three phases. In Phase I, the major focus will be on funds, facilities, clients and manpower. Phase II will focus on implementing management-program systems that are geared to the goals of documented client gains in independence, productivity and community acceptance. Phase III, where we are currently, necessitates developing the expertise required to integrate program services across agencies so as to facilitate a person's increased independence and productivity.

Although there is a great deal of work remaining to be done, the process of deinstitutionalization has lowered significantly the numbers of institutionalized developmentally disabled persons (Willer, Scheerenberger & Intagliata, 1978). In the recently published series of project reports and briefs of the Developmental Disabilities Project on Residential Services and Community Adjustment (Note 1) there is a wealth of descriptive information presented on public and community-based residential facilities for the retarded. According to the data presented, there is an obvious need for new and expanded community-based programs to serve those who are about to enter the community from institutions and from public schools. Such expansion will require both Phase I and Phase II activities, especially if we are to prevent repeating the problems associated with the lack of adequate support and follow-up services accompanying the rapid deinstitutionalization of the mentally ill (Bassuk & Gerson, 1978). And finally, let us not forget the people we have expediently "placed" in nursing homes, for the "forgotten institutionalized population" will need to be addressed in Phase IV.

Reference Note

1. Developmental Disabilities Project on Residential Services and Community Adjustment has published several project reports and report briefs concerning residential alternatives for mentally retarded persons. These are available from the Project, 209 Pattee Hall, 150 Pillsbury Drive, Minneapolis, Minnesota 55455.

References

Anthony, R. N. & Herzlinger, R. *Management control in nonprofit organizations.* Homewood, IL: Richard D. Irwin, Inc., 1975.

Bassuk, E. L. & Gerson, S. Deinstitutionalization and mental health services. *Scientific American,* 1978, *238,* 46-53.

Borst, D. & Montana, P. J. *Managing nonprofit organizations.* New York: Amacom, 1977.

Conroy, J. W. Trends in deinstitutionalization of the mentally retarded. *Mental Retardation,* 1977, *15,* 44-46.

General Accounting Office. Returning the mentally retarded disabled to the community: Government needs to do more. Washington, DC: United States Government Printing Office, 1977.

Grossman, H. J. *Manual on terminology and classification in mental retardation.* Washington, DC: American Association on Mental Deficiency, 1973.

Harper, R. S. Resources for MR/DD programs in rural settings. In R. L. Schalock (Ed.), *MR/DD services in rural America . . . It is time.* Washington, DC: EMC, 1980.

Heal, L. W., Sigelman, C. K. & Switzky, H. N. Research on community residential alternatives for the mentally retarded. In N. R. Ellis (Ed.), *International review of research in mental retardation* (Vol. 9). New York: Academic Press, 1978.

McDevitt, S. C., Smith, P. M., Schmidt, D. W. & Rosen, M. The deinstitutionalized citizen: Adjustment and quality of life. *Mental Retardation,* 1978, *16*(1), 22-24.

Moen, M. G. & Aanes, D. Eclipse of the family group home concept. *Mental Retardation,* 1979, *17*(1), 17-19.

O'Connor, G. *Home is a good place: A national perspective of community residential facilities for developmentally disabled person.* Washington, DC: American Association on Mental Deficiency, 1976.

Schalock, R. L. *Independent living screening test and remediation manual.* Hastings, NE: Mid-Nebraska Mental Retardation Services, Inc. 1975.

Schalock, R. L. *Independent living screening test standardization manual.* Hastings, NE: Mid-Nebraska Mental Retardation Services, Inc., 1979.

Schalock, R. L. A management information system for program delivery and evaluation. In R. L. Schalock (Ed.), *MR/DD services in rural America . . . It is time.* Washington, DC: EMC, 1980.

Schalock, R. L. A systems analysis approach to client and program evaluation. In Schalock, R. L. (Ed.), *A comprehensive service delivery system for persons with developmental disabilities.* Springfield, IL: Governor's Planning Council on Developmental Disabilities, 1978.

Schalock, R. L. & Gadwood, L. *Program handbook.* Hastings, NE: Mid-Nebraska Mental Retardation Services, Inc., 1979.

Schalock, R. L. & Harper, R. S. Placement from community-based mental retardation programs: How well do clients do? *American Journal of Mental Deficiency,* 1978, *83*(3), 240-247.

Schalock, R. L. & Harper, R. S. Three-track approach to programming in a rural community-based mental retardation program. In P. Mittler (Ed.), *Research to practice in mental retardation* (Vol. 1). Baltimore: University Park Press, 1977.

Schalock, R. L. & Harper, R. S. Training in independent living can be done. *Journal of Rehabilitation Administration,* 1979, *3*(3), 128-132.

Schalock, R. L., Harper, R. S. & Carver, G. What follows community placement and what is relevant community living skills training? Paper presented at the Thirteenth Annual Gatlinburg Conference on Research of MR/DD. Gatlinburg, Tennessee, March 12-14, 1980.

Schalock, R. L. & Karan, O. C. Relevant assessment: The interaction between evaluation and training. In T. Bellamy, G. O'Connor, & O. Karan (Eds.), *Vocational rehabilitation of severely handicapped persons: Contemporary service strategies.* Baltimore: University Park Press, 1979.

Schalock, R. L., Karan, O. C. & Harper, R. S. An evaluation-remediation model for serving people with significant handicaps. *Mental Retardation,* in press.

Scheerenberger, R. C. & Felsenthal, D. Community settings for mentally retarded persons: Satisfaction and activities. *Mental Retardation,* 1977, *15*(4), 3-7.

Sternlicht, M., Schalock, R. L. & Harper, R. S. The viability of group living homes: The implications of semi-institutional living. Paper presented at the 103rd annual meeting of American Association on Mental Deficiency, Miami, Florida, May 27-June 2, 1979.

Willer, B., Scheerenberger, R. C. & Intagliata, J. Deinstitutionalization and mentally retarded persons. *Community-Mental Health Review,* 1979, *3*(4), 1-12.

Placement Type and Client Functional Level as Factors in Provision of Services Aimed at Increasing Adjustment

Arne T. Bjaanes
The Center for the Study of Community Perspectives

Edgar W. Butler
University of California at Riverside, and
The Center for the Study of Community Perspectives

Brendan R. Kelly
Department of Developmental Services State of California

In the last two decades there has been a national trend toward deinstitutionalization and increased utilization of community residential facilities for persons with developmental disabilities (O'Connor, 1976). Concurrently, particularly in the last decade, there has been a parallel trend toward increased use of in-home placement, i.e., placement with natural parents and/or guardians. Community residential facilities have often been viewed as a homogeneous placement type with shared, similar characteristics (Bjaanes & Butler, 1974). There is, in fact, substantial variation among community residential facilities which is related to the various kinds of facilities (Butler & Bjaanes, 1977). Within different types of facilities, there are systematic differences in services afforded to the residents. There is, however, little in the way of systematic research relating differences in residential programs to client outcome and adjustment. Given the national trend toward increased utilization of community residential facilities (O'Connor, 1976), there is an urgent need for comprehensive and systematic study of program variation and the relationship of facility characteristics to client adjustment.

The Normalization Principle (Bank-Mikkelsen, 1969; Nirje, 1969; Wolfensberger, 1969, 1972) has been predominant in the emerging philosophical basis for deinstitutionalization. Proponents of normalization maintain that more normalized service environments will result in client progress and that habilitation will be enhanced. Although the need for more culturally normal service settings is generally accepted, questions have been raised concerning the appropriateness of the normalization principle for achieving client progress (Browning, 1975; Fram, 1974; Rhoades & Browning, 1977).

To claim that normalization will result in client progress or to question the appropriateness of normalization for achieving client progress misses an important part of the overall picture, i.e., *What are the optimal conditions for enhancing client development and growth*? The problem is, in part, due to a dual usage of the term "normalization," and a lack of distinction between what will be referred to as environmental normalization and client normalization.

Data reported in this investigation were collected under the auspices of the Department of Developmental Services, State of California, in conjunction with Operation PINpoint. Conclusions are those of the authors and do not necessarily represent the position of the state of California.

Environmental normalization is the process of developing culturally appropriate residences and services, devoid of the dehumanizing stigma so often attached to being mentally retarded. Included in this process are restructuring of the service system, training service providers, and changing prevailing attitudes toward developmentally disabled persons. The process focuses primarily on altering the environment and the life experiences of the mentally retarded. Normalizing the environment is a necessary, but not sufficient, condition for enhancing client development and growth.

Client normalization is the acquisition of skills necessary for assuming culturally normative social roles and responsibilities. This usage of normalization refers to programs aimed at client habilitation, including training in specific functional skills and the reduction of maladaptive behaviors. While environmental normalization focuses on environmental conditions, client normalization focuses directly on the functional characteristics of the client. Client normalization, however, cannot proceed without environmental normalization. The writers believe that environmental normalization without a systematic attempt to enhance client normalization is likewise inadequate. Achieving client normalization not only requires habilitation programs but also requires the provision of a culturally normative environment in which to exercise acquired skills and thereby achieve normalization in the broader sense of the term. Present emphasis is primarily on environmental normalization with relatively little stress on the processes required for individual or client normalization.

To achieve successful adjustment to placement in the community, or for that matter in any setting, systematic attention must be paid to functional deficiencies in clients and the provision of services directed at remediating those conditions. At the present, little is known either about service needs or service provision (O'Connor, 1976). The need for a comprehensive, multi-disciplinary, community-based service system, however, is clearly recognized (Grossman & Rowitz, 1973).

Problems in adjusting to community placement can be viewed in a number of ways. One way is to note failures to adjust to community placement defined by subsequent institutionalization or reinstitutionalization (cf. McCarver & Craig, 1974). Among factors frequently found to predict institutionalization are IQ, adaptive behavior failures, physical disabilities (Eyman, O'Connor, Tarjan & Justice, 1972) and disruptive behavior (Wolf & Whitehead, 1975). Using a different definition of "unsuccessful adjustment," specifically their clients' inability to maintain themselves in independent or semi-independent apartment living, Schalock and Harper (1978) noted a number of specific social and independent living skills which were related to failure. Thus, a number of client characteristics as well as the absence of specific skills have been identified as presenting frequent and significant barriers to successful community adjustment. Among these factors found predictive of failure to adjust to community life are low IQ, maladaptive behavior, deficient independent living skills, and physical disabilities. Assuming that these factors have an important relationship to failure in community placement, it can be argued that along with environmental normalization, client normalization must emphasize habilitative services focusing on those factors constituting barriers to successful community adjustment which are, in addition, amenable to remediation.

This paper examines three areas of client behavior in which deficiencies create problems in placement and adjustment: adaptive behavior, independent living skills, and level of functional competence. In each of these three areas a comprehensive state agency evaluation model is used to assess the degree to which placement patterns and levels of service are directed toward responding to the clients' needs. The focus is therefore on the degree to which a service system responds to problems of client normalization.

The Client Centered Evaluation Model

This paper is based on data collected during the field test of a comprehensive evaluation system being implemented by the Department of Developmental Services in California (Kelly, 1978). The sample population (about 6% of all clients served by the Department) was drawn from the caseloads of three Regional Centers serving diverse geographical areas. The 2,881 clients represented all diagnostic categories and age ranges. Placement types ranged from state hospitals to independent living settings. Although strict sampling procedures were not used, it was found that the population included in the study was relatively representative of the developmentally disabled population being served by the Department (Day & Lebrato, 1978). The functional level and service needs of clients were assessed using the Client Centered Evaluation Model (CCEM; Bjaanes, 1976).

The CCEM consists of three major modules. The first consists of a tracking, diagnostic, and demographic section. The second consists of 127 performance measurement items. The final module gathers data on need for and delivery of 52 types of service. All data, including the service element, are individualized. Thus, service delivery can be directly linked to client as well as to the placement facility in which the client is served.

Performance data from the CCEM were subjected to a factor analysis which yielded 11 functional dimensions. By combining highly intercorrelated dimensions into single dimensions, these 11 factors were reduced to 8 functional dimensions of client performance. Scores for each dimension were standardized to have a mean of 50 with a standard deviation of 10 (Day & Lebrato, 1978). Client typologies were developed using cluster analysis which yielded 11 distinct and homogeneous person types, i.e., "0" types with shared functional characteristics (Day & Lebrato, 1978). Table 1 provides summary descriptions of each "0" type.

Table 1

Summary Characteristics of Client "O" Types[a]

0 Type	Summary Characteristics
1	Severe mental retardation complicated by physical disability. Clients characterized by low scores on all dimensions except those dealing with emotional adjustment and maladaptive behavior.
2	Severe mental retardation complicated by emotional disability and extreme disruptiveness. Clients have extremely low scores on all dimensions except motor skills.
3	Severe mental retardation complicated by limited social and independent living skills. This group can be distinguished from the most severely impaired by their relatively average motor skills, adjustment to change and maladaptive scores.
4	Moderately disabled with deficient independent living skills and high social confidence. Clients are rated high in terms of their adjustment to change and the non-disruptiveness of their behavior. These clients are above average in social initiative. They are deficient in personal and community self-sufficiency.

5 Mental retardation complicated by emotional disability. Clients are slightly above average on all dimensions except the two emotional domain factors of adjustment to change and maladaptive behavior.

6 Mental retardation complicated by limited ability to cope with change. Clients are average with respect to the sample in all domains except the adjustment to change factor.

7 Mental retardation complicated by behavioral disruptiveness. Clients have lower scores in community living skills but are within the average range for the sample in all other dimensions.

8 Mental retardation with limited social skills. Clients have below average scores in self-help skills and community living skills. Scores in adjustment to change, social initiative, and communication skills also tend to be low.

9 Mildly disabled individuals with limited cognitive skills. Clients are rated above average on all dimensions except cognitive skills.

10 Mildly disabled. All members of this cluster have above average scores on all eight dimensions.

11 Potentially autonomous with mild disability. These clients score above average on all dimensions and have extremely high scores in self-help skills, community living skills, social initiative and communication.

[a]Adapted from Day and Lebrato (1978).

For the purposes of this analysis, the 11 "0" types were grouped into the three categories described in Table 1. Group A included client "0" types 9, 10, and 11. Group B included client "0" types 4, 6, 7, and 8. Group C included client "0" types 1, 2, 3, and 5. These groups, therefore, represent clients of different levels of mental and social disability, with Group A including those clients with the least impairment, Group C including those with the greatest impariment, and Group B including clients in an intermediate range. Table 2 shows the three categories into which the 2,881 clients were grouped and the mean score of each category on the 8 functional dimensions of client performance.

Table 2

Mean Scores on Eight Dimensions for Each Client Category[a]

Client Category	Maladaptive Behavior	Self-Hellp Skills	Community Living	Communi-cation	Cognitive	Motor Skills	Social Initiative	Adjust-ment
A (11,10,9)[a]	54.1	57.5	54.9	56.3	55.0	54.3	56.4	53.8
B (8,7,6,4)[a]	48.5	47.9	44.9	49.5	45.4	52.4	48.6	44.4
C (5,3,2,1)[a]	39.8	40.0	43.2	33.8	42.8	44.2	38.0	42.8

[a]"O" Type Membership in each Client Category.

The data reported here should be viewed with caution since they were collected during a field test operation and are based on sample regions of the state and not a scientific sample of clients. While the generalizability of these data may be limited, reliability estimates have been quite high (Day & Lebrato, 1978).

Relationship Between Client Characteristics and Placement Type

Four categories of placement facilities are commonly used in California. They include state hospitals, large care facilities, small care facilities, and in-home placement. State hospitals are major state operated residential facilities. Large care facilities provide services for sixteen or more residents and include large skilled nursing facilities and small convalescent type hospitals. Small care facilities, or board and care facilities, provide services to an average of three to six clients. In-home placement includes placement of the client with parents, relatives, or guardians. In most cases only one developmentally disabled person resides in such settings.

Table 3 presents the distribution of clients in four different placement categories. The majority (62.3%) of the clients in this sample were in in-home placement, 27.0% were in small care facilities, 4.3% were in large care facilities, and 6.3% were in state hospitals. The highest proportion of clients in in-home placement (69.4%) were those in the higher functional group, i.e., Group A. This group also had the smallest representation in state hospitals and large care facilities. In Group B, the intermediate group in terms of level of functioning, 58.6% were in in-home placement, 30.6% in small care facilities, 4.4% in large care facilities, and 6.3% in state hospitals. The most impaired group, Group C, had 49.9% in in-home placement, 21.8% in small care facilities, 11.5% in large care facilities, and 16.9% in state hospitals.

Table 3

Client Placement Distribution by Client Category

Placement Type	Client Category A		B		C		Total	
	n	%	n	%	n	%	n	%
State Hospital	27	1.9	53	6.3	103	16.9	183	6.3
Large Care Facility	18	1.2	37	4.4	70	11.5	125	4.3
Small Care Facility	389	26.9	255	30.6	133	21.8	777	27.0
In-Home Placement	1002	69.4	489	58.6	305	49.9	1796	62.3
Totals	1436	100.	834	100.	611	100.	2881	100.

Table 3 clearly shows that the greater the degree of impairment, the greater was the likelihood of hospitalization and the smaller the likelihood of in-home placement. There was a slightly different pattern in the usage of small care facilities. The intermediate level, Group B, had the greatest utilization of small care facilities while both Groups A and C had a lower utilization rate. Clearly, a greater proportion of the least impaired group was in in-home placement. Group B, the intermediate category, did not utilize in-home placements to the degree of Group A and did not utilize hospital placements to the extent that Group C did. This fits well with the intended function of small care facilities, i.e., they tend to serve those who cannot be, or are not, placed in in-home placement, but who are not impaired to the degree that hospitalization is required.

Group C, the most impaired group, was least likely to be placed in in-home placements or small care facilities and had the highest rate of placement in large care facilities and state hospitals. Placement patterns for large care facilities and state hospitals show a great deal of similarity and may function in similar ways. Both tend to provide around the clock, intensive care.

Previous studies indicate that maladaptive behavior, deficient self-help skills, and physical impairment are related to institutionalization, unsuccessful community placement and reinstitutionalization (Eyman et al., 1972; Schalock & Harper, 1978). Table 2 shows differences in functional levels among the groups on the CCEM. These differences are apparent in observing the differences between the mean scores on each functional dimension for groups. Thus, Group C, which had the greatest frequency of hospitalization and placement in large care facilities, also had the lowest mean scores on *all* functional dimensions. The dimension with the greatest observed difference was communication, with a difference in mean score of 22.5 between Groups A and C. (The sample mean for each dimension was 50 with a standard deviation of 10.) Mean differences in the social skills dimension was 18.4, self-help skills 17.5, and maladaptive behavior 14.3. The dimensions in which there was the least difference between Groups A and C were motor functions, 12.2, community living skills, 11.7, and adjustment to change, 11.0. Earlier publications (Eyman et al., 1972) have presented similar findings but have not included communication as a major factor of differentiating those who tend to be in in-home placements and those who tend to have the highest rate of institutionalization. In addition, the small difference in motor function levels appears to contradict earlier findings. In part, this may be due to changes that have taken place in placement practices in the time between earlier studies and the present one.

Client Needs and Available Services

The authors maintain that to achieve normalization in the broader sense of the term, it is necessary to emphasize client normalization. An important part of client normalization is the provision of services aimed at ameliorating socially deficient behavior. Furthermore, adjustment to placement can be enhanced through the provision of services aimed at specific behavioral deficiencies which are related to unsuccessful placement. In view of the findings described above, the authors examined four generic service categories targeted at those areas in which the greatest differences between Groups A and C were found. These were: a) Supportive Counseling, b) Independent Living Skills Training, c) Behavior Therapy, and d) Social Interaction Training.

a) *Supportive Counseling* is defined as regularly scheduled, goal-oriented intervention which is responsive to the decision making needs of the impaired individual or his family. The primary focus of this intervention is upon solving interpersonal problems such as acceptance of the disability, over-anxiety, overprotection, and the ability to deal with daily demands resulting from the client's disability.

b) *Independent Living Skills Training* is defined as an individualized program designed to enhance and develop skills required for independent living.

c) *Behavior Therapy* is defined as therapy specifically for the purpose of reinforcing desirable and adaptive behaviors and the reduction or elimination of maladaptive behaviors.

d) *Social Interaction Training* is defined as regularly scheduled programs aimed at developing and improving a person's interpersonal skills. Included is training in manners, communication, and appropriate social behavior.

The service element of the CCEM includes a number of different entries for describing each service. These include actual provision of service, service not required, service needed but not available, and service needed but temporarily unavailable to the client. This permits an analysis of actual service provision as well as the perceived service needs of each client. The service element of the CCEM is completed by the case manager, usually a social worker at the MSW level, who is responsible for the client.

Discussion of Findings of the Client Centered Evaluation

Generally the results of the Client Centered Evaluation supported the findings of Eyman et al. (1972) and Wolf and Whitehead (1975) that deficits in the areas of adaptive behavior, social skills, and self-help skills are strongly related to the likelihood of being institutionalized. However, the data further suggest that deficits in other functional areas, particularly communication, are also critical predictors of placement in an institution or large care facility. In the group with the highest rate of placement in state hospitals and large care facilities, the level of function in all 8 behavioral dimensions is substantially lower than that of the other two groups. In all behavioral dimensions, the mean level of function was the highest for Group A in which there was also the highest level of in-home placement. Generally, those with the lowest level of function were the most likely to be placed in state hospitals and large care facilities.

Since California does not yet have longitudinal tracking data describing placement history, the observed conditions cannot be directly attributed to either deinstitutionalization or institutionalization of those who are more severely impaired. Some inferences can be made, however. The major emphasis in California in the last decade has been on deinstitutionalization. Thus, it can be assumed that the observed patterns are in large part due to deinstitutionalization of clients in the higher functional groups. Even though there is a relatively high percentage of Group C clients placed in state hospitals and large care facilities, the majority of clients (62.3%) are in in-home placements with small care facilities accounting for another 27.0%. Of the total developmentally disabled population in this sample, only 10.6% are in large care facilities and state hospitals, attesting to the heavy emphasis on community placement.

While no data were collected to assess compliance with normalization principle requirements, it is generally assumed by normalization proponents that small, family-like residences and parental homes approximate the tenets of the principle to a greater degree than do state hospitals and large care facilities. If one accepts this assumption, then a majority of the clients in fact reside in more normalized environments. However, as maintained earlier, environmental normalization is only one part of the broader implications of normalization. Client normalization must also be taken into account. In this conceptualization, client normalization requires habilitation services aimed at enhancing clients' skills and reducing maladaptive behaviors.

Tables 4 through 7 contain information on the services needed by and provided to the three categories of developmentally disabled clients within the four placement types. Table 4 contains information on social interaction training; Table 5, independent living skills; Table 6, behavior therapy; and Table 7, supportive counseling. While there are many interesting comparisons in these tables, only some of the more significant patterns will be highlighted here.

Table 4

Perception of Need for and Provision of Social Interaction Training by Client Category and Placement Type

Client Category	State Hospitals				Large Care Facilities				Small Care Facilities				In-Home Placement				Totals			
	n	NR	P/S	%	n	NR	P/S	%	n	NR	P/S	%	n	NR	P/S	%	n	NR	P/S	%
A	27	5	22	81.5[a]	18	6	12	66.7[a]	388	222	166	42.8a	1002	655	347	34.6[a]	1435	888	547	38.1[a]
			21	95.4[b]			11	91.7[b]			143	86.1[b]			263	75.8[b]			438	80.1[b]
				77.8[c]				61.1[c]				36.8[c]				26.2[c]				30.5[c]
B	53	4	49	92.4[a]	37	11	26	70.3[a]	255	112	143	56.1[a]	489	328	161	32.9[a]	834	455	379	45.4[a]
			49	100. [b]			26	100. [b]			126	88.1[b]			132	82.0[b]			333	87.9[b]
				92.4[c]				70.3[c]				49.4[c]				27.0[c]				39.9[c]
C	103	19	84	81.5[a]	70	36	34	48.6[a]	133	64	69	51.9[a]	305	218	87	28.5[a]	611	337	274	44.8[a]
			80	95.2[b]			33	97.1[b]			53	76.8[b]			69	79.3[b]			240	87.6[b]
				77.7[c]				47.1[c]				39.8[c]				22.6[c]				39.3[c]

n = Number of clients.
NR = Clients who were judged as not requiring services.
P/S = P are clients deemed to require the service, S are clients actually served.
a = Percentage of clients judged as requiring the service.
b = Percentage of clients judged as requiring the service who are actually receiving the service.
c = Percentage of facility type clients actually receiving the service.

Table 5

Perception of Need for and Provision of Independent Living Skills Training by Client Category and Placement Type

Client Category	State Hospitals				Large Care Facilities				Small Care Facilities				In-Home Placement				Totals			
	n	NR	P/S	%	n	NR	P/S	%	n	NR	P/S	%	n	NR	P/S	%	n	NR	P/S	%
A	27	8	19	70.3[a]	18	5	13	72.2[a]	388	190	198	51.0[a]	1002	620	382	38.1[a]	1435	823	612	42.6[a]
			15	78.9[b]			12	92.3[b]			174	87.9[b]			266	69.3[b]			467	76.3[b]
				55.5[c]				66.7[c]				44.8[c]				26.5[c]				32.5[c]
B	53	15	38	71.7[a]	37	17	20	54.0[a]	255	165	90	35.3[a]	489	405	84	17.2[a]	834	602	232	27.8[a]
			37	97.4[b]			20	100. [b]			82	91.1[b]			68	80.9[b]			211	90.9[b]
				69.8[c]				54.0[c]				32.2[c]				13.9[c]				25.2[c]
C	103	33	70	68.0[a]	70	43	27	38.6[a]	133	91	42	31.6[a]	305	273	32	11.7[a]	611	439	172	39.2[a]
			70	100. [b]			25	92.6[b]			39	92.9[b]			26	81.2[b]			160	93.0[b]
				68.0[c]				35.7[c]				29.3[c]				8.5[c]				26.2[c]

n = Number of clients.
NR = Clients who were judged as not requiring services.
P/S = P are clients deemed to require the service, S are clients actually served.
a = Percentage of clients judged as requiring the service.
b = Percentage of clients judged as requiring the service who are actually receiving the service.
c = Percentage of facility type clients actually receiving the service.

Table 6

Perception of Need for and Provision of Behavior Therapy by Client Category and Placement Type

Client Category	State Hospitals				Large Care Facilities				Small Care Facilities				In-Home Placement				Totals			
	n	NR	P/S	%	n	NR	P/S	%	n	NR	P/S	%	n	NR	P/S	%	n	NR	P/S	%
A	27	14	13	48.1[a]	18	8	10	55.5[a]	338	353	35	9.0[a]	1002	895	107	10.7[a]	1435	1270	165	11.5[a]
			8	61.5[b]			10	100. [b]			23	65.7[b]			70	65.4[b]			113	68.5[b]
				29.6[c]				55.5[c]				5.9[c]				7.0[c]				7.9[c]
B	53	24	29	54.7[a]	37	17	20	54.1[a]	255	191	64	25.1[a]	484	365	119	24.6[a]	834	597	237	28.4[a]
			26	89.6[b]			18	90.0[b]			33	51.6[b]			84	70.6[b]			181	72.4[b]
				49.1[c]				48.6[c]				12.9[c]				17.3[c]				19.3[c]
C	103	33	70	68.0[a]	70	41	29	41.4[a]	133	73	60	45.1[a]	305	214	91	29.8[a]	611	361	250	40.9[a]
			65	92.9[b]			25	86.2[b]			31	51.7[b]			60	65.9[b]			181	72.4[b]
				63.1[c]				35.7[c]				23.3[c]				19.7[c]				29.6[c]

n = Number of clients.
NR = Clients who were judged as not requiring services.
P/S = P are clients deemed to require the service, S are clients actually served.
a = Percentage of clients judged as requiring the service.
b = Percentage of clients judged as requiring the service who are actually receiving the service.
c = Percentage of facility type clients actually receiving the service.

Table 7

Perception of Need for and Provision of Supportive Counseling by Client Category and Placement Type

Client Category	State Hospitals				Large Care Facilities				Small Care Facilities				In-Home Placement				Totals			
	n	NR	P/S	%	n	NR	P/S	%	n	NR	P/S	%	n	NR	P/S	%	n	NR	P/S	%
A	27	8	19	70.4[a]	18	1	17	94.4[a]	388	79	309	79.6[a]	1002	339	663	66.2[a]	1435	427	1008	70.2[a]
			16	84.2[b]			17	100. [b]			299	96.8[b]			584	88.1[b]			916	90.9[b]
				59.3[c]				94.4[c]				77.1[c]				58.3[c]				63.8[c]
B	53	32	21	39.6[a]	37	4	33	89.2[a]	255	90	165	64.7[a]	489	201	288	58.9[a]	834	328	506	60.7[a]
			18	85.7[b]			31	93.9[b]			164	99.4[b]			264	91.7[b]			477	94.3[b]
				39.6[c]				83.8[c]				64.3[c]				54.0[c]				57.2[c]
C	103	84	19	18.4[a]	70	24	46	65.7[a]	133	57	76	57.1[a]	305	105	200	65.6[a]	611	270	341	55.8[a]
			14	73.7[b]			46	100. [b]			75	98.7[b]			185	92.5[b]			320	93.8[b]
				13.6[c]				65.7[c]				56.4[c]				60.7[c]				52.4[c]

n = Number of clients.
NR = Clients who were judged as not requiring services.
P/S = P are clients deemed to require the service, S are clients actually served.
a = Percentage of clients judged as requiring the service.
b = Percentage of clients judged as requiring the service who are actually receiving the service.
c = Percentage of facility type clients actually receiving the service.

In general, a small proportion of clients in the lowest functioning group receive these four services in comparison to the two other groups. Group A has the highest mean score on the self-help dimension and has the highest proportion (32.5%) receiving independent living skills training. Group C, which is the lowest functioning group, and Group B have smaller proportions receiving such training (26.2% and 25.3%, respectively). Again a smaller proportion (52.4%) of clients in Group C receive supportive counseling than those in Group A (63.8%). When viewing the sample as a whole, social interaction training and behavior therapy present a different picture. In these, clients in the lower functioning group receive more services than do the two other groups. However, the pattern is by no means uniform across the different placement types.

Provision of independent living skills training in hospitals tends to be related to level of performance. A slightly higher proportion (69.8%) of those who are in the intermediate group receive training in comparison to those who are most impaired while only 55.5% of those in the least impaired group receive training. For all other placements types, the most severely impaired group also has the smallest proportion of clients in training. Only 8.5% of Group C clients in in-home placement receive independent living skills training. A similar pattern is observed in the provision of supportive counseling with the exception of Group C in in-home placement where 60.7% of the residents receive the service in comparison to 58.3% for Group A and 54.0% for Group B.

In hospitals there is a high level of provision of social interaction training with the intermediate group having the highest level (92.4%). There is little difference between Groups A and C. In large care facilities and in-home placements, clients in Group C receive the least amount of training. In small care facilities a higher proportion of Group C clients than Group A clients receive social interaction training. However, Group B, functioning at a higher level, also has a higher proportion (49.4%) of clients than either Groups A or C receiving such training.

The only relatively uniform service category is behavior therapy. In hospitals, small care facilities, and in-home placements the proportion of clients in therapy increases with the level of maladaptive behavior, i.e., the more the maladaptive behavior, the greater the proportion of clients in therapy. The exception is large care facilities where the group with the most maladaptive behavior also has the least proportion of clients receiving behavior therapy.

As was seen in Tables 4 through 7, when service data are analyzed, the general pattern tends to be that those who are the most severely impaired, and hence also in most need of habilitation services, are those for whom services are least likely to be provided. This raises the philosophical and moral dilemma: to whom should services be provided? Should services be provided to those for whom the greatest gain can be expected or to those with the greatest need for those services? Without consciously addressing the issue, it appears the California service system primarily has opted for the former course. This raises a thorny problem because, in so doing, the potential for the adjustment of the most severely impaired to community placement is seriously restricted. Consequently, in line with the authors' formulation of client normalization in the broader sense, the potential for normalization of lower functioning individuals is circumscribed and limited. This issue warrants a much closer examination both in practical as well as philosophical terms.

When service provision was compared across different placement types, the proportion of clients being provided with required services in small care facilities and in-home placements was generally lower than that in state hospitals and large care facilities for all client categories. Furthermore, the perception of service needed in in-home placements and small care facilities tended to be lower than in state hospitals and large care facilities, even when controlling for client level of function (a notable exception to this pattern was in the area of supportive counseling for members of the most seriously impaired group of clients who were living at home, possibly due to the inclusion of parental counseling under the "supportive counseling" dimension).

When small care facilities and in-home placements are compared, with the exception of behavior therapy, a greater proportion of clients in small care facilities receive services in comparison to those in in-home placement. A greater proportion of Group A and B clients in in-home placements were involved in behavior therapy programs than was the case with clients in smaller care facilities. However, the converse was true for the most seriously impaired group.

The service provided most frequently for in-home placements was supportive counseling. Even so, the level of provision of this service was lower than in either large or small care facilities, but generally higher than that provided in state hospitals. The comparatively high rate of utilization of supportive counseling can be, at least in part, attributed to the fact that parent counseling is included. Parental involvement with the disabled person is higher in in-home placement, and hence there is greater utilization of parent counseling.

When service patterns are viewed in conjunction with placement patterns, it is clear that the greatest proportion of developmentally disabled clients in this sample (89.3%) are placed in settings in which the least amount of service is provided. It is evident that the community service network called for by Grossman and Rowitz (1973) has not yet been adequately developed. Supportive counseling appears to be an exception to this observation, but even here the service level is low. What is clearly required are specialized services related to the functional needs of clients. Hospitals and large care facilities are providing these services at a substantially higher level than are small care facilities and in-home placements.

As earlier work suggested (Bjaanes & Butler, 1974), there is a great deal of variation within different placement types. While these differences are not taken into account in this analysis, it is also clear from the data presented here that there are clear differences between different placement types. Especially notable is the significantly smaller proportion of clients in in-home placement and small care facilities receiving required services than is the case with residents of state hospitals and large care facilities. When these findings are viewed from the broader perspective of normalization, developed in the introduction, the authors feel that while *environmental normalization* requirements may have been met in small care facilities and in-home placement, elements of *client normalization* are clearly lacking in these types of placement.

State hospitals and large care facilities may be less normalized in the environmental sense of the term, but they provide a substantially greater level of services to clients and thus, at least in part, provide a greater potential for *client normalization*. The authors believe *both* aspects of normalization must be achieved for client development to be maximized. Therefore, in state hospitals and large care facilities there are significant deficiencies in normalization as the term is used here. State hospitals and large care facilities in general tend to place greater emphasis on client normalization while in-home placement and small care facilities may place greater emphasis on *environmental normalization* with less attention in the service component of *client normalization*.

These observations lead to two conclusions. First, clients who are placed in state hospitals and large care facilities are being provided with a greater basis for skill development but do not have the normalized environment in which to exercise those skills. Clients placed in small care facilities and in-home placement may have the normalized environment, but they lack the direct services which focus on the development of competence. *Both* conditions create barriers to normalization in its broadest sense.

Adjustment to community placement may be measured, in part, by whether or not placement is successful, i.e., whether the individual is able to remain in the setting. Schalock and Harper (1978) found that problems with social behavior and deficient independent living skills were major factors in placement failure. Provision of habilitation programs focused on these problem areas will often enhance the ability of individuals to adjust. In general, these data suggest that these services are not being provided to the extent they are needed in small care facilities and in-home placement. Thus, a major factor in enhancing adjustment is presently lacking in these service settings.

Given the differences among the different placement types and among the clients themselves, it might be assumed that different placement types may be more appropriate for certain client types. At present, however, there are few longitudinal studies exploring relationships between placement characteristics and client development. There has beeen no research systematically examining the differential impact of environmental versus client normalization for clients of differing degrees of handicap. Nor have there been any studies which systematically examine client development when both criteria for normalization are used. Such research could have practical implications for the determination of what types of clients adjust more readily to which type of placement and service combinations.

Longitudinal studies must be conducted taking into account client characteristics, development, and adjustment, as well as the environment in which the clients live. That is, placement, services, and client attributes must be systematically studied in relationship to each other. Such studies must address both environmental normalization *and* client normalization concurrently.

Conclusions

The authors would again reiterate a cautionary note regarding conclusions drawn from this study. Although the sample and the data were part of a large scale field test, they appear to be representative and reliable. Nevertheless, given the nature of the project, conclusions and generalizations must be viewed as tentative at this time.

The majority of the clients in this sample are in community placement. There is a higher rate of utilization of state hospitals and large care facilities by those clients who are in the lower functional group. However, even in this category the majority of the clients are in some form of community placement.

In general, clients in the higher functioning group have a greater proportion of their members receiving services targeted at specific behavioral skills. Those who are in the lowest functioning group have the lowest proportion of clients receiving the services discussed in this study. Clients exhibiting a high level of maladaptive behavior also have the highest proportion receiving behavior therapy.

When service provision is compared across the different placement types, community placements, including small care facilities and in-home placements, have the lowest proportion of clients receiving services aimed at increasing level of adjustment. There is a greater proportion of clients in state hospitals and large care facilities receiving needed services.

There are systematic differences among state hospitals and large care facilities and community placement. In the former there appears to be a greater emphasis on components of client normalization while environmental normalization may be deficient. In the latter, there may be an emphasis on environmental normalization while aspects of client normalization are deficient.

To date the primary emphasis in the deinstitutionalization process appears to have been on environmental normalization with considerable lag in activities aimed at enhancing client normalization. As was shown in the Client Centered Evaluation in California, a large number of deinstitutionalized mentally retarded persons are not receiving basic services focusing on client normalization.

A comprehensive, community-based, interdisciplinary service system has as yet not been adequately developed. An exception to this is the provision of supportive counseling which represents a broad, generalized service. While this may, in part, be due to the relative novelty of community placement and the decentralization of services, it is important that these needs be addressed in programs which conceptualize normalization as including the client as well as the environment. Finally, there is an urgent need for systematic, longitudinal research focusing on *both* environmental normalization *and* client normalization.

References

Bank-Mikkelsen, N. E. A metropolitan area in Denmark: Copenhagen. In R. B. Kugel & W. Wolfensberger (Eds.), *Changing patterns in residential services for the mentally retarded*. Washington DC: President's Committee on Mental Retardation, 1969.

Bjaanes, A. T. *The Client Centered Evaluation Model: Final report*. Sacramento: California Department of Health, 1976.

Bjaanes, A. T. & Butler, E. W. Environmental variation in community care facilities for mentally retarded persons. *American Journal of Mental Deficiency*, 1974, *78*, 429-439.

Browning, P. L. *Several issues in mental retardation: A need perspective?* (Working paper No. 81) Eugene, OR: Rehabilitation Research & Training Center in Mental Retardation, Oregon University, 1975.

Butler, E. W. & Bjaanes, A. T. A typology of community care facilities and differential normalization outcomes. In P. Mittler (Ed.), *Research to practice in mental retardation: Care and intervention* (Volume 1). Baltimore, MD: University Park Press, 1977.

Day, D. & Lebrato, M. T. The analysis of rated competence and the classification of Operation PINpoint clients. In B. Kelly (Ed.), *Operation PINpoint; Part II*. Sacramento: California Department of Health, 1978.

Eyman, R. K., O'Connor, G., Tarjan, G. & Justice, R. S. Factors determining residential placement of mentally retarded children. *American Journal of Mental Deficiency*, 1972, *76*(6), 692-698.

Fram, J. The right to be retarded—Normally. *Mental Retardation*, 1974, *12*(6), 32.

Grossman, H. J. & Rowitz, L. A community approach to services for the retarded. In R. K. Eyman, C. E. Meyers & G. Tarjan (Eds.), *Sociobehavioral studies in mental retardation*. Washington, DC: , American Association on Mental Deficiency, 1973.

Kelly, B. *Operation PINpoint: Part II*. Sacramento: California Department of Health, 1978.

Nirje, B. The normalization principle and its human management implications. In R. B. Kugel & W. Wolfensberger (Eds.), *Changing patterns in residential services for the mentally retarded*. Washington, DC: President's Committee on Mental Retardation, 1969.

O'Connor, G. *Home is a good place*. Washington, DC: American Association on Mental Deficiency, 1976.

Rhoades, C. & Browning, P. Normalization at what price? *Mental Retardation*, 1977, *15*(2), 24.

Schalock, R. L. & Harper, R. S. Placement from community-based mental retardation programs: How well do clients do? *American Journal of Mental Deficiency*, 1978, *83*(3), 240-247.

Wolf, L. C. & Whitehead, P. C. The decision to institutionalize retarded children: Comparison of individually matched groups. *Mental Retardation*, 1975, *13*(5), 3-11.

Wolfensberger, W. *Normalization: The principle of normalization in human services*. Toronto: National Institute on Mental Retardation, 1972.

Comparative Adaptive and Maladaptive Behavior of Mentally Retarded Clients of Five Residential Settings in Three Western States

Sharon A. Borthwick
C. Edward Meyers
Richard K. Eyman

University of California, Los Angeles
Neuropsychiatric Institute Research Group at
Lanterman State Hospital and Development Center
Pomona, California

This paper describes some characteristics of the mentally retarded population of five categories of residential placement in three Western states. A table of comparisons (Table 1) is provided as a background for understanding the data regarding alternative placements presented in this volume and elsewhere. Hopefully these comparisons can help answer frequently asked questions related to differences among clients in various residential placements. For example, is it true that the mentally retarded clients still residing in institutions after years of effort toward deinstitutionalization have characteristics that make successful community placement unlikely, or at least considerably more difficult? Or do small family care homes generally get the "best" clients? Questions such as these are frequently asked in discussions of residential alternatives, but data have generally been lacking for those seeking to respond.

Our center routinely collects demographic and behavior data on mentally retarded people in several western states. Careproviders are asked to respond to statements about the adaptive and maladaptive behavior of clients in five residential settings, using a simplified version of the AAMD Adaptive Behavior Scale (described below). In order to present the comparisons in a manner most immediately meaningful, we provide not domains or factor scores, but the actual statements on the abbreviated Adaptive Behavior Scale (Nihira, Foster, Shellhaas & Leland, 1974) form, and the percentage of responses made in each category for each setting.

Sample

The sample consisted of 6202 people receiving services for the developmentally disabled (DD) during 1979 in three western states. Two of the states (Arizona and Nevada) use a centralized service delivery system, each responsible for the provision of services to all developmentally disabled clients in its state. The third state (California) contracts with several centers that are responsible for service delivery in a specified geographic area. Clients from one of these centers were included in the sample, a center serving a total population of one and a quarter million people. Although the agencies are intended to serve people with all types of developmental disabilities, 98% of the sample were identified as mentally retarded. All community and institutional residential placement decisions are

This study was supported in part by the National Institute of Child Health and Human Development Research Grants No. HD-04612, HD-05540, HD-7-2847, & DHEW, Developmental Disabilities Division, Office of Human Development, Grant No. 54-P-71117/9.

made by these service systems in the three states, in addition to providing other services.

The five placement alternatives compared in this report are 1) public institutions, 2) convalescent hospitals, 3) board and care homes, 4) family care homes, and 5) parental homes. Institutions are state facilities providing a comprehensive array of services primarily to severely mentally retarded residents. Convalescent hospitals are generally skilled nursing facilities, caring for nonambulatory severely and profoundly retarded persons. Board and care homes consist primarily of group homes and residential schools, usually providing such services as nursing care and schooling. Family care homes are licensed to care for six or fewer developmentally disabled persons of all ages and levels of retardation, although profoundly retarded persons are seldom found in them. Clients who reside with their own parents are provided services other than out-of-home placement by the service agency. The characteristics of the clients in these states were found to be similar with regard to IQ, age and sex. One of the states makes somewhat greater use of board and care homes and convalescent hospitals than the other two states, probably related to its being a considerably more urban state. Still, the data for the three states show no appreciable differences among states. For that reason we present one set of combined data.

Procedure

Information on adaptive and maladaptive behavior was obtained from the Behavior Development Survey (BDS), a shortened version of the AAMD Adaptive Behavior Scale (ABS)[1]. Adaptive behavior items on the short form appear exactly as they do on Part 1 of the ABS. Maladaptive behavior items on the short form have been slightly modified from their actual wording on the ABS, Part II; the questions are representative of the subdomain headings on the ABS. Additional items on the short form of BDS, but not on the ABS, which we considered to be of interest were ambulation, speech, prosthetics, and use of medications. Space precludes the presentation of all the items for which there are available data. Items from Part I of the ABS that are scored by counting checkmarks were eliminated, as the totals are not easily interpreted. All items selected for comparison were those considered to be of primary interest in placement decisions.

Results

Table 1 displays comparisons for each item. The percentage of clients who function or behave at each level is shown for each type of placement. Also included are comparisons of age and IQ.

Summary

It is apparent from the information in Table 1 that institutions and convalescent hospitals serve more severely handicapped clients, while other community placements serve people who are more able to care for themselves. In particular, self-care abilities such as bathing, dressing, toilet training and ambulation seem to

[1]The Behavior Development Survey (BDS) is a short research form of the AAMD Adaptive Behavior Scale, developed by the UCLA Mental Retardation Research Center, Research Group at Lanterman State Hospital. More complete information regarding the BDS is available upon inquiry from the authors.

Table 1

Comparative Percents of Selected ABS Item Categories and Other Characteristics of Residents in Five Residential Settings

Type of Behavior	*Type of Setting*[a]				
	I	C	B	F	H
Ambulation[b]					
Unable to walk	23	50	1	3	16
Walks only with help	4	15	2	1	4
Limps or walks unsteadily	17	16	16	17	14
Walks with no difficulty	56	19	81	79	66
Speech					
Makes no sounds	15	14	2	3	4
Speech is not understandable but makes sounds	46	46	11	15	20
Speech is very difficult to understand	11	7	13	18	15
Speech somewhat difficult to understand	14	20	29	30	27
Speech easily understood	14	13	45	34	34
Use of Table Utensils (a)[c]					
Feeds self with fingers or must be fed	19	34	1	3	15
Feeds self with spoon—considerable spilling	22	19	4	4	6
Feeds self with spoon—neatly	10	13	5	3	6
Feeds self with spoon and fork—considerable spilling	14	6	9	11	7
Feeds self with spoon and fork—neatly	24	11	21	29	18
Uses table knife for cutting or spreading	3	2	8	9	7
Uses knife and fork correctly and neatly	8	15	52	41	41
Drinking (3)					
Does not drink from cup or glass unassisted	19	37	1	3	14
Drinks from cup or glass unassisted—considerable spilling	24	18	7	5	8
Drinks from cup or glass unassisted—neatly	18	12	9	13	14
Drinks without spilling, holding glass in one hand	39	33	83	79	64
Toilet Training (5)					
Is not toilet trained at all	24	40	2	5	20
Frequently has toilet accidents during the day	12	9	4	3	3
Occasionally has toilet accidents during the day	26	19	9	15	11
Never has toilet accidents during the day	11	6	4	7	7
Never has toilet accidents	27	26	81	70	59
Bathing (8)					
Makes no attempt to wash or dry self	31	25	2	4	14
Cooperates when being washed and dried by others	25	40	6	9	13
Attempts to soap and wash self	8	9	3	6	7
Washes and dries self with help	9	7	9	16	8

[a]**Note.** I = Institution; C = Convalescent Hospital; B = Board & Care Home F = Family Care; H = Own Home.

[b]Item that was not extracted from the ABS

[c]Numbers in parentheses refer to item numbers on AAMD Adaptive Behavior Scale, Part I. (Nihira, Foster, Shellhaas & Leland, 1974).

Table 1 (Continued)

Comparative Percents of Selected ABS Item Categories and Other Characteristics of Residents in Five Residential Settings

Type of Behavior	*Type of Setting*[a]				
	I	C	B	F	H
Washes and dries self reasonably well with prompting	14	10	17	19	9
Washes and dries self completely without prompting or helping	5	5	7	10	8
Prepares and completes bathing unaided	8	4	56	36	41
Dressing (15)					
Must be dressed completely	23	22	0	3	14
Cooperates when dressed by extending arms or legs	16	40	3	5	13
Dresses self with help in pulling or putting on most clothes and fastening them	14	8	5	10	9
Dresses self by pulling or putting on all clothes with verbal prompting and by fastening them with help	16	10	7	12	9
Completely dresses self with verbal prompting only	9	5	9	10	5
Completely dresses self	22	15	76	60	50
Reading (37)					
Recognizes fewer than ten words or none at all	91	85	51	63	55
Recognizes ten or more words by sight	4	4	8	9	9
Reads various signs, e.g. "NO PARKING," "MEN," "WOMEN," etc.	2	3	16	12	11
Reads simple stories or comics	1	2	9	6	8
Reads books suitable for children seven years old	1	2	5	5	8
Reads books suitable for children nine years or older	1	4	11	5	9
Numbers (41)					
Has no understanding of numbers	73	63	23	30	34
Discriminates between "one" and "many" or "a lot"	10	11	10	9	7
Counts two objects by saying "one...two"	5	4	11	14	7
Mechanically counts to ten	4	7	12	12	10
Counts ten or more objects	5	7	16	18	16
Does simple addition and subtraction	3	8	28	17	26
Sense of Direction (18)					
Gets lost whenever leaving own living area	38	43	7	13	21
Goes around cottage, ward, or home alone	34	37	24	37	28
Goes around hospital ground or a few blocks from home without getting lost	20	14	18	21	16

[a]**Note.** I = Institution; C = Convalescent Hospital; B = Board & Care Home F = Family Care; H = Own Home.

[b]Item that was not extracted from the ABS

[c]Numbers in parentheses refer to item numbers on AAMD Adaptive Behavior Scale, Part I. (Nihira, Foster, Shellhaas & Leland, 1974).

Table 1 (Continued)

Comparative Percents of Selected ABS Item Categories and Other Characteristics of Residents in Five Residential Settings

Type of Behavior	*Type of Setting*[a] I	C	B	F	H
Goes a few blocks from hospital or school ground, or several blocks from home without getting lost	8	6	51	29	35
Room Cleaning (44)					
Does not clean room at all	81	84	24	21	41
Cleans room but not thoroughly	15	13	44	50	31
Cleans room well, e.g., sweeping, dusting and tidying	4	3	32	29	28
Personal Belongings (58)					
Not responsible at all—does not take care of personal belongings	72	68	11	16	32
Unreliable—seldom takes care of personal belongings	10	6	13	15	11
Usually dependable—usually takes care of personal belongings	12	12	41	40	31
Very dependable—always takes care of personal belongings	6	14	35	29	26
Food Preparation (47)					
Does not prepare food at all	90	85	51	51	48
Prepares simple foods requiring no mixing or cooking	9	12	32	37	27
Mixes and cooks simple food, e.g. fries eggs, cooks TV dinners	1	3	13	10	19
Prepares an adequate complete meal (may use canned or frozen food)	0	0	4	2	6
Table Clearing (48)					
Does not clear table at all	55	77	21	17	37
Clears table of unbreakable dishes and silverware	36	17	24	23	13
Clears table of breakable dishes and glassware	9	6	55	60	50
Job Complexity (50)					
Performs no work at all	72	80	16	18	39
Performs simple work, e.g. simple gardening, mopping floors	24	14	64	70	45
Performs a job requiring use of tools or machinery, e.g. shop work	4	6	20	12	16
Initiative (53)					
Will not engage in assigned activities, e.g. putting away toys, etc.	49	38	6	9	21
Will engage in activities only if assigned or directed	40	43	39	40	27

[a]**Note.** I = Institution; C = Convalescent Hospital; B = Board & Care Home F = Family Care; H = Own Home.

[b]Item that was not extracted from the ABS

[c]Numbers in parentheses refer to item numbers on AAMD Adaptive Behavior Scale, Part I. (Nihira, Foster, Shellhaas & Leland, 1974).

Table 1 (Continued)

Comparative Percents of Selected ABS Item Categories and Other Characteristics of Residents in Five Residential Settings

Type of Behavior	*Type of Setting*[a]				
	I	C	B	F	H
Asks if there is something to do, or explores surroundings	3	7	18	17	15
Initiates most of own activities, e.g. tasks, games, etc.	8	12	37	34	37
Interaction with Others (63)					
Does not respond to others in a socially acceptable manner	45	36	7	7	13
Interacts with others imitatively with little interaction	26	27	14	16	18
Interacts with others for at least a short period of time	18	17	29	29	26
Interacts with others in group games or activity	11	20	50	48	43
Threatens or does physical violence to others					
Frequently	12	4	3	2	2
Occasionally	36	19	25	22	16
Never	52	77	72	76	82
Damages own or other's property					
Frequently	13	2	3	5	2
Occasionally	30	12	20	22	15
Never	57	86	77	73	83
Disrupts other's activities					
Frequently	17	6	6	5	6
Occasionally	37	26	32	29	26
Never	46	68	62	66	68
Is rebellious					
Frequently	27	9	9	8	6
Occasionally	38	33	37	35	33
Never	35	58	54	57	61
Runs away or attempts to run away					
Frequently	6	2	2	1	1
Occasionally	15	4	8	5	6
Never	79	94	90	94	93
Displays stereotyped behavior, e.g. rocks back and forth					
Frequently	35	22	8	13	6
Occasionally	22	17	10	16	11
Never	43	61	82	71	83

[a]**Note.** I = Institution; C = Convalescent Hospital; B = Board & Care Home F = Family Care; H = Own Home.

[b]Item that was not extracted from the ABS

[c]Numbers in parentheses refer to item numbers on AAMD Adaptive Behavior Scale, Part I. (Nihira, Foster, Shellhaas & Leland, 1974).

Table 1 (Continued)

Comparative Percents of Selected ABS Item Categories and Other Characteristics of Residents in Five Residential Settings

Type of Behavior	*Type of Setting*[a] I	C	B	F	H
Removes or tears off own clothing					
Frequently	12	4	1	2	1
Occasionally	21	7	4	9	3
Never	67	89	95	89	96
Does physical violence to self					
Frequently	15	5	2	2	2
Occasionally	23	13	6	11	6
Never	62	82	92	87	92
Is hyperactive, e.g. will not sit still for any length of time					
Frequently	22	6	8	9	8
Occasionally	26	11	15	15	13
Never	52	83	77	76	79
Displays heterosexual behavior that is socially unacceptable					
Frequently	2	0	1	1	1
Occasionally	6	3	6	5	3
Never	92	97	93	94	96
Displays homosexual behavior that is socially unacceptable					
Frequently	3	0	1	0	0
Occasionally	8	3	4	4	1
Never	89	97	95	96	99
Displays other unacceptable sexual behavior, e.g. masturbates, exposes self					
Frequently	13	4	1	2	1
Occasionally	20	8	5	6	4
Never	67	88	94	92	95
Requires seclusion					
Frequently	1	0	1	1	1
Occasionally	8	5	5	7	4
Never	91	95	94	92	95
Requires restraint					
Frequently	2	6	0	1	0
Occasionally	9	9	4	4	4
Never	89	85	96	95	96

[a]**Note.** I = Institution; C = Convalescent Hospital; B = Board & Care Home F = Family Care; H = Own Home.

[b]Item that was not extracted from the ABS

[c]Numbers in parentheses refer to item numbers on AAMD Adaptive Behavior Scale, Part I. (Nihira, Foster, Shellhaas & Leland, 1974).

Table 1 (Continued)

Comparative Percents of Selected ABS Item Categories and Other Characteristics of Residents in Five Residential Settings

Type of Behavior	*Type of Setting*[a]				
	I	C	B	F	H
Percent of residents who use:					
Glasses	12	7	28	25	22
Hearing aid	2	0	2	3	2
Braces	5	5	1	2	3
Walker	3	6	1	1	2
Wheel chair	25	57	2	2	6
Is client receiving any regular medication?					
Yes	85	87	60	44	33
No	15	13	40	56	67
Mean Age—years	25.5	30.2	35.3	26.6	17.2
standard deviation	2.7	4.1	14.7	9.1	3.7
Mean IQ	26.0	21.9	45.4	39.8	51.7
standard deviation	5.6	19.7	17.1	4.8	5.0
Number of clients in sample	2048	684	461	984	2025

[a]**Note.** I = Institution; C = Convalescent Hospital; B = Board & Care Home F = Family Care; H = Own Home.

[b]Item that was not extracted from the ABS

[c]Numbers in parentheses refer to item numbers on AAMD Adaptive Behavior Scale, Part I. (Nihira, Foster, Shellhaas & Leland, 1974).

separate institutions and convalescent hospitals from other placements. A further distinction can be seen between convalescent hospitals and institutions in that clients residing in convalescent hospitals seem least able to care for themselves and are more likely to be nonambulatory. These differences in ambulation are also reflected by the percentage of residents requiring the use of braces, walkers and wheelchairs in each placement.

A noteworthy difference among the community-based placements is the higher percentage of low functioning clients residing at home, compared with board and care homes and family care. In contrast to hospital settings, where nearly all residents perform at lower levels, a substantial number of clients living at home *are* able to care for their needs. In other words, abilities of clients observed in parental home settings range from very low to relatively high functioning.

Although the differences are not great, people living in board and care homes seem most capable of functioning both in and outside of normalized residential settings when compared with residents in the other placement alternatives. They are more capable of handling self-help behavior, responsibilities in the home, reading and simple number concepts, and finding their way around the neighborhood.

Differences in maladaptive behavior among settings are dramatic. Institutions care for a much larger proportion of residents with behavior problems than do any of the other placement alternatives. This dimension of behavior seems to be an important discriminator between those in institutions and convalescent hospitals, who otherwise function at similar levels. Moreover, there are no major differences between any of the community-based settings with regard to maladaptive behavior.

Most (85%) of clients in institutions and convalescent hospitals receive some kind of regular medication; the average use of medication in other placements is only 45%. The only notable age difference among settings is that clients living at home tend to be younger (average 17 years) than in other settings (average 25-35 years).

Average IQs reflect what has already been observed in the adaptive behavior scores, i.e., clients in institutions and convalescent hospitals tend to be more seriously handicapped. Although residents in board and care homes seem to function at a relatively high level as a group, the wider range of abilities seen among residents of these facilities is especially noteworthy.

In summary, it seems that mentally retarded people are currently being placed in accordance with their overall functioning levels. More specific information such as ambulation levels, use of medication and physical aids, and presence of behavior problems also contributes to the placement process. Hopefully, the data presented in this report can serve as a reference for policy making and for decisions affecting the placement of mentally retarded clients.

Reference

Nihira, K., Foster, R., Shellhaas, M., & Leland, H. *AAMD* Adaptive Behavior Scale. Washington, DC: American Association on Mental Deficiency, 1974.

Service Paths Prior to Clinic Use by Mentally Retarded People: A Retrospective Study

Louis Rowitz

Illinois Institute for Developmental Disabilities
and
University of Illinois School of Public Health

In the study of frequencies of use of community services by handicapped people it has been the custom to count all the individuals who use a community service during one period or at one point in time. The characteristics of these users are analyzed and presented as one indicator of the true prevalence of the handicap being studied. One very interesting variable that is often excluded in these studies is the referral source for the individual who is being counted as an agency consumer. The inclusion of this one variable allows for a beginning of the study of the referral process and with this information it is possible to track an individual from one service provider to another.

The above discussion is a rather simplified version of a quite intricate and complex process of service use. In effect, the continuum of care cycle, which is the dynamic representation of the referral process, is a series of service links from the first realization that help is needed for an individual through a number of contacts with several service providers who define, diagnose or label the problem and then determine some course of action for the possible amelioration of the problem (Rowitz, 1974b). If the process were a unidimensional one with a referral from service provider one to service provider two, it would be possible to study more easily the continuum of care cycle. However, the cycle is extremely complex and is multidimensional. The continuum of care cycle is sometimes discussed under the rubric of client-centered tracking systems.

There are three ways to undertake the study of the referral process (Rowitz, 1974a). A prospective study can be undertaken beginning at birth and carried through the life cycle of the mentally retarded individual. This type of study implies an early identification of mental retardation. This is not presently a realistic option. A second possibility relates to drawing a cohort of mentally retarded individuals in the service system at a particular point in time and following this cohort for several years. This option is possible but quite expensive and difficult to implement. A third type of study is a retrospective one which asks individuals to recall all the services they used prior to the use of the present service. The problem with this approach is that it relies heavily upon memory. Despite the limitations inherent in retrospective studies it is believed that this type of research will give some insights into the dynamic aspects of the referral process. Moreover, it will give information on the diversity of services that handicapped individuals use in the community. The present research was based on the retrospective analysis of all service contacts reported by the mothers of a large sample of retarded individuals prior to the use of a state operated outpatient clinic for retarded children. The intent was to look at the service paths that mentally retarded people might utilize when they remained in their home communities.

It is hoped that the study of the continuum of care cycle will begin to help us unravel some of the questions about whether shopping around or service hopping might involve duplication of effort. Other questions relate to whether it will become possible from this type of research to begin to reveal inadequacies either in the services provided or in the methods of referral. Moreover, it will be useful to begin to determine the factors which affect referral as well as gain information on the sources that the family uses to seek out specific types of services. Some beginning answers to these questions will be explored in this chapter and some issues that need to be studied in the future will be posed.

Some Definitions

Since this chapter will be using several concepts that may not be familiar to the reader, a series of definitions may help.

(1) *Referral*: The recommendation and/or transfer of an individual from one service provider (person or agency) to another.

(2) *Referral source*: An individual or agency that recommends the transfer of an individual from one service provider or agency to another.

(3) *Service contact*: The presentation of an individual to a service-providing agency that sets up a service record or adds to an existing service record within that agency. A service contact may be short term or long term.

(4) *Service path*: A unidimensional series of connected service links (referral from source one to source two in a direct, time related sequence). Each path may contain a number of service contacts.

(5) *Continuum of care cycle*: A longitudinal series of service contacts from initial contact for a specific problem or set of problems through a final disposition and/or resolution of these problems. For a given client, the cycle will contain multiple service paths. The data can also be aggregated for a sample of individuals to see how the process works at a community level.

(6) *Client-centered tracking system*: The data-related operationalization of the continuum of care cycle which centers on the needs of the service recipient within the service system. Intragency tracking relates to the elapsed time between initial referral to a treatment facility, first face-to-face contact with the service provider and the final disposition of the case as well as the number of contacts within the various components of the particular facility (Rowitz, Adams, & Barrett, 1974). Interagency tracking allows for a description of all contacts a client makes while in the community service system(s) from initial referral through the latest change in status.

(7) *Administrative prevalence*: A term used to refer to all the recipients of service within a given agency or series of agencies (service system) during one period or at one point of time. Referrals will only become part of the administrative prevalence figure if they are accepted for service by an agency or individual.

Review of Literature

Very little research has been done specifically on the referral process. The few studies that are available give some beginning insights into the study of the continuum of care cycle. Mercer (1973) studied the labeling process in the public schools by investigating the process of referral of students as they moved towards being labeled as mentally retarded persons. Eight stages were identified from initial enrollment in the public school system, through referral by teachers and principals for special evaluation and testing, then to the labeling process and finally the possible vacating of the status of retarded person when the individual leaves the school.

In a study of retarded children in Detroit, Jaslow and Stehman (1966) looked at the types of service advisors individuals saw by order of contact and by advice to make a commitment to a residential institution. The researchers found that those who were or were not committed tended to see a medical advisor early in the sequence of service use. In the committed group, almost nine out of ten families reported that their first contact was medical, but by the fifth contact, the majority were seeing non-medical sources. Only individual contacts were studied so an overall analysis of service paths was not possible.

Another approach to the study of service use that can have an impact on research on the referral process is the study of all reported services rendered to mentally retarded individuals in a specified geographic area. Rowitz, O'Connor and Boroskin (1975) reported on patterns of service use by severely and profoundly retarded individuals in a western state. Over 90% of the profoundly retarded persons in the service system were in public residential institutions. Forty-eight percent of severely retarded persons were living in their parental home, a relative's home or legal guardian's home, and another 35% were living in a state residential institution. Patients in institutions tended to get similar services regardless of social characteristics. As the service options in the community increased for severely retarded individuals, differences in types of services received were noted for different racial and ethnic groups. The above study is important in that it showed that different types of services were received by clients in different types of treatment settings. Access to the settings differed by type of retardation and other social characteristics of service users.

Since the present study takes place within the context of a state operated clinic for mentally retarded individuals, it is important to look at other research on the use of mental retardation clinics. The context of the clinic may be one of the important factors helping to explain the system of referrals over time which eventually leads to the use of a clinic. Specialty clinics tend to have a strong medical orientation. It appears that mental retardation clinics have this same bias (Grossman & Rowitz, 1973). There are three locations in which social epidemiological studies of clinics have taken place. These studies have also covered a wide time span.

Wortis and Wortis (1968) studied patients who were seen over a ten year period in a mental retardation specialty clinic at a Jewish hospital in Brooklyn. The authors found that a high proportion of the clinic patients were severely retarded. The clinic seemed to see very few mildly or moderately retarded patients and very few black patients in spite of the fact that the area surrounding the hospital mainly contained black families. It was found that the patients who were referred to the clinic were predominantly from middle income, skilled worker families. As was expected, Jewish children were overrepresented in the clinic population. Wortis and Wortis identified it as a middle class use pattern for the clinic located in a lower class area.

The second major clinic study took place in an outpatient clinic in a university hospital in the State of Washington (Justice, Campbell, O'Connor, & Sabotta, 1970). The study sample consisted of 282 children and their families who were seen in the clinic between 1961 and 1966. The racial distribution and the occupation of fathers of clinic cases were not significantly different from the general distribution of these racial and occupational groups in the population as a whole. An underrepresentation was found among widowed parents and there was a high percentage of married parents, which was not unexpected since the clinic sample tended to be young. There was an overrepresentation of clients from poorer families in the community. Whereas the Wortis and Wortis study found a middle class use pattern in the New York clinic, Justice and his colleagues found a lower class use pattern in the Washington study.

Finally, there are a number of reports in the literature based on a large state-operated outpatient clinic in Chicago, the setting of the present study. Rowitz (1973) studied all cases admitted to the Illinois State Pediatric Institute from the opening of the clinic in 1962 until 1970. During this period the clinic was the only state-operated clinic in the Chicago metropolitan area. Male admissions predominated in every admission year. In the early years there was a middle class utilization pattern with a significant increase in lower class admissions over the study period. Private medical referrals predominated during the early 1960's, whereas public medical referrals began to predominate during the late 1960's. Nonmedical referrals were not very prominent. In fact, some unpublished data from this study demonstrated that nonmedical referrals were less likely to follow through on their referrals to the clinic than referrals who had been sent to the clinic by some medical source. Rowitz concluded that clinic use patterns do not seem to remain stable over time. It is necessary to determine the environmental factors that affect the patterns of service use. For example, the study clinic was pressured to admit cases from an area adjacent to the clinic which was a lower class catchment area. This began to affect the use of the clinic by the late 1960's.

The data from Rowitz (1973) were submitted to a discriminant function analysis (Rowitz & Lei, 1975) comparing the demographic characteristics of city and suburban clinic users. Black admissions were overrepresented in the city relative to their proportion in the city as a whole and lower class individuals were also overrepresented in the clinic population. The suburban clinic use pattern differed from the city pattern in that suburban admissions tended to approximate the characteristics of suburbia as a whole. In the stepwise discriminant function analysis, race was found to be the best predictor. Employment and occupational status, type of family structure and certain medical referral agents also discriminated the city and suburban clients to varying degrees.

A follow-up study of the Illinois State Pediatric Institute was done for the period 1970-71. These data are discussed in some detail in the present research. Rowitz (1980) looked at the original identifiers of mental retardation in a clinic population of almost 500 people during one admission year. It was found that the great majority of these community clinic clients had been originally identified as being mentally retarded by a private physician or a public or private health related agency. Clients identified by private physicians were found on reevaluation to be more often less severely retarded than were the clients identified by public health related agencies. It was also found that nearly half of the admissions had been identified as mentally retarded prior to clinic admission. Thus, it appeared that users of a state clinic, which was generally perceived as a medical service resource, were clients who had been identified as mentally retarded by another medical service resource or physician.

The two sets of studies reported above—the referral studies and the clinic service use studies—give some evidence of the complexities involved in the study of the continuum of care cycle. Attempts to look at the dynamic aspect of referral were seen in the Mercer and the Jaslow studies. The Western State Study was an attempt to look at all services received by clients in one state as of a given date. The clinic studies showed that service population characteristics differ by location and by time periods. The present study looks at the service contact history of clinic clients. This research begins to integrate the concept of referral with a specific service type.

Study Population and Setting

All new clients accepted for admission between July 1, 1970 and June 30, 1971 (N = 498) to the Illinois State Pediatric Institute outpatient clinic in Chicago were included in the study population. An interview was completed with the parent of the child admitted (usually the mother or mother surrogate). In those few instances where an interview was not possible, an attempt was made to find as much out about the client as possible from the case record which included information on social background and former service contacts of the client. The interview took place on the first day of service and occurred before any service was rendered. In effect, the interview took the place of the intake interview.

The interview which took an average of forty-five minutes was quite extensive. It included general questions on the social background of clients as well as detailed information on the referral and medical history of the new case. Each respondent was asked to answer the following question: "From the time when you felt there might be something wrong with your child, where did you go for help?"

Sixty-two percent of the clients were male. In terms of age at time of admission, 36% were between 0 to 4 years of age; 30% between 5 to 9; 20% between 10-14; and the remainder (14%) were over 15 years of age. Relative to the age percentages previously reported by Rowitz (1973), there was an increase in the percentage of older clients (10-14 years). Sixty percent of the study population lived in Chicago. Sixty percent were white, 30% were black, and 6% were Hispanic. It was found that the percentage of clients by race and place of residence was stable during the study year in comparison to the changes noted by Rowitz in previous years. Relative to income, 33% of the sample had incomes between $5000 to $9000, 21%, less than $5000, and 24%, over $10,000. Some of the sample (22%) were not willing to report income. On the whole, there was evidence of increasing usage of the clinic by people from lower socioeconomic levels in comparison to previous years. Relative to service history, clients identified as mentally retarded by physicians had more service contacts between identification and the use of the study clinic than any other previously labeled clients. Individuals identified as mentally retarded by public or private health and mental health related agencies and by social agencies received fewer services prior to state clinic use than physician identified clients, but slightly more services than school identified clients.

The Illinois State Pediatric Institute is a State of Illinois, Department of Mental Health and Developmental Disabilities facility, located west of the downtown section of Chicago. The clinic's name was changed to the Illinois Institute for Developmental Disabilities in 1974. Its outpatient service was one of the few existing state operated service and evaluation centers for mentally retarded persons in the northeastern counties of the state. The mandate of the Institute was to serve mentally retarded individuals from birth to age 21. Occasionally people were admitted who were over 21 years of age. Those requesting service and living in the Chicago metropolitan area were admitted on a "no decline" basis.

Methodology

Except for a review of a selection of sample cases, the present study relates primarily to the study of the first three service paths used by a population of clinic users rather than individual service contacts. A given service path may involve only one service contact or it may contain several contacts. A number of assumptions were made about service paths in order to expedite the present analysis. First, contacts between agencies (interagency tracking) were stressed rather than contacts or services received within agencies (intragency tracking). Second, a service path was defined as a continuous series of service contacts with a referral from one source to the next source in the chain (''Continuous Path,'' Figure 1). Time as a variable was included only as a method for determining order of service contacts and not the amount of time spent in a given service agency. Every time that a parent or parent surrogate initiated a new contact without a designated prior referral, a new path was started. Third, if one agency referred an individual to several different agencies, each referral became the beginning of a new service path (''Branching Paths,'' Figure 1). Fourth, it was possible for a client to be in more than one service path at any given time (''Overlapping Paths,'' Figure 1). A path terminates when no more service is delivered by service providers within that path. Specifics related to service termination were not investigated in the present study.

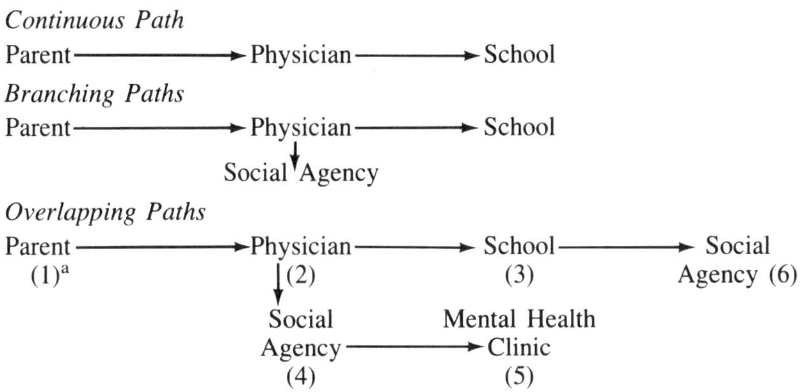

[a]Numbers refer to the time sequence of services in the path

Figure 1. An example of possible service paths.

Since some clients had as many as nine service paths, it was decided to limit the present analysis, except for some case history analysis, to the first three service paths because it became necessary to recode the data after the analysis of each individual path. Moreover, 86% of the clients in the study population had three service paths or fewer prior to the use of a state operated outpatient clinic.

Another major problem related to the classification of service paths. Service paths were classified according to the types of contacts in each path. The original breakdown showed 74 different types of service paths. The 74 paths were collapsed into 6 summary groups in order to make the cells of the tables large enough to allow for statistical analysis: (1) physician, (2) public health and mental retardation related agencies, (3) private health and mental retardation related agencies, (4) all nonmedical service providers (social, educational, etc.), (5) medical combinations (physician, public and private health related combinations), and (6) medical-nonmedical combinations. Where clarification of the findings was necessary, the original data on the 74 groups were investigated to find the source of some of the differences found in the 6 summary classification groups.

Case History Analysis

Since the aggregation and summary of information of 498 people will lose some of the dynamic aspects of the use of services by the study clients, a few examples of the continuum of care cycle in action will be presented. First, 30 percent of the sample had only one service path. An example to show this related to a set of twins from an Hispanic background. Both twins had one service path which was continuous.

Path 1 Parent → School → Study Clinic

This would be an example of the simplest form of service path. To categorize the path, it was labeled a medical-nonmedical service path.

A number of cases had a series of continuous service paths with no apparent connections between the paths. An example case related to a six year-old Puerto Rican child. She was not in school at the time of the study and she did not speak English. The mother and father were separated. Two other children were in the household. The client was diagnosed as profoundly retarded by the study clinic. This client had four different service paths. Path 1 occurred in Puerto Rico; Path 2 in New York; and the final two paths in the study city. Three paths duplicated each other.

Path 1 Parent → Public Health Related Agency (Public Health)
Path 2 Parent → Public Health
Path 3 Parent → Public Health
Path 4 Parent → School → Study Clinic

Path 1 occurred in Puerto Rico when the subject was three. The mother reported that she went to the hospital because her child was having seizures. The hospital told the mother that there was nothing wrong with the child. Two years later, the mother took the child to a hospital in New York for the child's seizures (Path 2). The mother was told the child had epilepsy. A third parent-public health contact was initiated by the child's parents in the study city. Finally, when the child reached six, the mother tried to enter her into school. The school referred the child to the study clinic for evaluation (Path 4) where the child was diagnosed as profoundly retarded and epileptic. In summary, the first three paths were categorized as public health paths and path four was called a medical-nonmedical service path.

The next case related to a branching path example. This client was a five year old male at the time of admission to the study clinic and he showed no evidence of speech. His mother had never been married to the child's father. However, she was married to her third husband at the time of admission. When the client was four, the mother took the child to a private children's hospital at the advice of a friend. The hospital told the mother her son was severely retarded. She was referred to a public health related agency (city health agency). The mother reported that she received no information from this referral. The children's hospital then referred the mother and child to the study clinic (Path 2). Graphically, this branching path would look as follows.

Path 1 Parent (1) → Friend → Private Hospital (3) → Public Health Clinic (4)

Path 2 Private Hospital (3) ↓ Study Clinic (5)

Both paths are medical combination paths.

Overlapping paths are much more difficult to show graphically since the time sequence becomes more critical. Within the following example, service had been received by the client in two service paths concurrently. The case that demonstrates these overlapping paths was that of a thirty-one year old woman. With much documentation, seven service paths were identified. Dates are included for better historical reference.

Path 1	Parent →	Public Health Hospital (1943)		
Path 2	Parent →	Private Clinic (1950)		
Path 3	Parent →	Physician (1955) →	Psychiatrist (1955) →	Psychologist (1955)
			↓	
Path 4			Public Mental Hospital (1956)	
Path 5	Friend →	Private Sanitarium I (1957)		
	↓			
Path 6	Private Sanitarium II (1959)			
Path 7	Parent →	Public Mental Hospital (1970) →	Public Mental Retardation Hospital (1970) →	Study Clinic

This woman had been institutionalized several times. During her younger years she attended public as well as private schools. She graduated from elementary school and also went to high school for a time. Relative to her service history, there is evidence that she received many different diagnoses over the years. For Path 1, she went to a public university hospital because of slow speech development. The parents were told that nothing was wrong and no disposition was made. Path 2 occurred seven years later, according to the mother, when the client was ten. She was taken to a private clinic to determine the reason for slowness in speech. The parents were told the client was "slow." Five years later, the client's family doctor noted that the client was "imagining things." She was referred to a psychiatrist who said that the client had psychiatric problems. He referred the client to a psychologist for testing, then she went back to the psychiatrist. A year later the psychiatrist referred the client to a state mental hospital (Path 4). She stayed in the hospital and was eventually discharged. Over the next few years, she was placed in two private psychiatric hospitals. Path 7 related to a number of service contacts the client had in the several months prior to admission to the study clinic for evaluation. The client had been placed in a public mental hospital where it was decided that the client was actually mentally retarded. She was transferred to a public mental retardation facility. This latter facility referred her to the study clinic for evaluation of her retardation. At this time she was still a resident of the public institution. After evaluation at the clinic, a further placement was being contemplated in a private residential facility for retarded women. This case was extremely complex showing branching as well as overlapping service paths. There was further information in the study interview to show that the parents shopped around for appropriate services for their daughter.

Each case presented unique possibilities for a service path analysis. A summary look at the service history of a given client can help both in the planning of more efficient delivery of services as well as better coordination of services on a case by case level. The more information that can be collected on the operation of the continuum of care cycle, the easier it will be to understand the dynamics of service delivery in the community. Whereas the present analysis has been centered on the provision of direct services to mentally retarded individuals, the eventual inclusion of all sorts of indirect services and changing residential alternatives will complicate the service path analysis path but should give much greater information to the administrator, clinician and researcher on the dynamics of community living for the mentally retarded individual.

Analysis of Service Paths

As mentioned earlier, clients in the study (N = 498) had as few as one path in some instances and in one case as many as nine paths. Number of contacts within a service path also varied greatly. It was necessary to summarize all contacts in a service path into a general path classification. Table 1 presents data on the social characteristics of clinic users at the time of admission to the study institution by type of service path that was used by clients when problems were first perceived. In general, there was a greater percentage of males than females in each service path classification. The smallest percentage of females (17.2%) was seen in the mixed medical-nonmedical service category. Clients who used a straight physician service path were younger on the average when they came to the study clinic than clients who began service with any other providers. Of clients who used private health related paths, a greater percentage of individuals were under five years of age (41.1%) in comparison with clients who used public health related services (24.7%). Those clients who used a private and public medical path combination (medical combination) were younger (33.8% under five) than clients who used a medical-nonmedical path combination (23.4% under five). Older outpatient clients tended to use nonmedical services first.

Overall data showed that 49% of whites used physicians or private health services on their first service path compared with 26% of the blacks. Blacks tended to predominate in the use of public health related services whereas whites tended to predominate in the use of private physicians and private health related services. Whites and blacks tended to use nonmedical services in similar proportions. Hispanic clients tended to use nonmedical services to a greater extent than any other service combination.

The analysis of level of mental retardation was confounded by a number of factors. The level of mental retardation reported in Table 1 was the level determined by the Illinois State Pediatric Institute rather than the service contacts in Path 1. However, some interesting findings should be noted. Higher functioning clients and clients with questionable etiology predominated among physician path users and nonmedical path users. There were greater percentages of moderately, severely, and profoundly retarded individuals in public health, private health and medical combination service paths than in physician or nonmedical service paths.

The last category of Table 1 refers to the occupation of the client's father relative to type of first service path. Among physician path users there was a large

Table 1

Social Characteristics of Clinic Users by First Service Path (N = 498)[a]

	First Service Path Classification											
	Physician		Public Health		Private Health		Non-Medical		Medical Combinations		Medical-Non-Medicals	
	N	%	N	%	N	%	N	%	N	%	N	%
TOTAL	133	100.0	81	100.0	58	100.0	66	100.0	74	100.0	64	100.0
SEX												
Male	79	59.4	50	61.7	36	62.1	39	59.1	37	50.0	53	82.8
Female	54	40.6	31	38.3	22	37.9	27	40.9	37	50.0	11	17.2
AGE IN YRS.												
0-4	78	58.6	20	24.7	24	41.4	9	13.6	25	33.8	15	23.4
5-9	25	18.8	28	34.6	13	22.4	23	34.8	22	29.7	28	43.8
10-14	18	13.5	15	18.5	12	20.7	17	25.8	21	28.4	14	21.9
15-19	8	6.0	8	9.9	4	6.9	13	19.7	2	2.7	5	7.8
20+	4	3.0	9	11.1	5	8.6	2	3.0	4	5.4	2	3.1
RACE												
White	112	84.2	30	37.0	29	50.0	27	40.9	51	68.9	40	62.5
Black	16	12.0	43	53.1	21	36.2	27	40.9	17	23.0	18	28.1
Hispanic	5	3.8	5	6.2	5	8.6	7	10.6	3	4.1	1	1.6
M.R. LEVEL												
Border.	13	9.8	13	16.0	4	6.9	12	18.2	5	6.8	13	20.3
Mild	29	21.8	11	13.6	11	19.0	21	31.8	11	14.9	16	25.0
Moderate	29	21.8	19	23.5	10	17.2	9	13.6	14	18.6	8	12.5
Severe	17	12.8	9	11.1	9	15.5	8	12.1	16	21.6	3	4.7
Profound	13	9.8	17	21.0	16	27.6	3	4.5	15	20.3	9	14.1
Normal	18	13.5	10	12.3	0	0.0	9	13.6	10	13.5	13	20.3
FATHER'S OCC.												
Profess.	13	9.8	0	0.0	7	12.1	4	6.1	4	5.4	6	9.4
Manager	19	14.3	2	2.5	3	5.2	3	4.5	5	6.8	5	7.8
Clerical	12	9.0	4	4.9	4	6.9	3	4.5	10	13.5	3	4.7
Craftsman	31	23.3	9	11.1	7	12.1	12	18.2	6	8.1	9	14.1
Operative	19	14.3	12	14.8	7	12.1	5	7.6	9	12.2	7	10.9
Priv.Hhd.	6	4.5	6	7.4	6	10.3	6	9.1	11	14.9	3	4.7
Laborers	6	4.5	9	11.1	3	5.2	11	16.7	10	13.5	7	10.9
No Father Present	27	20.3	38	46.9	20	34.5	21	31.8	17	23.0	23	35.9

[a]Missing data prevented the including of 22 respondents in this table

percentage of clients whose fathers were craftsmen or foremen (23.3%) in addition to clients whose fathers were professionals, managers or clerical workers (33.1%). A large percentage of users of public health services (46.9%) came from households without fathers present at the time of admission to the study clinic. A large percentage of users of nonmedical services (31.8%) also showed no father present in the household at the time of the study. It was impossible to determine occupation of father at the time of the use of services during the first path.

Table 2 shows the distribution of the second service path matched against the first service path. Seventy percent of the respondents (N = 349) had at least two reported service paths. Clients with only one path were not included in Table 2. Of those clients with a physician first path, the majority had a physician second path

Table 2

Service Path 1 by Service Path 2 (N = 349)[a]

Service Path	Path 2 Classification: Total		Physician		Public Health		Private Health		Non-Medical		Medical Comb.		Medical-Non Med.	
	N	%	N	%	N	%	N	%	N	%	N	%	N	%
Physician	109	100.0	30	27.5	10	9.2	10	9.2	29	26.6	16	14.7	14	12.8
Public Hlth.	60	100.0	5	8.3	13	21.7	11	18.3	18	30.0	7	11.7	6	10.0
Private Hlth.	54	100.0	7	13.0	21	38.9	10	18.5	7	13.0	4	7.4	5	9.3
Non Medical	28	100.0	1	3.6	6	21.4	5	17.9	7	25.0	3	10.7	6	21.4
Medical Comb.	54	100.0	5	9.3	18	33.3	2	3.7	14	25.9	7	13.0	8	14.8
Med. Non-Med.	44	100.0	7	15.9	5	11.4	2	4.5	19	43.2	1	2.3	10	22.7

[a]127 Cases had only 1 path

(27.5%) or a nonmedical second path (26.6%). Of those with a public health first path, most had either a nonmedical (30.0%) or public health (21.7%) second path. Private health clients tended to use public health services (38.9%) on the second path. Nonmedical Path 1 clients tended to use nonmedical services (25.0%) or public health services (21.4%) on Path 2. One interesting finding for all groups was the large proportion of clients (26.9%) who used only nonmedical services on the second path.

In Table 3, service Paths 1 and 2 are combined into 6 summary groups. The social characteristics of clients at the time of admission to the study institution can then be seen on the basis of this new combination. Males tended to predominate in all service path combinations. Of those clients with two service paths those for whom both were physician paths (60.0%) or both were private health related service paths (58.8%) showed a large percentage of clients under five years of age. As shown in Table 3 all clients with two nonmedical service paths were from age 5 through 14 at the time of the study. Except for a lack of clients in the late adolescent years, public health service users tended to be represented in all other reported age groups. Clients with mixed medical combination service paths tended to fall primarily in the age groups under fifteen (81.9%) at the time of the study. Whites predominated in all paths except the public health path (38.5%). With regard to mental retardation level as diagnosed by the study clinic, those clients with two physician paths showed a large percentage of moderately retarded clients (36.7%) or clients later judged to be normal (20.0%). Public health clients tended to be classified mildly (30.8%), moderately (30.8%) or profoundly retarded (30.8%) at the time of the study. In the private health sector, clients tended to be either mildly (29.4%) or profoundly retarded (29.4%). Nonmedical path users were found on the average at the mild or moderate levels of mental retardation (85.8%) with the remainder normal. Medical combination path users tended to show more moderately, severely and profoundly retarded clients (65.5%).

With regard to reported occupation of father, physician path clients tended to be from managerial (30.0%) or craftsmen (20.0%) families. With regard to all other path combinations except private health, there was a large percentage of clients without a father present at the time of the study.

The final table looks at Paths 1 and 2 combined and compared with service Path 3. At this point only 190 (38.2%) of the cases had 3 paths prior to admission to the study clinic. Of those clients with a physician first and second path, 38.9% had a physician third path and another 22.2% had a nonmedical third path. Of those with a public health first and second path, 55.6% had a public health third path. Those outpatient clients with a private health first and second path had primarily a public health (40.0%) or a physician (26.7%) third path. Those with a mixed medical first and second path showed primarily a nonmedical third path (34.6%) or a public health third path (20.5%). Detailed demographic comparisons of the three combined path classifications are not shown since the cell frequencies were too small.

Table 3

Social Characteristics of Clinic Users by First and Second Service Path Combined (N = 498)[a]

	Path 1 and 2 Combined Classification													
	Physician		Public Health		Private Health		Non-Medical		Medical Cimbin.		Medical Non-Med.		No* Second Path	
	N	%	N	%	N	%	N	%	N	%	N	%	N	%
TOTAL	30	100.0	13	100.0	17	100.0	7	100.0	116	100.0	166	100.0	149	100.0
SEX														
Male	18	60.0	9	69.2	12	70.6	4	57.1	60	51.7	110	66.3	98	65.8
Female	12	40.0	4	30.8	5	29.4	3	42.9	56	48.3	56	33.7	51	34.2
AGE IN YRS.														
0-4	18	60.0	4	30.8	10	58.8	0	0.0	45	38.8	43	25.9	58	38.9
5-9	7	23.3	4	30.8	2	11.8	3	42.9	22	19.0	60	36.1	49	32.9
10-14	4	13.3	3	23.1	2	11.8	4	57.1	28	24.1	37	22.3	23	15.4
15-19	1	3.3	0.	0.0	1	5.9	0	0.0	13	11.2	16	9.6	11	4.0
20+	0	0.0	2	15.4	2	11.8	0	0.0	8	6.9	9	5.4	6	4.0
RACE														
White	28	93.3	5	38.4	13	76.5	4	57.1	66	56.9	101	60.8	83	55.7
Black	2	6.7	6	46.2	3	17.6	1	14.3	42	36.2	51	30.7	43	28.9
Hispanic	0	0.0	2	15.4	1	5.9	2	28.6	5	4.3	6	3.6	12	8.1
M.R. LEVEL														
Border.	1	3.3	0	0.0	0	0.0	1	14.3	10	8.6	24	14.5	26	17.4
Mild	4	13.3	4	30.8	5	29.4	2	28.6	13	11.2	45	27.1	29	19.5
Moderate	11	36.7	4	30.8	0	0.0	3	42.9	28	24.1	25	15.1	23	15.4
Severe	3	10.0	1	7.7	2	11.8	0	0.0	19	16.4	28	16.9	9	6.0
Profound	1	3.3	4	30.8	5	29.4	0	0.0	29	25.0	19	11.4	16	10.7
Normal	6	20.0	0	0.0	0	0.0	1	14.3	15	12.9	14	8.4	20	20.1
FATHER'S OCC.														
Profess.	2	6.7	0	0.0	5	29.4	1	14.3	6	5.2	12	7.2	10	6.7
Manager	9	30.0	1	7.7	0	0.0	1	14.3	6	5.2	14	8.4	8	5.4
Clerical	4	13.3	0	0.0	2	11.8	0	0.0	8	6.9	11	6.6	12	8.1
Craftsman	6	20.0	0	0.0	1	5.9	3	42.9	16	13.8	26	15.7	27	18.1
Operative	3	10.0	0	0.0	3	17.6	0	0.0	21	18.1	21	12.7	11	7.4
Priv. Hhd.	2	6.7	2	15.4	3	17.6	0	0.0	9	7.8	11	6.6	13	8.7
Laborers	2	6.7	3	23.1	1	5.9	0	0.0	9	7.8	13	7.8	20	13.4
No Father Present	2	6.7	6	46.2	2	11.8	2	28.6	40	34.5	55	33.1	43	28.9

[a]22 had no service path information

Table 4

Service Path 1 and 2 Combined by Service Path 3 (N = 190)[a]

Service Path 1 and 2 Combined	Path 3 Classification													
	Total		Public Physician		Private Health		Non-Health		Medical Medical		Medical Comb.		Non. Med.	
	N	%	N	%	N	%	N	%	N	%	N	%	N	%
Physician	18	100.0	7	38.9	2	11.1	0	0.0	4	22.2	1	5.6	4	22.2
Public Hlth.	9	100.0	1	11.1	5	55.6	1	11.1	0	0.0	0	0.0	2	22.2
Private Hlth.	15	100.0	4	26.7	6	40.0	2	13.3	1	6.7	2	13.3	0	0.0
Non Medical	1	100.0	0	0.0	1	100.0	0	0.0	0	0.0	0	0.0	0	0.0
Medical Comb.	78	100.0	4	5.1	16	20.5	12	15.4	27	34.6	7	9.0	11	14.1
Med. Non-Med.	69	100.0	7	10.1	8	11.6	4	5.8	29	42.0	5	7.2	16	23.2

[a]286 Cases had only 2 paths

Conclusions

It was this purpose of this paper to look at a population of mentally retarded individuals who are using a specified type of community service—a community mental retardation clinic. Rather than focusing on the services received in the clinic, the present study retrospectively asked questions regarding how the client and his parent reached this specialty clinic. With deinstitutionalization and the attempt to prevent institutionalization in the first place, it becomes important to investigate how clients move through the various service delivery systems that have developed to serve mentally retarded individuals.

The concept of "continuum of care" has been used to refer to the use of services by a client over time. From the vantage point of various reporting agencies, this same process has been called "client-centered tracking." Tracking may be of two general types. Intragency tracking relates to the elapsed time between initial referral to a treatment facility, first face-to-face contact with the service provider and final disposition of the case as well as the number of contacts within the various service components of the particular facility (Rowitz, Adams, & Barrett, 1974). Measures of quality of care can be built into the intramural tracking system. Rather than concentrating on the intramural tracking side, the present study began the complex study of the interagency tracking problem. Interagency tracking allowed for a description of all contacts a client made while in the community service system(s) from initial referral through the latest change in status. In addition to plotting service contacts, this tracking approach should include elapsed time between services and the particular type of service rendered in the various facilities in order to check on a client's progress over time. Different criteria for evaluation and accountability may need to be determined for residential as contrasted with nonresidential services.

The present study did an interagency tracking analysis in a retrospective manner. A retrospective analysis has many difficulties in that the approach has to rely on the memory of the respondents. Checks were possible in the present study. Since the clients were generally relatively young, backup information to support the client's reports was included in the case records. Ideally, future studies using this approach should try to do the study prospectively.

How an individual enters the service system initially appears to have an impact on the entire continuum of care cycle. The great preponderance of clients in this study entered the service system with a medical contact and, in fact, were first identified as mentally retarded by a medical service contact. In general, contacts with nonmedical services for this clinic population tended to come later than the first path for most clients. It also became clear that service use is not continuous and is made up of a number of starts and stops. Moreover, the social and professional characteristics of the service providers probably also affected the cycle of service use for individual clients.

A number of impressions of how the continuum of care cycle works can be gleaned from the present study. Evidence of "shopping around" or "service hopping" was apparent in many cases. When parents were unhappy with the diagnosis given or the prognosis given for their child's problems, they tended to go elsewhere. Much service duplication was noted. Repetition of tests and diagnostic procedures was apparent even among many of the younger clients. Each service provider had its own favorite battery of tests and tended to use them regardless of whether the tests had been performed earlier. A criticism of duplication of service needs to be tempered by evidence of some error in the diagnosis of a child's problems by community service providers.

Many parents reported going for specialized services to a community agency and having been referred elsewhere for that service. A number of agencies could not afford to provide a comprehensive array of services and made referrals to agencies or individuals which could provide the needed service. It was also clear from reports of parents that some service providers did not know where to send the individual for specialized service. Clients and their parents relied on professionals to have knowledge of these services. When this knowledge was not available, some people kept hunting until they found the necessary service or relied on friends to tell them what to do or where to go. Many private family physicians were aware of some medical specialty service to which to refer an individual but were not aware of a number of possible nonmedical service providers which could provide the needed service. It is important to note that once an individual enters a service system defined as medical, there is a strong tendency to continue to use that system for service for specific problems regardless of whether or not the problem is medical in origin.

The present study, limited to interagency service paths, could not explore all aspects of the problem. In order more fully to understand the grief people with a retarded child experience in seeking help, the expensive duplication of clinic effort, and the increasing complexity of service delivery networks, many more questions need study. First, the information sources that the individual uses to determine how and why to enter the service delivery system need to be explored. If a parent is the initiator of a service path, information on the mechanics behind the use of specific service agencies needs determination. For example, health insurance may play an important role for the individual in the decision to use a medical resource rather than a nonmedical resource for specific problems such as mental retardation. Perhaps pressure from outsiders such as a school may also precipitate the use of a service. However, this external pressure may or may not be mentioned when a service contact is made.

A second issue is specific to intragency tracking. This study did not look at this issue at all. However, this is a very important part of the study of the continuum of care. In addition, services within agencies are affected by agency service priorities, existing treatment programs, external funding and treatment outcomes. The temporal aspect also needs to be considered. For example, a mother with other young children may not accept an appointment at an hour when her other children may be coming home from school.

Relative to interagency tracking, the same issues as discussed above are important. In addition, issues of location and transportation may affect the use of services. Cost is also critical. In a large urban area, the proliferation of services needs to be studied. A given agency may make referrals to agencies within a specific geographic subdivision of the city. Suburbanites may have to come to the city for service when specialized services do not exist in their home communities. The mechanics of movement through a complex service system need to be explored. This may mean that the system will also have to be studied in order to better understand the service paths possible within it.

In the present study, it was not possible to explore the issue of short versus long term service. The question of multiple service contacts and the use of several different services in a limited time period needs to be explored in more detail. The use of services as affected by the acceptance of diagnosis by the parent or client needs exploration. Finally, the effect of age and life cycle phase as a factor in service delivery needs extensive study. As more and more mentally retarded individuals spend their lives in their home communities, it will be necessary to investigate the changing needs for service as people get older.

In conclusion, this chapter has begun to unravel some of the mystery of how people use services in the community. It has concentrated on the cases admitted to one type of facility. Further research will have to expand the context of the present study to gain more information on the elements involved in the process of referral and the continuum of care cycle.

References

Grossman, H. J., & Rowitz, L. A community approach to services for the retarded. In R. K. Eyman, C. E. Meyers, & G. Tarjan (Eds.), *Sociobehavioral studies in mental retardation*. Washington, DC: American Association on Mental Deficiency, 1973.

Jaslow, R. I., & Stehman, V. A. *The decision to commit: A study of Detroit's retarded children*. Lansing, MI: Michigan Department of Mental Health, 1966.

Justice, R. S., Campbell, M. M., O'Connor, G., & Sabotta, E. A look at the population served by a university clinic for retarded children. *Mental Retardation*, 1970, *78*(3), 43-46.

Mercer, J. R. *Labeling the mentally retarded*. Berkeley, CA: University of California Press, 1973.

Rowitz, L. Changing perspectives in social epidemiological research. *Mental Retardation*, 1974, *12*, 3, 21-23. (a)

Rowitz, L. Social factors in mental retardation. *Social Science and Medicine*, 1974, *8*, 405-412. (b)

Rowitz, L. A socioepidemiological analysis of admissions to a state operated outpatient clinic for retarded children. *American Journal of Mental Deficiency*, 1975, *80*, 165-171.

Rowitz, L. Original identifiers of mental retardation in a clinic population. *American Journal of Mental Retardation*, 1980, *85*, 82-86.

Rowitz, L., Adams, J., & Barrett, T. An approach to the evaluation of clinical services. *Mental Retardation*, 1974, *12* (4), 6-9.

Rowitz, L., & Lei, T. Differentials in characteristics between city and suburban admissions to a state clinic for retarded children. *American Journal of Mental Deficiency*, 1975, *80*, 165-171.

Rowitz, L., O'Connor, G., & Boroskin, A. Patterns of service use by the severely and profoundly retarded individuals: A preliminary analysis. In C. C. Cleland & L. W. Talkington (Eds.), *Research with profoundly retarded*. Austin, TX: Western Research Conference and the Brown Schools, 1975.

Deinstitutionalization: Phase II

Tadashi Mayeda
Patricia Sutter

University of California, Los Angeles
Neuropsychiatric Institute Research Group
at Lanterman State Hospital and Developmental Center
Pomona, California

For nearly 15 years the predominant social policy in mental retardation has been to deinstitutionalize mentally retarded persons as a means of providing a more normalized and more normalizing environment. According to Scheerenberger (1976, this volume), deinstitutionalization is being implemented and institutional populations are decreasing. From the viewpoint of increased numbers of mentally retarded persons now residing in community settings rather than in institutions, deinstitutionalization can be considered to be succeeding.

The deinstitutionalization process, however, has been implemented in the absence of systematic empirical documentation of its effectiveness. For example, only partial information is available on the programmatic qualities of community-based residential care settings and knowledge of the availability, utilization, and effectiveness of other community services also is incomplete.

Research evidence suggests, however, that the needs of some community placed clients have not been met. Edgerton (1967, 1975, this volume) has described the difficulties encountered by mildly retarded persons residing in the community.

Client failure in community placement, as defined by return to the institution, also has been a topic of concern for many years. In 1919 Fernald calculated the failure rate for community residential placement to be 36.1% (cf. Lakin, Bruininks & Sigford, this volume). More recently, Eagle (1967) estimated the failure rate for community residential placement at 39.5% and further indicated that during the immediately preceding five years the rate of residential placement failure had increased to 52%. These data suggest that successful deinstitutionalization is becoming more difficult and that an examination of contributing factors is in order.

The purpose of this paper is to consider some of these factors as they apply to deinstitutionalization processes that rely for their success on the provision of generic community services. While some deinstitutionalization efforts have involved the creation of a comprehensive network of services in the community to accommodate deinstitutionalized clients, it is more commonly the case that once placed in the community clients must rely on services provided by the existing community service network. It is from within this type of deinstitutionalization system that community placement success or failure must be judged.

This study was supported by OHD-DHEW Developmental Disabilities Grant Number 54-P-71117/9.

The authors wish to express appreciation to Robert Newton for assistance in data summarization and analysis.

A consideration of deinstitutionalization as it has proceeded in one such large system, the State of Hawaii, may serve to illustrate some of the difficulties inherent in the process. As one of the early proponents of deinstitutionalization, Hawaii has sought to implement a deinstitutionalization policy since the 1960's. The experiences of this state may well be representative of other states where deinstitutionalization has long been a goal, and also may be predictive of the difficulties and barriers to be faced by states now in the early phases of deinstitutionalization.

Deinstitutionalization in Hawaii has followed a pattern proceeding from the placement of relatively self-sufficient and problem-free clients to clients who function less well. Yanagi (1979) states that, in spite of active placement efforts, the client population of Hawaii's state institution for the mentally retarded is now being reduced at a slower rate than in previous years because of difficulty in finding community placements for lower functioning clients. In addition, a greater number of recently placed clients are proving to be unsuccessful in community care, and as a result, readmissions have increased each year for the past several years.

Hawaii community placement and readmission data are presented in Figure 1. As can be seen, during the mid-1970's the number of clients placed in the community was substantially greater than the number of clients readmitted to the institution. By 1978, however, client placements and client readmissions were nearly equal in number and in 1979 readmissions exceeded placements.

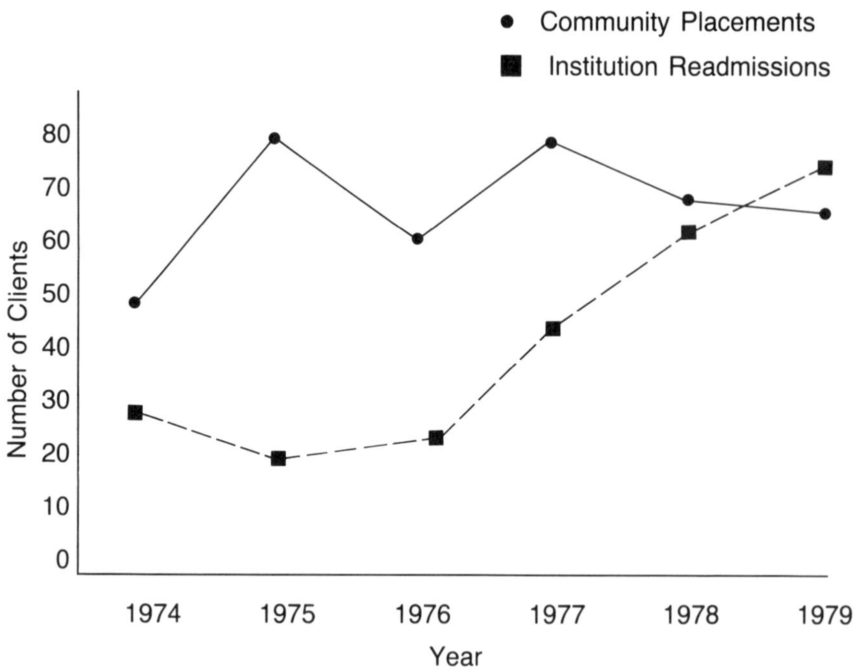

Adapted from Yanagi, 1979

Figure 1. Total number of community placements and readmissions for clients being deinstitutionalized from Waimano Training School and Hospital, Pearl City, Hawaii. (Adapted from "Why We Need Waimano" by G. Yanagi, *Hawaii Health Messenger,* 1979, *42*(3).

A systematic effort has been put forth to determine the reasons for client failure in community placement and return to the institution. The results of several studies indicate that reasons for return are related to the characteristics of the clients themselves. Client maladaptive behavior and health problems account for almost all returns, with behavior problems being by far the most frequently cited reason for readmission to the institution.

Clients who failed in community care and were returned to the institution were found to manifest significantly higher frequencies of behavior problems of an acting-out nature (e.g., aggression, property destruction) than clients who were successful in community placement (Sutter, Mayeda, Yanagi & Yee, 1980). These data are consistent with other studies that have found behavior problems to be a major factor in placement failure (Bishop, 1957; Brown, Windle & Stewart, 1959; Keys, Boroskin & Ross, 1973; Pagel & Whitling, 1978; Windle, 1962).

Placement failure also was found to be related to the compatability of careproviders and clients in terms of the match between the expressed preferences of careproviders in managing clients with behavior problems and the actual behavior problems exhibited by clients in their care. Unsuccessful careprovider/client pairs were found to have been significantly more mismatched for maladaptive behaviors than were successful careprovider/client pairs (Sutter, Mayeda, Yee & Yanagi, 1980).

The recent increase in readmissions to the state institution in Hawaii and the results of inquiries into reasons for return raise a question as to the characteristics of the institutionalized clients now available for placement. These clients may differ substantially from those who have previously been deinstitutionalized and from community-based clients. The purpose of the present study was to compare the characteristics of clients now considered to be candidates for community placement with the characteristics of clients already in community care. Significant differences in the characteristics of these two groups would indicate a difference in client needs that must be met by the community services if community placement is to be successful.

Method

The client samples consisted of 446 mentally retarded, community-based clients and 162 mentally retarded, institutionalized clients who had been identified as potential candidates for community placement. All clients were 18 years of age or older at the time of the study.

The Community Client Group (N=446) consisted of all Hawaiian clients residing in state-licensed, community residential facilities. The majority of these clients resided in small community homes licensed to provide residential services to a maximum of five mentally retarded, mentally ill, or geriatric clients. Small community homes generally are owned by the careprovider who manages them. The remainder of the clients resided in larger residential facilities which often are not operated by the owners.

The Placeable Client Group (N=162) consisted of institutionalized clients who had been identified as potentially placeable based on an assessment of their current level of functioning and physical health status. Client level of functioning was assessed using the Behavior Development Survey (BDS), a five-factor modified version of the AAMD Adaptive Behavior Scale (Nihira, Foster, Shellhaas & Leland, 1974). Clients were first selected based on relatively low frequencies of maladaptive behavior and an absence of serious health problems. This client group was then reviewed for placement potential by institution direct-care staff familiar with the clients. The final sample consisted of the 162 clients who were deemed placeable by virtue of both their BDS scores and the clinical judgement of staff.

The Community Client Group and the Placeable Client Group were compared on demographic variables such as age, sex, and level of retardation, and on level of adaptive behavior as measured by the BDS. The first three factors of the BDS, Domains I-III, measure adaptive behavior skills in three distinct areas of development, personal self-sufficiency, community self-sufficiency, and personal/social responsibility. The last two factors, Domains IV and V, measure maladaptive behavior directed toward others and toward self, respectively.

Results

Table 1 presents a comparison of the demographic characteristics of the clients in both groups. As can be seen, the institution clients considered to be good placement candidates were primarily male, tended to be younger, and were more severely retarded than the clients already residing in the community. Mann-Whitney U tests for differences between the two groups in age, sex, and level of retardation all were significant ($p < .0001$).

Table 1

Demographic Characteristics of Institutionalized Placeable Clients and Community Based Clients in Percent*

Client	Sex		Age				Mental Retardation Level				
Group	M	F	18-25	28-37	38-47	48+	Borderline	Mild	Moderate	Severe	Profound
Placeable Clients	64	36	39.5	29.0	11.1	20.3	0.0	4.9	14.8	29.6	50.6
Community Clients	44	56	11.9	19.7	22.0	46.4	4.5	26.7	34.8	26.0	7.8

*Discrepancies in totals due to rounding error

The Placeable Client Group also scored significantly lower than the Community Client Group on all five BDS domains. Placeable Clients were significantly less proficient in all areas of adaptive developmental behavior (BDS Domains I-III) and exhibited a significantly higher frequency of maladaptive behavior (BDS Domains IV and V). BDS mean domain scores and the probability levels attained are presented in Table 2. For BDS Domains I-III high scores correspond to greater competence in adaptive behavior skills while high scores for Domains IV and V correspond with an absence of maladaptive behavior.

Table 2

Mean BDS Scores for Institutionalized Placeable Clients and Community Based Clients

	Placeable Clients	Community Clients	$p=$
I.(Fundamental self-help skills)	26.2	39.8	.0000
II.(Independence beyond immediate needs)	10.8	26.7	.0000
III.(Self-direction and socialization)	8.2	16.0	.0000
IV.(Acting-out behavior)	11.4	12.2	.0000
V.(Self-stimulation, autistic behavior)	6.6	7.5	.0000

Discussion

The implications of the study become clear when one considers the nature of the deinstitutionalization process. Deinstitutionalization can be viewed as proceeding in phases with the highest functioning, most problem-free clients always being selected from among those available as the best placement candidates.

In the first phase of deinstitutionalization, the clients selected for placement are relatively self-sufficient and problem-free. These clients do not require extensive supervision or training and readily can be accommodated by community careproviders who have no special training either in teaching developmental skills or managing problem behaviors.

During the second phase of deinstitutionalization, however, the clients considered to be the most placeable are not as high functioning and, while largely free of serious physical disabilities and medical problems, exhibit more behavior problems than those clients first deinstitutionalized. Theoretically, the final phase of deinstitutionalization would involve successful community placement of very low functioning clients, many of whom have serious health problems requiring skilled nursing care.

The results of this study suggest that Hawaii is in the second phase of deinstitutionalization. The clients now considered to be prime candidates for community placement are significantly lower functioning and have significantly more behavior problems than clients already residing in the community. These results are consistent with other research showing that the more severely retarded, with their attendent developmental deficits and maladaptive behavior, still reside in institutions (Borthwick, Meyers & Eyman, this volume; Eyman & Borthwick, 1980).

The lack of proficiency in self-help and social skills and the high manifestation of maladaptive behaviors which characterize the placement candidates in this study may well be predictive of community placement failure. Reported difficulties in finding placements and increasing institution readmission rates indicate a lack of community readiness to provide the services needed by these lower functioning clients.

It would appear that the deinstitutionalization efforts of Hawaii, and perhaps of other agencies involved in second phase deinstitutionalization activities, are approaching asymptotic levels. Recently community placements have been equaled or exceeded by institutional readmissions and the institutional population may be stabilizing. The question then arises as to how to promote continued successful deinstitutionalization.

Several avenues of approach might prove beneficial. A good first step would seem to be the simple acknowledgement that successful deinstitutionalization is becoming more difficult to realize and that deinstitutionalization rates are likely to decline.

By taking into consideration the decreased number of placements available to lower functioning clients and the increased probability of placement failure which has been noted, more realistic projections could be made of the rate at which institutional populations can be reduced. Appropriate adjustments in unrealistic placement expectations would ease the pressures to deinstitutionalize now being experienced by many agencies and perhaps would avert unsuitable community placements for which the probability of failure is high.

In addition, the community must recognize that a large proportion of the clients for whom placement is now being sought have developmental deficits and behavior problems that are much greater than those of clients placed during earlier phases of deinstitutionalization. If successful placements are to be made, the community must adapt to the changing requirements for service provision as dictated by the characteristics and needs of this new incoming population.

The development of effective programs and services, however, may be difficult to achieve. A common recommendation for improving placement success, for example, is to provide in-service training to careproviders on the development of client self-help and social skills and on the management of client behavior problems. Hawaii does, however, provide a variety of in-service training courses to careproviders as well as follow-along services and respite care. In spite of these efforts, and a very active deinstitutionalization program, the State has not been able to achieve projected deinstitutionalization goals.

It seems apparent that second phase deinstitutionalization is accompanied by a series of problems and barriers for which solutions are not readily apparent. A refinement of current policies and practices, however, might be expected to increase both placement success and placement setting availability.

One potential area of improvement lies in the placement process itself. Once the decision has been made to deinstitutionalize a client, social workers and other placement agency staff seek a community home setting appropriate to the needs of the client. Placement is made through mutual approval of agency staff and the careprovider involved and is based primarily on a clinical judgement of appropriateness of client to home.

A refinement of the placement process in which client behavioral characteristics are carefully matched to the expressed preferences and tolerances of prospective careproviders for specific client behaviors might be expected to improve the rate of placement success. Matching careproviders and clients for maladaptive behaviors is particularly crucial since it has been shown that careprovider/client incompatability in this area is related to placement failure (Sutter et al., 1980). More important, this same study found that even clients with a large number of behavior problems (five or more per client) could be successful in community care if placed with careproviders who indicated a willingness to manage the behavior they exhibited. These results are consistent with those of Eyman and Call (1977), who likewise found a substantial number of behavior problem clients apparently residing successfully in the community.

In addition, an evaluation of the effectiveness of support programs already being provided to the community might prove beneficial. For example, evaluations of on-going in-service training to careproviders could determine 1) the appropriateness of training program content, 2) the extent to which careproviders apply what they have been taught, and 3) whether hands-on assistance in the application of what has been presented would be beneficial to careproviders. Modifications of in-service programs based on the obtained information could result in careproviders who are better trained and more confident of their ability to provide care successfully to lower functioning, more problematic clients. Similar evaluations of follow-along and respite care services might likewise be expected to improve these community support mechanisms.

However, the results of this study and clinical experience suggest that during second phase deinstitutionalization even drastic measures are not likely to restore (or to maintain) either the placement rates or the degrees of placement success that are common to the early phases of the process. The writers believe that deinstitutionalization goals should be reevaluated based on a consideration of the characteristics of the clients available for placement and on the capabilities of the community to provide the services they need. A realistic assessment of placement feasibility would seem to be essential to further successful deinstitutionalization.

References

Bishop, E. Family-care: The patients. *American Journal of Mental Deficiency,* 1957, *61,* 583-591.

Brown, S., Windle, C., & Stewart, E. Statistics on a family care program. *American Journal of Mental Deficiency,* 1959, *64,* 535-542.

Eagle, E. Prognosis and outcome and community placement of institutionalized retardates. *American Journal of Mental Deficiency,* 1967, *72,* 232-243.

Edgerton, R. *The cloak of competence.* Berkeley: University of California Press, 1967.

Edgerton, R. Issues relating to the quality of life among mentally retarded persons. In M. Begab & J. Richardson (Eds.), *The mentally retarded and society: A social science prospective.* Baltimore: University Park Press, 1975.

Eyman, R., & Borthwick, S. Patterns of care for mentally retarded persons. *Mental Retardation,* 1980, *18,* 63-66.

Eyman, R., & Call, T. Maladaptive behavior and community placement of mentally retarded persons. *American Journal of Mental Deficiency,* 1977, *82*(2), 137-144.

Fernald, W. After-care study of the patients discharged from Waverly for a period of twenty-five years. *Ungraded,* 1919, *5,* 25-31.

Keys, V., Boroskin, A., & Ross, R. T. The revolving door in the MR hospital: A study of returns from leave. *Mental Retardation,* 1973, *11,* 55-56.

Nihira, K., Foster, R., Shellhaas, M., & Leland, H. *AAMD Adaptive Behavior Scale.* Washington, DC: American Association on Mental Deficiency, 1974.

Pagel, S., & Whitling, C. Readmissions to a state hospital for mentally retarded persons: Reasons for community placement failure. *Mental Retardation,* 1978, *16*(2), 164-166.

Scheerenberger, R. *Public residential services for the mentally retarded.* Madison, WI: National Association of Superintendents of Public Residential Facilities for the Mentally Retarded, 1976.

Sutter, P., Mayeda, T., Yanagi, G., & Yee, S. Comparison of successful and unsuccessful community placed mentally retarded clients. *American Journal of Mental Deficiency,* in press.

Sutter, P., Mayeda, T., Yee, S., & Yanagi, G. *Community placement success based on client behavior preferences of careproviders.* Manuscript submitted for publication, 1980.

Windle, C. Prognosis of mental subnormals. *American Journal of Mental Deficiency Monograph Supplement,* 1962, *66,* 1-180.

Yanagi, G. Why we need Waimano. *Hawaii Health Messenger,* 1979, *42*(4).

Deinstitutionalization and Community Adjustment: A Summary of Research and Issues

K. Charlie Lakin
Robert H. Bruininks
Barbara B. Sigford

University of Minnesota

Each contributor to this volume has joined many other researchers who over the past 60 years have sought to add some useful information and ideas to the study of the readjustment process of persons released from institutions for the mentally retarded and/or persons placed in community-based facilities from non-institutional residences. None of these authors assumes that the process is easily understood, or that any one solution to either the methodological or programmatic problems will ever be singled out. The authors have undertaken the consideration of this complex social phenomenon with the assumption that insight into a complex problem can be gained from sharing observations based on its systematic study. As the reader has no doubt noted, the papers in this volume have raised more issues than offered solutions. Still the authors may find some solace in the old truism, "Progress begins with getting a clear view of the obstacles."

Even before we consider the obstacles to successful social reintegration faced by formerly institutionalized mentally retarded persons, we are compelled to consider the problems inherent in the ways researchers approach their study of the adjustment process. Generally speaking, the most important of these obstacles can be placed in one of two broad categories: conceptual issues and methodological issues.

Conceptual Issues

By conceptual issues we are referring to problems which lie outside the social phenomena being investigated, but which affect what is learned about it by shaping what is being observed. Leading the list of conceptual issues are the semantic problems which Bachrach addressed in her paper in this volume. There is no question we are living in a period of "euphemania," a period of concerted searching for words of positive valence to apply to persons, programs and things about which we care. Such efforts are not to be scorned, but we must be cautious about assuming that new words indicate new realities. We would cite as an example how "inmates of institutions for the idiotic and feeble-minded" have, through a number of semantic transformations, become "residents of public residential facilities for the mentally retarded" within the past few decades with a number of recent court decisions apparently questioning whether the changes in the realities of "residence" have been sufficiently substantive.

Among the primary semantic barriers to understanding the realities of community adjustment and community care and services are those very terms themselves: "community," "adjustment," "care," and "services." As Bachrach noted, the word "community" has come to be used so loosely in the literature concerning the mentally disabled that it has lost its original meaning and has become synonymous with "noninstitution." Bachrach and Bjaanes, Butler and Kelly, also in this volume have amply cautioned us against the danger of investing a geographical relocation, from a residential facility funded directly by the State (public) to one funded indirectly (community), with the assumption of better or more appropriate care. Still, now that community and institution have become the primary "buzz-words" of deinstitutionalization, much of our literature treats them as though they convey clear meaning more than stimulate emotional response. Obviously, if we are ever to hope that our research on the extra-institutional adjustment of mentally retarded people can be of use in addressing the real life problems involved in this process, we must maximize the degree to which that research is science-oriented, as opposed to semantics-oriented. It is not an easy task, but it is essential. Meaningful categorization is one of the most important elements of scientific analysis, and perhaps the most elusive one for social scientists.

As was pointed out earlier in the paper by Lakin, Bruininks, and Sigford, the notion of "adjustment," with its numerous operational definitions, is every bit as problematic as is the term "community." The breadth of conceptualization of "adjustment" has spanned from complete self-sufficiency to simply not being remanded to an institution within a specified period of time. While such a wide range of operational definitions of adjustment does not inherently lead to confusion (if the operations are made explicit), it does lead to problems in comparability and consistency of research findings. Furthermore, it does not recognize the fact that for all of us, adjustment is a matter of degree and of personal preference which may vary from time to time and from one area of life to another. This notion has been a consistent theme of the research and writing of Edgerton (1967; this volume), and the fact that it may pose a special problem for researchers and service providers makes it no less a reality of life. Beyond this, the notion of adjustment as it has been operationalized in previous studies implies a standard or norm by which the adjustment of mentally retarded persons can be determined—that is by which one can separate those who are "adjusted" from those who are not. Such a standard can be most easily criticized in that even among non-mentally handicapped persons adjustment is at best ill-defined and represents no particular pattern of behavior, but rather a wide range of socially tolerable activity. Perhaps more importantly such a conceptualization of adjustment fails to appreciate the fact that life experiences of deinstitutionalized mentally retarded persons have been (and often remain) vastly different than those of "normal" people. When we consider the adjustment of deinstitutionalized persons we should be guided by Hansberry's plea in *A Raisin in the Sun*: "When you starts measuring somebody, measure him right. . . . Make sure you done taken into account what hills and valleys he come through before he got to wherever he is" (1959, p. 125). Seltzer, Sherwood, Seltzer, and Sherwood (this volume) discuss these issues as they relate to mentally retarded people and suggest an alternative conceptualization of adjustment.

Furthermore, investigators who have reviewed numerous studies for variables which consistently predict successful or unsuccessful adjustment have been, for the most part, hopelessly bogged down not only by the wide range of definitions of adjustment, but also by the fact that adjustment is an interactive process. All aspects of the environment contribute to the eventual adaptation made by the retarded individual. People caring for the retarded person are called upon to make adjustments as well. When they are willing and able to make adjustments to accommodate undesirable or demanding client characteristics, carepersons enhance the likelihood that their wards will remain in community-based placements (Sutter & Mayeda, this volume). While the notion of reciprocal adjustments between the released resident and significant others in his or her life and the interactions of individual and environmental variables present complex problems to researchers, overlooking this reality can only lead to more research which fails to catch enough of real life to be usable.

Finally we are haunted by the term "care" and its modern equivalent "services"—services being countable, while care is not! Although often treated as though they were synonymous, the two terms present very different conceptualizations of that which is given to dependent persons by the people or the society upon which they are dependent. Choosing one or the other of these notions of social provision can only lead to certain misconceptualizations. For example, as Bjaanes, Butler, and Kelly point out many more formal services are provided to people in institutions than persons outside. In fact, nearly every activity within the total institution can be designated as a service of one form or another. That does not mean, however, that "care" is better. In fact, the entire deinstitutionalization movement has been based primarily on the assumption that care will be improved by placing mentally retarded persons in smaller, community-based residential facilities. On the other side of the coin, however, there really are such things as services, that is, organized programs, activities, and other provisions of the society which are countable, funded not only to increase the opportunity for mentally retarded persons to adjust to the society in which they live, but also to affect the quality of care they receive. In short, then, it seems that to equate the concepts of care and services may be a mistake, but no larger than the mistake of dealing with one without simultaneous concern for the other.

Methodological Issues

In addition to the conceptual issues plaguing research on deinstitutionalization are important issues related to the research methodologies employed by those persons attempting to learn about and describe to others important aspects of the phenomenon. The paper by Taylor and Bogdan in this volume has provided a distinction between the dominant paradigm of studying social phenomena, the "quantitative method," and a less frequently used methodology with a rich tradition of application in anthropological and sociological research, the "qualitative method." These authors have also provided an excellent discussion of the assumptions made by researchers viewing social phenomena from each perspective. Both paradigms have earned the status of being "scientific" within a particular cohort of trained researchers, and each, therefore, has the effect of shaping the observations of those who employ them. It is extremely important that students of social phenomena learn to recognize and openly discuss the benefits and liabilities of each in social investigations. Only then can each be appreciated by those schooled in the other, and can researchers become more sophisticated in utilizing the most appropriate method, or blend of methods, given a particular research problem. The only real obstacle to a wide range of useful approaches to researching the community adjustment process is the unenlightened perspective of more than a few that there is *a* scientific method for studying psychological or sociological questions. If there is any lesson to be learned from the study of the impact of scholasticism on the emergence of modern Western thought, it is that little human progress is possible when the road to that progress, our observations, are systematized by the toleration of only one world view. As the Nobel prize-winning physicist, Percy Bridgman, is quoted by C. Wright Mills (1961, p. 58) as having said: "There is no scientific method as such, but the vital feature of the scientist's procedure has been merely to do his utmost with his mind, *no holds barred*!"

The majority of recent studies of deinstitutionalization of mentally retarded persons have been quantitative in nature, broad in scope, retrospective and of brief duration, usually measuring dependent variables at only one period in time. Today there is a strong need to balance previous research endeavors with new approaches stressing observational investigations of specifically designated aspects of the adjustment process over the period during which they are occurring. The papers by Bercovici, Berkson and Romer, and Edgerton in this volume have well shown the usefulness of such research in exploring the realities of extra-institutional life as a mentally retarded person.

Another crucial issue facing researchers is to what degree the clients of the residential services system should be employed as primary informants about their own lives. As Wyngaarden and Gollay pointed out in this volume, the inclusion of mentally retarded subjects is not only possible, but adds a dimension to the research on extra-institutional living which is simply unobtainable in any other way. Such an approach, however, is fraught with an abundance of problems related to the reliability and validity of responses, as Sigelman and her associates so clearly related in this volume. These researchers have, however, outlined those approaches to gathering information from residents of non-institutional settings which appear to be most methodologically sound, and they stand behind a cautious application of the assumption that we can learn much from our subjects simply by asking them.

Research Questions

Having presented some of the fundamental conceptual and methodological issues evident in the research conducted in this field, we now turn to important topical areas addressed by the papers contained in this volume for which additional study would clearly be beneficial. In outlining these areas we will attempt to identify some of the more notable research and writing related to each.

Assessing Treatment Environments: Search for Facility Characteristics Which Affect the Quality of Care

In the recent literature on residential care for mentally retarded people, a gross dichotomy of residence types is often employed with the underlying assumption that one type is preferable to the other. Specifically public residential facilities, or institutions, are usually treated either implicitly or explicitly as inferior places to live when contrasted to community residential facilities. Further research, however, is necessary to explore the nature of different residential environments and delineate their impact on the persons living in them. Attention must be paid in this research to the mechanisms by which characteristics of the environment affect quality of life. It will be important in this research to define clearly both the independent variables—characteristics of the environment such as size, organizational patterns, staff attitudes, and explicit and implicit care modes (e.g., custodial, health maintenance, family living, independence training)—as well as the dependent variables—measures of quality of life such as "care," services provided, and satisfaction of residents. Dependent variables measured are particularly likely to reflect our professional or personal biases and philosophy and thus must be carefully scrutinized.

One of the most serious difficulties in researching "community" (non-public) residential facilities derives from the fact that the term encompasses a large number of vastly different modes of care-providing. Not only can systematic differences be found in program content of community-based residential facilities (Bjaanes, Butler & Kelly, this volume), but as Borthwick, Meyers and Eyman (this volume) clearly demonstrated there are also systematic differences in the characteristics of residents among different types of non-public residential facilities. Unfortunately the term "community facility" has come to be used as though it had a uniformly understood meaning. The fact of the matter is, however, as a term it is extremely vague. As Bachrach noted, in its broadest and most common definition, it means simply all non-public residential facilities. When such a definition is employed, as it was in the recent Developmental Disabilities Project on Residential Services and Community Adjustment (DDP, 1978), one notes that over half the mentally retarded persons in "community facilities" in 1977 lived in settings with over 30 residents. To what degree states have, by releasing residents from their own large institutions and funding their placement in facilities of over 30 residents, protected them from the long recognized impersonal, and culturally abnormal aspects of institutionalizational living is a question worthy of consideration.

Whatever the ultimate answer to such a question, it can hardly be negated that the size of a residential facility influences its organization in ways that must naturally influence the way in which services (or care) are provided to residents. Still little is actually known about how the size of a facility operates to affect its patterns of care. Cleland (1965) in a review of institution size as related to quality of care, concluded that for the most part the conviction that residential facilities were most effective as treatment environments when of limited size was based on very little objective evidence. Since that time, a number of conflicting studies have shown place of residence to be interrelated with a number of outcome measures, including motivation to interact with adults (Zigler, Butterfield, & Capobianco, 1970), level of aspiration (Rosen, Diggory, & Werlensky, 1966), withdrawal from intrinsically non-stimulating tasks, imitation and behavioral variability (Balla, Butterfield, & Zigler, 1974), and verbal mental age (Schroeder & Henes, 1976; Tizard, 1964).

In a review of this literature, Balla (1976) considered quality of care research within four areas: resident-care practices, behavioral functioning, rate of discharge, and residents' involvement with family and community. While Balla concluded that "resident-care practices seem to be more resident-oriented in smaller, community-based facilities than in large central institutions" and therefore that "it is reasonable to conclude that the quality of life for the retarded person is, *on the average,* better in small community-based facilities," he was firm in cautioning that "it seems equally reasonable to conclude that it is the type of institution, rather than its size per se, that is the primary determinant of care practices" (p. 120, emphasis added). For the most part research on the effects of the size of a residential facility on its residents is mixed and there appears to be as much variation among facility types as there is between large and small facility groupings.

The findings of extensive variability among programs within a particular classification is a frequently found phenomenon in educational research. Light (1979) and Glass (1979) have noted that in educational research studies variation across sites within models often greatly exceeds between-model variation. It is quite plausible to assume, therefore, that considerable difference in the characteristics and qualities of environments exists within size groups and residential models as the work of Intagliata, Willer and Wicks (this volume) suggests.

The recognition that rather global factors such as facility size seem only to operate to affect resident and caretakers' behavior in indirect ways has led a number of researchers to examine carefully the social environments of residential facilities through direct observational techniques. For the most part these researchers have centered their work in large institutions (e.g., Goffman, 1961; Braginsky & Braginsky, 1971). One notable exception is the work of King, Raynes, and Tizard (1971) in their study of residential care for children in England. Using a scale which attempted to quantify many of the concepts developed by Goffman (1961) in his analysis of "total institutions," these researchers measured child management practices in large, intermediate, and small facilities providing residential services to mentally handicapped children. The scale they devised (*The Revised Child Management Scale*) focuses on four categories along which the "totalness" of care facilities is assessed: "rigidity," "block treatment," "depersonalization," and "social distance." Each category has several specific questions which are designed to assess the degree of "child-orientation" versus "institution-orientation" of facilities. For example "rigidity" refers to the degree of routinization of the lives of residents and is assessed by questions such as, "Do children get up at the same time on weekends?" and "Do they use the yard or garden at set times?"

The study of King and his associates showed that the *Revised Child Management Scale* was able to discriminate successfully between types of facilities. A clear tendency was evidenced for smaller facilities to be more child-oriented than the larger facilities. The size of the living unit, however, produced no such differences. Neither were differences found with regard to the variables of staffing ratios, and degree of handicap of residents.

Perhaps even more important than these general findings concerning facility size was the discovery of a clear relationship between the child-orientation of a facility and its organizational structure. In child-oriented units there was less division of labor, more direct involvement with the children by supervisors, more program autonomy at the living unit level and more flexibility in terms of staff scheduling. In addition the researchers were able to correlate child management practices to types of training received. The organizational and training factors outlined by the authors are important examples of how information gained from objective scales may eventually be utilized. It is relatively easy to develop objective scales which can discriminate one type of setting from another, but such measures become useful when they help understand the processes by which one facility becomes, for example, "child-oriented" and another "institution-oriented." Size, one might conclude from this research, does not affect the child-orientation of a facility so much as it affects organizational structure which in turn affects the nature of its orientation toward residents.

Clearly, although the scale developed by King, Raynes, and Tizard is an important beginning for the study of community-based residential facilities, it would seem that the further development of such scales may benefit from more direct observational studies of the social climate of these facilities. While smaller residential facilities may overcome many of the impersonal, and at times dehumanizing, qualities of many larger facilities, the various forms of organization found among community residences may create either similar or new impediments to the delivery of humane care and habilitative services, a possibility discussed in a number of papers in this volume.

An earlier study by Bjaanes and Butler (1974) provides one example of the use of behavioral measures in assessing the effects of facility types on the behavior of their residents. These researchers examined two board and care facilities (with 30 and 50 residents) and two home care facilities (4 and 6 residents) all for adults, comparing them on dimensions of physical environment, support to client, attitudes toward clients, and behavior of clients. The last dimension was broken down into active and passive leisure, work and chores, personal activity and social interaction. Questionnaires were used to evaluate the supportive and attitudinal dimensions, environmental ratings were used to assess the physical setting, and an observation schedule was developed to assess the behavioral dimension.

Although based on relatively short periods of observation in each of the four settings, the authors noted large and systematic differences in the independent behavior among residents in the two types of facilities and concluded that the board and care facilities were more conducive to the promotion of independent behavior than were the family care settings. The authors hypothesized that long-term followup would show that specific types of community care environments would be associated with different outcomes in social behavior. This research also suggested, as has that of D'Amico, Hannah, Milhouse and Froleich (1978), Eyman, Demaine and Lei (1979), and Stebbins (1931), that geographical location is an important factor in the social participation and integration of mentally retarded adults.

Another method of research effective in assessing the social environment of residential facilities was used by Moores and Grant (1976) in studying verbal and non-verbal interactions in hospitals for the mentally handicapped in England. In their research an observation schedule was developed to measure both the frequency and nature of interactions among residents and staff. Among types of social interactions the authors coded non-verbal, commands, teaches, converses, encourages, transacts, and discourages. In addition the researchers coded the interactions according to their purpose from the institutional standpoint, e.g., supervising, social, and teaching. This research showed the observation schedule clearly discriminated between the frequency and types of interaction taking place within the two hospitals. It also showed substantial variations in the frequency of positive (teaches, encourages, and converses) versus negative and neutral interactions, and interactions filling a social or training function versus those involved in organizing and directing the residents of the institution. In all cases differences favored the same institution (probability levels were less than .001 for three comparisons and .005 for the other). Unfortunately the differences between the two institutions which might explain such differences were not isolated by these researchers. Groups of variables worthy of investigation in explaining such differences include: 1) organizational (e.g., division of labor, bureaucratization), 2) social psychological (e.g., role perceptions of staff, staff morale), 3) programmatic (e.g., goals and programs of facility, types of training given staff) and resident characteristics (e.g., real and staff-perceived degrees of handicap and potential, resident responsiveness). This type of research has considerable potential for isolating those intra-facility factors related to quality and effectiveness of care, especially if the effects of staff-resident interactions are studied over a period of time.

Another direct-observation study which revealed considerable variation among apparently similar residential facilities (group homes) was conducted by Landesman-Dwyer, Stein and Sackett (1976). This research of behavioral and environmental variations across homes showed major interfacility differences in the frequency of such basic experiences as unstructured activities, organized activities, household maintenance, time spent out of house and general social behavior. In this latter area, for example, the residents of one home spent 21.4% of their time engaging in activity categorized as "general social" as opposed to only 4.7% in another home. Although this study reconfirmed the differences among facilities referred to as "group homes," the authors did note that

> since the observational data were collected at only one point in time no meaningful conclusions about the *progress* of an individual can be made. Similarly without an adequately matched set of control subjects who live in other places—such as institutions, or boarding homes—no valid principles can be derived about the impact of a given type of residential program on the clients, nor is there a comparison of different group home programs. (p. 30)

Similar observations have been made by a number of experienced researchers contributing to this volume, including Gollay and Seltzer, Sherwood, Seltzer, and Sherwood.

A number of ways have been outlined above to assess the social climate of residential facilities. In addition, the paper by Berkson and Romer in this volume describes their observational techniques for studying the social climate of residential facilities. Their findings interpreted for a fictitious policy-maker show clearly the practical utility of such research.

Any method of direct observation has its strengths and more importantly, perhaps, each is a gross over-simplification of the social setting. Many factors shape the environment which pose difficulties in attempts at objectification. For one, the social setting involves both residents and staff, and each group reciprocally affects the other, as individuals in one group affect other members of that group. Resident responsiveness will shape staff attempts to interact, as well as vice versa. In some settings (just as some homes) independent activity will be more valued than structured teaching/learning activities. In some facilities (e.g., nursing homes) staff responsiveness is more likely to be determined on the physical needs of residents rather than on perceived social needs. In some settings the focus may be on developing skills while others focus on "kindness" and making the environment a happy place to live. In short the assessment of the social climate of community residential services is complex. But it is this very complexity which has made a number of writers plead for research that is grounded in an environmental context.

In 1977, Brooks and Baumeister made a strong argument for research which was "ecologically valid," that is, treated environment as a vitally important variable in the behavior of developmentally disabled persons. Measures of adaptive behavior, they argued, should be based on direct and naturalistic observations of developmentally disabled persons and should be especially sensitive to the social and programmatic interactions taking place in that environment. To demonstrate how little of this type of research is actually taking place, Berkson and Landesman-Dwyer (1977) noted that less than 5% of published research on severely and profoundly retarded persons over a 20 year period was based on direct observation. Obviously little will be learned about factors which affect the quality of care and habilitative training in residential facilities until many more observers "take to the trenches." Harry Harlow's (1957) admonition that "complex problems evade effective experimental analysis far less frequently than experimentors evade complex problems" (p. 485) may be especially appropriate at this time in the study of community-based residential services.

Community facilities have been developed on the assumption that they will overcome the more negative aspects of institutional life. While institutions take on a number of negative aspects because of the requirement that they manage a large number of handicapped residents in a confined and isolated space, operate a large organization and provide total life care for the residents, smaller facilities, too, have social and economic realities which may affect their responsiveness to client needs. Edgerton (1975) has noted regimentation and condescending treatment of persons in community facilities and suggested that fundamental rights are often denied those in non-institution settings. In addition one must note that a primary, unwritten rule in the social service enterprise is that one tries to keep "good" clients whenever possible; they are cheaper, more easily managed, and more gratifying to work with. The degree to which these factors keep persons in more restrictive residential facilities than they require has not been fully considered. To a greater degree in future research, "quality of care" must be measured by the degree it promotes the movement of residents toward less restrictive living arrangements, rather than simply maintaining them in extra-institutional settings. Understanding more about the types of programs and incentives that bring about such movement is vital not only in fulfilling the basic promises of community-based services and in providing program placements for other persons needing them (cf. Schalock & Harper, this volume), but is imperative to making community-based services more cost-effective.

As Willer, Intagliata and Wicks noted in this volume, researchers have virtually ignored the 20% (Sigford & Bruininks, in preparation) of persons released from public institutions who return to their natural home. They also alerted the reader to the discrepancy between the supportive services available to natural families as opposed to surrogate families. They noted that the more frequent utilization of our culturally ideal residential environment, the natural home, may depend on reducing this discrepancy in available services, as well as on a fuller acceptance of the natural home as a viable placement option on the part of professionals. However, since only about 3% of all persons "eligible" for classification as developmentally disabled are actually in residential programs (Bruininks, Hauber, Hill & Kudla, this volume; Scheerenberger, this volume), and since presumably home care support, once offered, would also need to be made available to families whose disabled member had never left home, it must be expected that a hard look will be taken by legislators at the potential expenditures involved in creating sizable incentives for natural home care. For that matter it is not clear that the types of services and incentives government agencies can offer would appreciably affect the level of extra-familial placement. This is an area ripe for joint scrutiny by service professionals and economists (cf. Bruininks & Krantz, 1979).

As yet very little participant observation research has been conducted in community-based residential facilities. The reason for this is not self-evident since descriptions of the social climate of total institutions using qualitative methods were so instrumental in shaping today's dominant philosophy of extra-institutional residential placement. As Bercovici noted in this volume, "institutional" treatment is not limited to institutions. Qualitative methods with their emphasis on holistic description of social settings are especially suitable to transcending our predispositions about what realities lie behind the, by now, semantically loaded terms "institution" and "community residence." In one of the few participant observation studies of community-based residential services, Kasanovich (1980a) concluded:

> I have already stressed the historical continuities of basic responsibilities Government has in relation to the retarded in the Civic Body . . . These interact to render a service system that is constituted *and* mandated to provide for the care and protection of the retarded, and only thereafter to address rehabilitative/devel-

opmental goals. Care is today paramount, even as it was in the past . . . Even though Government has adopted an entirely new service delivery philosophy (normalization) ostensibly antithetical to institutional service, yet the agents of actual service delivery employ models and priorities of perception and organization and tools for programmatic interaction that emerged out of service delivery accomplished in the total care environment of the state hospital. Faced with working with clients in new geographical, group-size, and service charter environments, service vendor organizations have drawn heavily upon the institutional legacy, and created human environments akin to those found in the state hospital. (pp. 123-124)

Such an observation, based on 18 months of full-time field-work, should challenge researchers to consider how much of the generally accepted differences among public and non-public facilities are based on prepossession. Since one of the primary goals of the large scale modifications in the residential services system in the past years has been to alter significantly the patterns of care associated with public institutions, to some extent improved quality of care effected by these modifications must be assessed by whether substantive changes actually have taken place. Our research should examine carefully the degree to which the "new" residential services system truly differs from the "old" one.

Normalization: Search for Means of Encouraging Normal Life Patterns

In 1969, Nirje put forth the concept which has in the past decade spread through the residential services system with unprecedented rapidity and unbridled acceptance. The concept, "normalization," according to Nirje's most recent definition, means "making available to all mentally retarded people patterns and conditions of everyday living which are as close as possible to the regular circumstances and ways of life of society" (1976, p. 231). As formulated by Nirje the "normalization principle" emphasizes the right of mentally retarded persons to experience "life conditions as normal as possible, respecting the degrees and complications of the handicap, the training received and needed, and the social competence and maturity attainable" (1976, p. 232). While at first reading such a "principle" seems to present a laudable model of respect for the individual's right to some semblance of a normal life, the clause which follows reconfirms the power given others to determine "how normal" through clinical judgments of degrees and complications of handicap, training received and needed, and social competence and maturity attainable.

The programmatic derivative of such a service model is no doubt something similar to what is now available, that is, a multitude of possible placement options into which retarded persons are placed on the basis of available space, cost and clinical judgments such as those mentioned above. Three points ought to be made in regard to this state of affairs. First, of course, is that the social status and personal power of mentally retarded persons remain unchanged from those days preceding the general acceptance of the normalization principle within the developmental disabilities services system, even though its clients' place of residence may have changed. Second, there is the insidious danger of assuming that the development of multiple placement options has led to matching clients with the facility most appropriate given the retarded person's characteristics, training and needs, or that the establishment of a "principle" which dictates such a policy necessarily transcends the bureaucratic and programmatic impediments to its realization. Third, there is a tendency for researchers to study the "normativeness" of residential options on the basis of what may be largely extraneous variables. Research and discussion in this area show a strong proclivity for using distinctions on the basis of facility "type" (e.g., boarding homes, groups, foster homes, institutions) or size as independent variables. Ultimately better independent variables must be drawn from the social aspects of the setting, since the "patterns and conditions of everyday living" (from Nirje's definition of normalization) of dependent persons are largely a function of the way their lives are directed (or not directed) by primary caretakers, which is in turn affected by client characteristics (Landesman-Dwyer, Stein, & Sackett, 1978), administrative policies (Bercovici, this volume), as well as "type," size and location of the residence (Butler & Bjaanes, 1978; Gollay, Freedman, Wyngaarden, & Kurtz, 1978).

In recent years normalization has become the dominant philosophic concept in the examination of the residential services system. In discussing the normalization principle one must not overlook one of the special ironies of this particular postulate: concurrent to its rise as a dominant philosophy among those interested in residential services for the mentally retarded, has been the realization that what is culturally normative family life in our society probably would not pass right to treatment challenges if natural homes were governed by a State Department of Mental Health. Among the many bits of information which suggest true normalization is not at all a lofty goal is Gerbner and Gross' (1976) report that "nearly half of the 12-year-olds in their research sample watch an average of six or more hours of television a day." Among the American adults the writers "estimate that one-third of all American adults watch an average of four or more hours of television a day" (p. 42). Still, whether one wishes to assess the extent to which facilities provide opportunities for "truly normal" or "idealized normal" life patterns, the questions are researchable once one has a measure of normal or ideal behavior in residential settings. Some preliminary work has already been done, all of which is based on idealized "normal," that is, it assumes that certain types of behavior are preferable to others without consideration of whether these actually reflect typical behavior patterns in the society.

Optimal provision for social integration of retarded persons has long been held as a goal for residential facilities. In judging the idealness of a residence, the "normalization principle dictates the promotion of integration so that residents will intermingle with typical citizens in typical activities" (Wolfensberger & Glenn, 1975, p. 3). Furthermore, the residence should have relatively few inhabitants (Wolfensberger & Glenn, 1975). These two characteristics were also suggested by Stebbins' (1931) presentation of the Parole Employers Score Card discussed earlier in the paper by Lakin, Bruininks, and Sigford. However, some research has suggested that the realization of one of these programmatic requirements of the normalization principle may at times be negatively affected in the realization of the other. For example, the work of Butler and Bjaanes (1974) and Landesman-Dwyer, Stein and Sackett (1978) suggests that the amount of unstructured social activity outside a residential facility is affected by the restrictiveness of that facility, which in turn is related inversely to size. Such unplanned interactions in the implementation of social programs with multiple goals are not, of course, uncommon. It has long been noted that programs providing economic assistance to needy persons while attempting to encourage the development of economic independence of these same persons often find that the goals, though commendable, are not necessarily harmonious.

Not only do small facilities not necessarily ensure the social integration of their residents, but they apparently do not necessarily increase "family" interactions.

In their study of foster homes in Canada, Murphy, Penner, and Luchins (1972) concluded that not only did most residents not interact with "typical citizens," they did not even interact with members of the foster family. The authors, in fact, failed to see much advantage of the foster home over the institutions where these persons had formerly lived. The same qualities of regimentation and depersonalization were attributed to both types of facilities. However, Intagliata, Willer and Wicks, and Lei, Nihira, Sheehy and Meyers (this volume) have balanced such strident criticism of some facilities with small numbers of residents with the documented observation that within a particular category of facilities some placements are clearly better than others and positively affect both residents' social abilities and their degree of community participation.

Whatever the problems in guaranteeing a "normalized" life through community-based placement, it is clear that the vast majority of involved decision-makers, legal, legislative and programmatic, accept the vastly greater potential of community-based residential programs to live up to the principle of normalization. A landmark in the formal recognition of this potential was the *Wyatt vs. Stickney* (1972) federal court decision in Alabama. Among the standards set for minimally adequate habilitation in the decision was one which virtually made at least administrative adherence to the normalization principle binding on that state (and presumably others):

> Residents shall have a right to the least restrictive conditions necessary to achieve the purposes of habilitation. To this end, the institution shall make every attempt to move residents from: (a) more to less structured living; (b) larger to smaller facilities; (c) larger to smaller living units; (d) group to individual residence; (e) segregated from the community to integrated into the community living; (f) dependent to independent living (1972, p. 396).

As noted before, in some cases one of these subpoints will not be harmonious with others. Clearly planning must focus on a system of residential steps clients can take toward maximum independence and look toward ways that careproviders can be taught to be involved in and rewarded for taking part in the growth of their wards. If there is one thing the research of the effects of deinstitutionalization clearly shows it is that generally accepted principles and even laws standardize very little of the day to day realities of a residential facility (or a natural home for that matter). Those realities lie much more directly in the hands of careproviders, and those attitudes, training, personal characteristics, opportunities and goals for their clients which relate to the promotion of "normalized" life patterns, either "true" or "idealized" normal, have been studied very little.

In addition, in our considerations of normalization we must never forget that freedom to choose activity (or inactivity) is also a normal part of life in our society. For example, Birenbaum and Re (1979) raise the question of how much the provision of an opportunity to participate in community activities will influence whether residents will choose to do so. Judging from the results of their follow-up study of persons in a large community facility, Matthews' comments, written in 1922, seem to remain highly descriptive of the activities of most persons who have resided for any length of time in community facilities for the mentally retarded:

> Few of them want, or expect excitement. They are satisfied with the "movies" once or twice a week, and an occasional visit to the theater. . . . On the whole their evenings are short, and most of them are spent at home with a Victrola or games, or with books or papers (p. 340).

The reader is invited to compare Matthews' comments with the observations of Birenbaum and Re, made 57 years later:

> Few residents ventured out at night, with 83% spending their time either watching television, listening to records, taking care of their rooms or engaging in personal hygiene (p. 328).

Theoretically, at least, intermingling is enhanced by living in an area with at least a moderate population density. The vast majority of community-based residential facilities appear to be so situated (Bruininks et al., 1979; Gollay et al., 1978), although regional differences are notable, as are the differences among the various types of facilities (Bruininks, Hill, & Thorsheim, 1979). Although strictly residential areas would seem preferable for enhancing normal life patterns among developmentally disabled persons, it is also true that they are often distant from commercial, recreational, and social opportunities. Optimizing the opportunity for integration may often mean not residing in areas which seem "ideal normal" by middle class standards, especially among persons who are restricted by personal ability or public availability in their travel. Secondly, as pointed out by Berkson and Romer (this volume), developmentally disabled persons tend to socialize primarily with other developmentally disabled persons. While those desirous of changing these patterns might look to emersion in the normal community through removal from "subcultures" of mentally handicapped persons as one means, there is little evidence that public support of normalization has gone so far that the handicapped will be welcomed or even tolerated in "non-deviant" social circles. There is great danger that intuitive notions of normal, as "normal neighborhood" will isolate handicapped individuals in normal physical settings totally void of the other normalities of social life.

Beyond this, it would seem perfectly understandable if it were discovered that large numbers of mentally retarded people did not desire substantial intermingling with non-handicapped persons. Certainly, the label mentally retarded and its confirmation through residence in a facility for the retarded is not likely to enhance the tendency to interact with other persons residing in the neighborhood. Edgerton (1967) minced no words in describing the effect of that label on the lives of the subjects in his research:

> The label of mental retardation not only serves as a humiliating, frustrating, and discrediting stigma in the conduct of one's life in the community, but it also serves to lower one's self-esteem to such a nadir of worthlessness that the life of a person so labeled is scarcely worth living (p. 145).

If there is any truth at all to such an observation, how reasonable is it to assume that persons whose retarded identity is maintained by their residence are likely to enjoy a harmonious unrestrained relationship with others in the community? This is a question for which qualitative investigation, in which researchers emerse themselves in the daily lives of their subjects, is of crucial importance in understanding the impact of placement in community residential facilities. It is essential also that these studies seek to identify important factors in the realization of a social integration which goes beyond physical proximity. Careful evaluation of ongoing programs with goals related to social integration is another means to this end. Clearly in the area of normalization there are enormous dangers that programming based on the values/perceptions of planners and care providers will be antithetical to the best interest of those persons in whose names the programs are instituted. Throughout history, and social services have been no exception, people often have proven to be most dangerous and most coercive when acting in the name of "principles." "Normalization" is not immune to such an outcome and clearly without considerable caution, many well-meaning social servants will, with the best of intentions, pave many roads to hell in their dedication to this "principle." Principles simply do not assure their own wise application. Now that normalization has become axiomatic, the specific propositions based on it which influence considerably the lives of persons in residential facilities need careful scrutiny.

Stigmatization: Search for Understanding of the Effects of Stigma on the Lives of Clients.

The past 20 years have seen considerable growth in the literature regarding identity and symbolic factors (e.g., where one lives) which might be directly related to the lives of persons residing in the various residential facilities for the mentally retarded. A good deal has also been written about the social and cognitive development which allow persons to take the perspective of others by Mead (1934) and Piaget (1928) and those following their paths. A far too limited, but convincing, body of research has documented the negative products of such thoughts when persons officially identified as mentally retarded symbolically weigh the effects of such a label on the perceptions of those around them (cf. Edgerton, 1967). Much more has been written about the effects that stigmatizing labels have on the perceptions of significant others in the lives of the labeled (c.f. Hersom, 1974; Kirk, 1972). For the most part, however, research has not gone beyond identifying the problems created for the stigmatized individual by these symbolic social processes.

The questions may be asked, "How important is the problem of symbols, of stigma, of identity?" To the researcher the answer to this question may depend on his/her particular perspective and interests. From the point of view of the individual, however, when personal identity, self-satisfaction, and even happiness itself are seen as a symbolic matter deriving from a conceptualization of one's "place" in the world through taking the perspective of others, symbols become very important. To affect one's symbolic self, one's identity, is to affect the person. While residential facilities for the mentally retarded have a primary social function of protecting the physical well-being of their residents, this well-intentioned concern may be at times detrimental to the identity of many who receive residential services. Anyone bright enough to have a vague idea of the meaning of "mentally retarded," "retarded," or one of the many other terms of clinical science and public playgrounds, knows it is not something good "to be." And anyone bright enough to know it is not something good to be would prefer not to be it. How a continuum of residential services (without assuming one already exists) could be put to use in balancing the physical as well as the symbolic needs of the individual has been very lightly considered in the research on residential facilities for the mentally retarded. As Gollay pointed out in this volume, very little of the community adjustment research has even attempted to understand the perspective of the residents. And as Bercovici noted in this volume, many persons in residential facilities are well aware of the negative valence their place of residence puts on their lives.

In Edgerton's (1967) follow-up of 48 persons released from a California state institution for the mentally retarded, the author noted that a significant goal of the persons studied was to pass as "normal" in the eyes of their new reference group, those normal people living around them. As time separated them from the "institutional phase" of their lives, however, this preoccupation became considerably less pervasive. By the time they were recontacted 12 years later by Edgerton and Bercovici (1976), few of these persons indicated that they remained actively concerned with keeping others from "finding out." As time separated them from the formal denunciation of being mentally retarded which having lived in a place for "that kind of person" represented, the stigma dissipated. Would the same thing have happened had the wide range of facilities which have since been opened been available for the community placement of these persons at the time of their release? This is an extremely important question to which research ought to be addressed. If the range of services that are now provided maintain in dependent, socially discredited roles persons who might have otherwise achieved a greater level of independence, no matter how unappealing their life style might be to middle-class perceptions, there is a strong potential of doing disservice to a person's chance for positive self-regard. Since social service agencies are often motivated to keep their "best" clients, this may not be an uncommon phenomenon at all. Judging from Edgerton and Bercovici's (1976) follow-up report of released institution residents, self-sufficiency (economic independence) appeared less important to the development of positive self-regard than did independence from those social constructions (e.g., clinical diagnosis, residence in facilities for special classes) which tend to confer perjorative social status.

Of course all such thoughts can be at best treated as hypotheses, given that they derive from a sample of rather mildly handicapped persons released from a large institution directly to independent living. Study of the many variations on this theme should be encouraged, as should be direct replication. For example, would the same social perceptions be observed among more seriously retarded persons who have greater difficulty with symbolic thought? And if so, at what general level of mental ability does the perception of stigma fall beyond the retarded person's conceptual skills?

Because of the dearth of participant observation studies in community facilities, the issue of the perception of stigma among persons residing in them has not been sufficiently addressed. From a social psychological perspective, however, one might hypothesize that the degree to which living in a particular facility is interpreted by the resident as communicating to the general public a negatively valued status would have a powerful influence on the quality of his social interactions and the satisfaction derived from them. In addition, some persons in residences for the mentally retarded have to face directly the fact that a few of the neighbors do not want a facility for "their type" in the neighborhood. Studies by O'Connor (1976) and Baker, Seltzer, and Seltzer (1974) report that approximately one-third of community facility openings meet opposition. While these studies found that opposition waned substantially once the facility was in operation, the impact of these confrontations on the persons living in these facilities was not addressed. Certainly the reduction of opposition once a facility is *fait accompli* does not mean that the residents will come to be or feel accepted and well regarded. The writers, however, could find no discussion in the mental retardation literature of the long-term effects of this forced integration.

In a study of 42 retarded residents who remained in a large community residence (63 persons) for a period of four years, Birenbaum and Re (1979) found 57% indicating they would rather live elsewhere. The most frequent choice among alternatives was an apartment of their own. To what degree such a choice was motivated by a desire to live in a non-retarded way was not probed by the authors, but reflections on Edgerton's work lead the reader to wonder if "guilt by association" might be one motivating factor. As Bergman (1975) observed about a person who unhappily lived in and finally left a community home, "It seems as though he wants to completely disassociate himself from anything or anyone related to institutions, retardation, community homes or even concerned individuals" (p. 106).

Bercovici, in her paper in this volume, presents examples of how two residents in care facilities for the mentally retarded perceived the distinction between retarded and normal to hinge on whether one lives "out there" or "in here" (in a facility for the mentally retarded). It seems important that future research begin to expand the sample of the residential population on which evidence of stigma has been collected, attempting to measure the intellectual and demographic characteristics of those who feel it and the alternatives to the care provision which produces it. For example, particularly worthy of study would be the effects of different care models on the perception of stigma. Do models where there are fewer retarded people than normal people in a dwelling affect the identity of the retarded people? Are foster home placements with one or two wards more effective in reducing stigma than congregate care? How effective is increasingly independent living in increasing positive identity?

Finally we must realize that for many mentally retarded persons in residential programs daily contacts are almost exclusively with other retarded persons in their residence and their day programs (cf. Berkson & Romer, this volume) and their primary caretakers. According to Goffman (1963) a person becomes stigmatized when others perceive in him/her "attributes that make him different from others ... in the extreme a person who is quite thoroughly bad, or dangerous, or weak. He is thus reduced in our minds from a whole and usual person to a tainted, disoriented one" (p. 3). For the most part, then, given the social realities of mentally retarded persons in residential facilities, it is the stigmatization by facility staff which is most directly relevant to the lives of persons residing in such facilities. Well-taught of the limitations of mentally retarded persons, it is often extremely difficult to take persons who have been seen as "tainted, disoriented" and expand them in our minds to a "whole." The effects of stigma, too, go beyond just the perceived dependency associated with "mental retardation" as a generic construct. Certain types of mentally retarded persons are seen as less adaptable than others, and individual staff vary in their own expectations which in turn greatly affects their clients. Kasanovich (1980b) has documented a number of the effects of staff expectations ("threshold of tolerance") in a program designed to train mentally retarded people for independent apartment living. About the effects of individual staff expectations on the lives of clients, he noted:

> The primary counselor is therefore the human agent who can push clients to move out, or progress faster, or decide that they are not progressing at the level or rate which they should be and therefore that they would be "better off" outside of the program . . . So strong are these differences in staff's tolerance thresholds that 40% of all differences among clients in the number of months spent in the training program are explained by the counselor caseload to which they are assigned. (p. 70)

Obviously the social stigma of dependence and non-adaptability of mentally retarded persons operates differently on different carepersons. In the best interests of the clients, however, professionals must learn much about the "real" skills required for different types of community-based living and make much more enlightened judgments about whether clients possess them. A far more debilitating stigmatization may be taking place within residential facilities than occurs outside.

Selecting Appropriate Residences: Search for Decision Models for Placement and Client Training

The writers can find no better way to begin this section than by quoting a statement made by Stanley Davies more than a half-century ago regarding this same topic of community adjustment.

> In reviewing this process of socializing the feeble-minded, one thing stands out: it resolves itself as does any process of assimilation or socialization into a matter of rapprochement between diverse social elements, in this case . . . the citizenry on the one hand, and the feeble-minded in question on the other. It is a process in which all the approach is not on the side of the feeble-minded . . . Let us see in what ways society must adapt itself to the feeble-minded (Davies, 1923, p. 195).

In his 1979 survey of public residential facilities Scheerenberger (1979) noted that the 172 facilities reporting estimated that 14,992 residents were ready for alternative placement, but the anticipated number who would be placed in the 1979-1980 fiscal year was only about one-half that number (7,853). Even disregarding the issue of quality of placement, it is clear that there exists today a severe quantitative shortage of alternatives to public institutions. Given how little is known about the nature of care provided in community facilities, however, it may well be a blessing in disguise that there now exists a chance to improve the placement process before complete and wholesale liquidations of public institutions take place, and residents are disbursed to wherever there is a "bed."

Issues related to matching the characteristics of a community residence to the particular characteristics of the individual requiring residential services are complex. As far back as 1937, Doll and Longwell were proposing that the Vineland Social Maturity Scale be used to assess those persons being considered for community placement. This recommendation was based on their findings of correlation between average social maturity score of those persons in various residential settings and the level of independence perceived as necessary in each of those settings, i.e., parolees had the highest group rating, colony residents the next highest, and boarding care (family care) and institution residents the lowest. Never, however, did the writers attempt to assess these settings in regard to the level of social competence and particular life skills required to reside in them successfully.

Among community residential facilities the problem of finding clients who can perform in accordance with the basic prerequisites of the individual setting seems crucial. Unlike public facilities, few community facilities are called upon or prepared to take everyone with total disregard for the personal characteristics of potential residents. Despite this different reality, very little published research is available on the selection or training of mentally retarded persons to meet the requirements of a particular residential alternative. Three notable and documented programs have been reported.

Recently, Schalock and Harper (1978, this volume) have reported on a program which systematically attempted to train candidates for placement in those skills needed for successful supervised or independent apartment living. After an analysis of skill areas and a delineation of specific subskills necessary for success in the program, clients were assessed for the presence of these skills. In those areas in which the client was deficient, a specific program of directive teaching was implemented. The results of this program demonstrated that these particular clients were generally able to learn those skills necessary for partial or complete independent living (87% remained in this type of placement after two years). The validity of the task analysis procedure was supported by the fact that the degree of mastery of subskills in four of the training areas (personal care, clothing care/use, community utilization, and functional academics) was strongly related to success in the placement.

Another program of a similar nature was reported by Seevers (1975). This program used a group home setting to train mild and moderately retarded young adult women to move into more independent living arrangements. As in the program described by Schalock and Harper (1978, this volume) training was based on a program developed from an initial assessment of client skills in the areas of self-help, communication, socialization, occupation and personality. Again considerable success was noted in a directive teaching procedure focusing on independent living skills. However, regarding the social integration of the program's graduates, Seevers (1975, p. 64) noted that they "have continued to rely primarily upon the group home houseparents and residents for affective and social needs. The normal 'community' is a misnomer in terms of affective support. The affective domain of developmental growth seems to be the crucial and primary domain affecting success or failure for residents."

A third program established on a similar model is described by Kasanovich (1980b, 1980c). Though somewhat different than the two programs described above in that clients were being trained for independent apartment living while actually living in an apartment complex operated by the training agency, the training model was again directive teaching of specific skills needed in independent living. Skill areas included apartment maintenance, food preparation, money management, grooming, health, vocational and social/leisure. Of particular interest in the evaluation of this program was the fact that seven of ten trainees with IQs below 50 and the one trainee with an IQ below 40 all achieved independent living status with 1½ to 6½ years of training.

The importance of these studies in regard to the suitability of a placement is that they demonstrate that the behavioral requirements of different settings can be specified and that success within the environment is predictable according to the degree the clients meet these requirements. It is a simple idea but one which seems to be overlooked in most research and, quite likely, in most placements. Such an idea might also be amplified so as to include the placement agency's requirements for a suitable placement from the perspective of those charged with the client's welfare (c.f. Sutter & Mayeda, this volume) and even, ideally, the clients themselves. Factors which might be considered in this regard include not only physical aspects of the environment, but also the type of developmental programming offered by a facility. The fact that one sees so little research like that done by Schalock and Harper, Seevers, and Kasanovich points out one of the greatest myths of residential care: despite the rhetoric, there is very little "continuity" and the sum total of the residential variations can be called a "system" only in the loosest sense of the term. As Bergman (1975) has pointed out the selection of an individual for community placement is usually determined by a decision by someone at the institution that he is "ready," with little or no specification of for what exactly he is "ready." At the other end of the "system," and usually with little or no coinvolvement with those who declared the resident ready, someone attempts to locate "a bed," often constrained to be far more concerned about availability than suitability.

Since the personal characteristics of residents are so seldom related to the institutional requirements of the settings in which they are placed, it should not be surprising that there have been notably inconsistent findings when major demographic variables have been examined for their relationships to adequate adjustment to the community. After an exhaustive review of research findings relating client characteristics to community adjustment, McCarver and Craig (1974) could conclude little but that the literature concerning the post-institutional adjustment of the mentally retarded is replete with inconclusive, discrepant, and contradictory findings. Among the client variables examined and the authors' conclusions about the relationship of each to community adjustment (i.e., avoiding return to an institution) were:

1) "Intellectual level . . . The largest number of studies concerning intelligence on community adjustment have found no meaningful relationship" (p. 171).

2) "Academic ability . . . On the basis of the reviewed studies, it would seem that the level of academic achievement is not strongly related to community adjustment, if at all" (p. 173).

3) "Age at release . . . At least 10 studies have reported that older subjects were more successful, 5 have suggested that younger subjects exhibit better adjustment, and 9 have found that age did not differentiate between successful and unsuccessful cases" (p. 169).

4) "Diagnosis . . . No studies to date have convincingly demonstrated that residents of any diagnostic category are more or less successful than those of other categories" (p. 170).

5) "Personality . . . The results suggesting a positive relationship between the adequacy of a resident's personality and outcome on community placement should be considered as only suggestive findings" (p. 173).

6) "Personal appearance . . . Three studies have found good personal appearance is positively related to success, while a fourth found no correlation (p. 175).

It would be a tiring litany to continue to cite the authors' conclusions on the other "personal" variables they examined. On physical handicaps, vocational skills, psychomotor measures, sterilization and social skills, the authors also find the evidence of a relationship with community adjustment in some studies contradicted by the findings of others. Obviously the striking variability among the studies reviewed by McCarver and Craig is most likely related to differences in what was required for a successful adjustment in the setting where those studied had been placed. In the case of IQ, for example, if the requirements for a successful adjustment of all released residents had been equal, then IQ might have been considerably more predictive. Two recent studies (Bell 1976; Schalock & Harper, 1978) support this notion, although Kasanovich (1980 c) notes that more extensive training may often compensate for relatively lower general ability.

The fact of the matter is, however, that individual placements vary tremendously in the types of behavior that are expected and are tolerated of the persons residing in them. And as Sutter and Mayeda (this volume) and Lei, Nihira, Sheehy and Meyers (this volume) point out, the development of systems which help match clients' characteristics with caretakers' tolerance for those characteristics promises to be much more fruitful research than attempting to predict placement success from client characteristics alone. Along these same lines researchers need to address the effectiveness of training programs such as those described by Intagliata and Willer (this volume) in enhancing caretakers', and potential caretakers', tolerance of and effectiveness in dealing with specific client behaviors.

At a time when states are setting goals such as the release of all ambulatory residents of public institutions (as is the case in Minnesota) much more research needs to focus on procedures which will enhance the reciprocal adjustments required of both residents and staff. As noted by Mayeda and Sutter (this volume), Scheerenberger (this volume) and Borthwick, Meyers and Eyman (this volume) the "best candidates" for deinstitutionalization today are considerably more handicapped and more difficult to care for than was the case in earlier years in the deinstitutionalization movement. Some writers question whether deinstitutionalization can go much further, while others point out that much greater social challenges have been met through a true commitment to do so. Whether that commitment exists among those persons concerned with residential services has not yet been fully demonstrated, but clearly the realization of the goals of deinstitutionalization with the institution residents of today will require much careful study of the needs of clients and staff, and of ways these can be met in mutually beneficial ways.

The writers certainly do not, however, see any research which supports a need for more studies on the relationships between client characteristics such as IQ and adjustment to the specific expectations of the thousands of community facilities. The payoff from this sort of research has been very low in the past and does little to meet the needs of the residential service system today, which, with or without the help of a research base, will continue to follow a policy of deinstitutionalization.

Two Cross-Cutting Factors: The Importance of Time and Concerned Others

Two other factors which are essential to the study of the community adjustment process have been discussed in this volume and in related writings: time and concerned others ("benefactors"). They are factors of indispensable importance to the lives of all human beings and we need not marvel at their relevance to the lives of deinstitutionalized persons. Neither, however, can they be discounted as mundane. They are of crucial importance to understanding the process of extra-institutional adjustment.

Time. In this volume Bell, Schoenrock, and Bensberg emphasize the importance of time as a factor in the adjustment process of mentally retarded persons returning to community life: "relationships between community functioning [as operationally defined in their research] and ability occurred most frequently after 10 months in the community and almost never during the first five months." However, not only did time relate to signs of increasing social integration and independence (e.g., community interaction, homemaking activities, phone contacts with friends), but time also related to the number of adjustment problems which needed to be confronted by the clients. In other words, it appears that as time passes some residents of community facilities may gradually increase the level of social participation which in turn reciprocally increases the problems they face. Such qualitative changes in life patterns, as these writers point out, can be studied only with research which treats time as a crucial variable in a process of adjustment.

Other writers (e.g., Cobb, 1972) have noted the importance of the passage of time to the lifestyle of released institution residents. Birenbaum and Re (1979) reported that after an initial enthusiastic plunge into community activities, the residents they studied slowed down substantially in the number of extra-facility activities, "settling into comfortable and conventional routines" (p. 329). Edgerton and Bercovici (1976), returning 12 years later to Edgerton's (1967) original sample, found that with time the burden of the mental retardation label had considerably dissipated and that these persons were no longer overwhelmingly concerned with signs of normality such as being employed. It was also found that only a minority of these persons with the passing of time continued to rely on the concerned others who were seen as crucial in the early stages of the adjustment process. Clearly the inclusion of a longitudinal component to any research or community adjustment is vital to developing a clear picture of the adjustment process.

Concerned others—"benefactors." The formal concept of "benefactors" was first outlined by Edgerton (1967), although the paper by Lakin, Bruininks, and Sigford in this volume noted that the importance of special help provided by family and concerned others to the released institution resident has been formally recognized for over 60 years. Edgerton (1967) in his study of persons released from a large state institution for mentally retarded persons concluded that "in general, the ex-patient succeeds in his efforts to sustain a life in the community only as well as he succeeds in locating and holding a benefactor" (p. 204). With the passage of time, however, the importance of a benefactor lessened considerably so that 12 years later (Edgerton & Bercovici, 1976) only about one-third of the original subjects were judged to be as dependent on benefactors as they were at the time of the original study.

Other research has emphasized the importance of benefactors. Henshel (1972) in studying the adjustment of both Anglo- and Mexican-American ex-patients found benefactors to be important to the community life of both groups, although among the Chicanos the role was more likely to be performed within a friendship network than in a more clear-cut, helper-helpee relationship. Gollay (1976) reported that among released residents 86% of those who remained in community placements had friends interested in their welfare as opposed to only 46% of those who were eventually returned to an institution. Such a finding suggests that while locating a benefactor may not be absolutely crucial to mentally retarded persons who are sheltered to some degree within a community-based residence, the benefactor may retain importance. How benefactors may function so as to decrease the probability for reinstitutionalization has not been extensively studied. It is, of course, possible that the resident characteristics which are related to readmission to the institution also have a negative effect on the likelihood of forming a friendship, creating only the illusion that the factors are directly related.

For residents in supervised community living arrangements the role of the private party who invests himself in the retarded person's welfare may largely be taken over by the "professional benefactors" employed by the various facilities. But Edgerton (1975) has questioned the effectiveness of staff members in fulfilling the benefactor role as he conceptualized it studying persons living independently. According to Edgerton (1975) the institutionalization of the role caused many community facility residents to be "caught up in elaborate and tenacious dependence relationships" (p. 132) in which the client's interests did not necessarily receive primary consideration. Among the more highly supervised facilities where professionals fulfill many of the functions of the beneficient counselor and advocate, outsiders may still fulfill the role of friend, providing the residents social experiences which they might not otherwise have had. In as yet unpublished data, the Developmental Disabilities Project on Residential Service and Community Adjustment at the University of Minnesota found that nearly 60% of its sample of residents of non-public residential facilities had some sort of special friend (excluding family) who shared time with the resident without financial compensation (Hill & Bruininks, 1980). Little has been written, however, about how such contacts are established or maintained, or about what effects they have on the lives of the mentally retarded persons in these facilities. With agencies such as the National Association for Retarded Citizens actively recruiting persons to serve as volunteers for mentally retarded persons, a growing recognition of the important roles such persons can fulfill in advocacy and enhancement of non-institutional life experiences, and a maturing apprehension of the limits of formal social programming, researchers should begin systematically to treat benefactors and concerned others as important factors in understanding extra-institutional adjustment.

A Conference Discussion

The original drafts of many of the papers contained in this volume were presented at a topical conference on the community adjustment of developmentally disabled persons living in residential facilities other than state-operated institutions. In addition to the presentation and discussion of the papers, two structured discussion sessions were held involving all conference participants. The purpose of these sessions was to allow active researchers in the area of residential services the chance to discuss with one another those questions and issues which seemed particularly relevant to them in their own work. What follows is a brief description of some of these discussions.

Research Questions

One of the discussion groups attempted to formulate a list of important research issues and questions for future studies of community adjustment. Unfortunately insufficient time was available to complete this list or to rank order possible issues on the dimensions of importance and feasibility. Questions identified as important for further study were:

1) What gaps in community services exist for persons released to community placements (including the natural family)?

2) For persons who are returned to institutions, what differences exist in the services provided the individual in the two different settings? Were any of these differences involved in the decision to readmit the individual to the institution?

3) At the time of release, what is the predicted "goodness of fit" between the characteristics of the released person and the characteristics of the receiving placement? How relevant was this prediction to adjustment at some time after release has occurred? How might "goodness of fit" be improved?

4) How do physical characteristics of retarded persons influence interactions with persons in the community and services provided to persons in non-institutional settings?

5) What "behavior problems" are perceived as most jeopardizing successful placement by significant others in the residential facilities? Do these perceptions vary according to placement type and/or characteristics of the residents and staff? How could such information be utilized in improving placement decisions and pre-release training programs.

6) In what manner do relationships with the natural family influence community adjustment?

7) To what extent are changes in the behavior of released persons associated with actual environment changes or the effects of novelty (i.e., Hawthorne Effects)? Is there a period of time after which behavior patterns stabilize sufficiently to be assessed as the residents' types, styles, or levels of "community adjustment?"

8) What aspects of institutional pre-release preparation or specific types of training affect the level of community adjustment, and to what type of placement?

9) In what ways do relationships with friends, peers, staff, and benefactors affect the quality of life and adjustment of released residents?

10) Who is responsible for coordinating the provision of services and how effectively are such services planned and coordinated? What system modifications are needed in this area?

11) How do the characteristics and attitudes of case managers in both the new residential placement and the releasing facility influence the person's community adjustment?

12) What are the feelings of the released resident regarding placement in community residential and service programs? What program "qualities" most greatly affect these feelings?

13) What is the nature and strength of the relationship between the person's self-perception and different aspects of post-institutional adjustment?

14) What is the nature of the relationship between changes in behavior of released persons as reported by caregivers and direct measures of behavior? How reliable are caretaker reports when compared with direct observation measures?

15) How do the lives of severely and profoundly retarded persons in community placements differ qualitatively from those of severely and profoundly retarded persons in state-operated facilities?

16) How do severely and profoundly retarded persons in community settings differ from those in institutional settings? Do persons returned differ significantly from those who are not released? What system modifications are needed based on these differences?

Subject Selection

One of the most problematic issues in conducting research on community adjustment is the criteria for use in selecting subjects. Discussants at the conference perceived several factors as being important, namely:
(a) characteristics of the residential setting;
(b) nature of pre-release preparation;
(c) location of the residential setting; and
(d) personal characteristics of released residents. Each of these factors and their implications, either for selecting persons for study or for areas of study is discussed below.

Characteristics of residential setting. It was concluded that environmental characteristics have been given relatively little attention in studies on the community adjustment of retarded people, yet, this factor was perceived to exert major influence on the adjustment of released residents. Discussants felt characteristics of the setting to which the subject is released—including size, homogeneity in the characteristics of residents, staffing patterns and staff characteristics, developmental programming and quality of care—were important factors to consider in studies of community adjustment. While some discussants felt characteristics of the placement setting were important considerations in selecting persons for study, most felt such factors should be the focus of study rather than the basis for selection.

Nature of pre-release preparation. In a penetrating study, the General Accounting Office (1977) identified the lack of pre-release preparation as a significant impediment to deinstitutionalization of mentally disabled persons. Discussants at the conference agreed regarding the importance of this issue, and felt that the scope and quality of training received by persons prior to release should be assessed carefully, but should not be used as a factor in selecting persons for study.

Location of residential setting. Characteristics of the community were considered important factors to consider in future studies of released residents. This area was cited as one of the most important factors determining whether an individual was able to remain outside the institution. Specific mention was made of the density of population (urban-rural), and important features of the community service delivery system (e.g., availability of needed services, type of organization, availability of advocacy and benefactor relationships). Again these factors were considered as important areas for study, but less important as criteria for selection.

Personal characteristics of residents. Discussants regarded personal characteristics of residents as the most important consideration in selecting persons for study. The criterion considered most important for selection was severity of mental retardation, followed by age. A major gap in current research was judged to be knowledge regarding the adjustment of severely and profoundly retarded and elderly retarded persons. Discussants felt additional information was also needed on the extra-institutional lives of young adults and persons in middle age. Additional factors identified as possibly important criteria for selection were: sex, degree of mobility, secondary disabilities, length of stay in an institutional setting and number of placements within the institution prior to release.

Further discussion revolved around the process of selecting persons for study. Broad consensus was reached in three areas: (1) the importance of studying the adjustment process of released residents with a prospective design; (2) the value of studying the interaction of environmental and personal characteristics, and (3) the importance of including group living, natural family and nursing homes as possible settings.

Research Methods and Procedures

In the discussion of research methods, it was acknowledged that the ultimate choice of methods depended primarily upon the research questions guiding the study and the characteristics of the subjects; certain research methods are inherently better suited for certain types of research questions or subject populations. Thus, participants tended to consider important research questions as well as methodological strategies. Discussants concluded that too little attention had been given to studying physical and social environmental influences on adaptation within the person's immediate residence, neighborhood, day placement and general community. This orientation was characterized as studying adaptation and adjustment in "real life" or naturalistic settings. Secondly, it was suggested that use of multiple methods of gathering data would lead to more valid findings than the use of a single approach.

The group reached consensus on a number of conclusions regarding needed methodological approaches, including:

1) The need for more and better conceptualized focus on environmental assessment and observation. It was agreed that attention should be given to measuring the adaptation of the environment to the needs and characteristics of subjects as well as the adaptation of subjects to environment.

2) Attention should be given to examining the content of individualized program plans and their implementation.

3) Use of participant observation and other forms of qualitative research methods should be increased in studying the process of adaptation and adjustment.

4) Greater focus should be given to gathering data on aspects of the subject's life in settings other than the residential facility.

5) Behavioral assessments should be gathered in preference to subjective opinions regarding the subject's behavior and capabilities.

Conclusions and Recommendations

In the closing session of the conference a plenary session involving participants was held for the purpose of formulating conclusions and recommendations regarding research on the community adjustment of retarded people. The session was conducted in an informal, brain-storming session in which participants generated statements that were recorded, generally verbatim, on large charts. No evaluative discussion of these statements was conducted during the session.

Following the conference the statements were compiled into categories and edited slightly to decrease ambiguity. These statements were then sent to conference participants for review, editing and rating for importance. Generally, all the statements received relatively high ratings.

Presented below in rank order are those statements rated as "very" or "above average" in importance by at least two-thirds of the discussion participants. (The reader is urged to realize that this is not an attempt to establish research agendas for others, but merely to point out some of the salient issues in research on extra-institutional placement of mentally retarded people as viewed by a sample of persons actively involved in its study.)

General Conclusions about Future Research

1) More attention should be given in research and policy development to understanding and expanding the residential service options for persons who are already in community-based settings.

2) An adequate model of the network of community and residential services is needed for analyzing the experiences of people during the deinstitutionalization process.

3) A standard and operationalized taxonomy of residential services, with categories that carry coherent variance, is needed.

4) Research should be more targeted and less broad in its scope and goals.

General Recommendations about Research Methodologies and Measurement

1) There is need for more longitudinal and prospective studies.

2) There is need to articulate, acknowledge, and solve the procedural and methodological problems that we have encountered in research efforts on community adjustment.

3) We should have more intensive and ethnographic approaches to complement the present large-scale surveys.

4) Studies should address formative issues in program evaluation so that results can be used to improve services.

5) Our research should more often include the client as respondent, by whatever means are effective.

6) There is need to develop and use common evaluation measures (e.g., measures of client adjustment) for use in research on deinstitutionalization and residential services.

7) It is important to accept natural and pluralistic outcomes and goals of clients in judging extent of adjustment.

8) Our present measures and analyses are inadequate to assess deinstitutionalization in terms of interaction between the person and the environment, and to capture the interactive process new methodologies are needed. This approach requires consideration of such phenomena as changes in environments brought about by clients as well as changes in clients brought about by environments.

General Recommendations about Research Questions and Issues

1) Social interactions involving a community of interested persons and relationships are crucial in community adjustment and should be researched in more detail with the goal of strenghtening social opportunities where they are weak.

2) We must avoid equating recidivism with failure to adjust as outcome variables in conducting future studies, and develop more individualized indices of adaptation to the community.

3) Most mentally retarded people experience degrees of success and difficulty, and it is necessary to clarify those degrees.

4) The differential impact upon client function of different environments should be examined.

5) It is essential to assess what services are needed by clients, regardless of whether or not they are available in the area in order to measure "need." (Assumptions about who can benefit from what kinds of services must be made explicit.)

6) Studies should examine the impact of deinstitutionalization upon clients in terms of:

a. Natural progress in absence of change in environments,
b. Differential life histories of persons,
c. Differential sequences of environmental change and their impact upon the individual.

7) In studying deinstitutionalization, the differential impact of particular placements should be distinguished from the impact of the deinstitutionalization process itself.

8) It is important to articulate and refine the goals we have in conducting research on community adjustment (i.e., prediction, description, understanding, and control of change).

A POSTSCRIPT

This volume has provided a discussion of research concerning the residential facilities where tens of thousands of mentally retarded persons live their daily lives. While we have written our papers for this volume with the impersonal, assumed objectivity typical of researchers approaching a problem scientifically, we all know that mental retardation is a social construct. We know, too, that the creation of categories such as mental retardation, which is so much a part of our professional writing and thinking, has often placed a wall between "them" and those of us who profess concern about their welfare. The impenetrability of this wall far exceeds its substance. Too often we have been guilty of allowing ourselves to be sufficiently removed from the lives of these persons to make careers out of studying and writing about them without sharing in the realities of their lives or without much concern for how what we do can possibly have a positive effect on their lives.

The broader study of community adjustment is an important aspect of evaluating the status and impact of our public policies on people whose development is retarded. It is, to use the words of Coleman, "policy research [which] is designed as a guide to [social] action" (1972, p. 2). In conducting such research we acknowledge that the most important outcomes of social policy are often unexpected and contrary to the desired goals of that policy. The history of our society's policies regarding mentally retarded persons is replete with examples of how, in the absence of systematic scrutiny, sheer *belief* that what we are doing is appropriate has led to faithful adherence for years to counterproductive treatment models. A major theme stated throughout this volume is the need for new and refocused directions in our research, not only to increase understanding and to improve opportunities for retarded people, but also to assess carefully the social consequences of what we do in attempting to reach these goals.

From the past century of research with institutionalized populations, it is abundantly clear that for the most part "we have missed the forest for the trees." We blithely entered institutions, psychometrically isolated subjects from their environment, and compared them with a host of noninstitutionalized groups with the sure result of discovering that "they" were different. But we overlooked the salient qualitative aspects of institutional life and, in missing the "forest," our research tacitly encouraged the status quo, and by default supported programs for thousands of people which were less than any person deserves.

Today we stand in the early years of a massive change in social philosophy and public policy which focuses on the conditions in which mentally retarded persons live. It is a movement, backed by billions of dollars, that contends that better and better knowledge of the characteristics of mentally retarded persons is not required to improve the way we treat these persons. It is a spirit which says that "they," as well as we, have human rights and that the recognition of these rights may not be tied to past or future research findings.

In a way all this puts the researcher in the field of mental retardation at a crossroads, because the social philosophy and policy which is responsible for deinstitutionalization did not evolve, for the most part, out of the research findings of mental retardation professionals. Its primary impetus came from a broader emphasis on human rights and exposés on how dependent persons were being treated in our society. As researchers we must ask ourselves if we can change as quickly as our residential service system is changing and begin to look carefully at a new, or at least different, form of care which will become more and more common with or without our participation. The persons whose work is presented in this volume have opted to take an active part in this form of social policy research, not because they necessarily believe that a better clinical understanding of mental retardation is not important, but because they believe that it is in the direct examination of this new social policy that our services can best be improved.

Whether one approaches the life problems of persons designated as mentally retarded on a tightly-designed, highly controlled experiment or in a more open-ended investigation, researchers need to continually ask themselves, "Why are we doing this research?" Given the vast number of questions raised by contributors to this volume, one reason that is no longer sufficient is, "because it has never been done." There are simply too many other questions of importance to governmental policy, direct programming, and the daily lives of mentally retarded persons, their families and their caretakers for us not to be concerned about the real life significance of what we do. Much more of our research on mental retardation must be tied to the criterion of potential relevance in the foreseeable future. And whatever type of research we undertake we must commit ourselves to never again being part of one of the most classic examples of intellectual myopia of this century: studying the characteristics of mentally retarded persons in residential environments without simultaneously observing the characteristics of those environments.

We possess imperfect knowledge about the people we call mentally retarded, about social behavior, and even about ourselves, but perfect knowledge is not required to improve social policies and programs. Clearly researchers cannot continue solely in traditional paths of research and ever give back to this system any measure of what they draw from it in terms of personal gain. They cannot justifiably continue to use monies which could be used to provide care to do research which does not have relevance to the giving of that care. Neither can they quit doing research. Researchers must continue to evaluate and often challenge the soundness of present day practices if there is to be any hope that they will become better in the future.

We must humbly proceed, but alongside our traditional research practices we must make much more room for, in fact encourage, new conceptualizations of what constitutes research. We need to look carefully at new or alternative models of care and look for those extremes of caregiving from which we might derive inspiration and rededication. Above all we must remember that the kind of residential care received in the future can be determined to a large degree by the way that those in the socially privileged role of researcher define their responsibility to their subjects today. The prospect should be both stimulating and humbling,and that responsibility should weigh much more heavily than that of maintaining any particular research tradition.

References

Baker, B. L., Seltzer, B. G., & Seltzer, M. M. *As close as possible*. Cambridge, MA: Behavioral Education Projects, 1974.

Balla, D. A. Relationship of institution size to quality of care: A review of the literature. *American Journal of Mental Deficiency*, 1976, *81*, 117-124.

Balla, D. A., Butterfield, E. C., & Zigler, E. Effects of institutionalization on retarded children: A longitudinal cross-institutional investigation. *American Journal of Mental Deficiency*, 1974, *78*, 530-549.

Bell, N. J. IQ as a factor in community life-style of formerly institutionalized retardates. Mental Retardation, 1976, *14*, 29-33.

Bergman, J. S. Behavioral programs. In J. S. Bergman (Ed.), *Community homes for the retarded*. Lexington, MA: D. C. Heath & Co., 1975.

Berkson, S. & Landesman-Dwyer, S. Behavioral research on severe and profound mental retardation (1955-1974). *American Journal of Mental Deficiency*, 1977, *81*, 428-454.

Birenbaum, A., & Re, M. A. Resettling mentally retarded adults in the community: Almost 4 years later. *American Journal of Mental Deficiency*, 1979, *83*, 323-329.

Bjaanes, A. T., & Butler, E. W. Environmental variation in community care facilities for mentally retarded persons. *American Journal of Mental Deficiency*, 1974, *78*, 429-439.

Braginsky, D. D., & Braginsky, B. M. *Hansels and Gretels: Studies of children in institutions for the mentally retarded*. New York: Holt, Rinehart & Winston, 1971.

Brooks, P. H., & Baumeister, A. A. A plea for consideration of ecological validity in the experimental psychology of mental retardation: A guest editorial. *American Journal of Mental Deficiency*, 1977, *81*(5), 407-416.

Bruininks, R. H., Hauber, F., & Kudla, M. *National survey of community residential facilities: A profile of facilities and residents in 1977*. Minneapolis: Department of Psychoeducational Studies, University of Minnesota, 1979.

Bruininks, R. H., Hill, B. K., & Thorsheim, M. J. *A profile of foster home services for mentally retarded persons in 1977*. Minneapolis: Department of Psychoeducational Studies, University of Minnesota, 1980.

Bruininks, R. H., & Krantz, G. C. (Eds.). *Family care of developmentally disabled members: Conference proceedings*. Minneapolis: University of Minnesota, 1979.

Butler, E. W., & Bjaanes, A. T. Activities and the use of time by retarded persons in community care facilities. In G. P. Sackett (Ed.), *Observing behavior* (Vol. 1): *Theory and applications in mental retardation*. Baltimore: University Park Press, 1978.

Cleland, C. Evidence on the relationship between size and institutional effectiveness: A review and analysis. *American Journal of Mental Deficiency*, 1965, *70*, 423-431.

Cobb, D. Preparing the mentally deficient child for community adjustment. *American Journal of Mental Deficiency*, 1951, *58*, 554-672.

Coleman, J. S. *Policy research in the social services*. Morristown, NJ: General Learning Press, 1972.

D'Amico, M. L., Hannah, M. A., Milhouse, J. A., & Froleich, A. K. Evaluation of adaptive behavior: Institutional vs community placement and treatment for the mentally retarded. Paper presented at the annual conference of the American Personnel and Guidance Association, Washington, DC, 1978. (Available from National Clearinghouse, Stillwater, OK.)

Davies, S. P. *Social control of the feebleminded*. Utica, NY: State Hospitals Press, 1923.

(DDP) Developmental Disabilities Project on Residential Services and Community Adjustment. *1977 national summary between public and community residential findings* (Brief #3). Minneapolis: Department of Psychoeducational Studies, University of Minnesota, 1978.

Discussion. Journal of Psycho-asthenics, 1918, *23*, 95-103.

Doll, E. A., & Longwell, S. G. Social competence of the feeble-minded under extramural care. *Psychiatric Quarterly*, 1937, *11*, 450-464.

Edgerton, R. B. *The cloak of competence: Stigma in the lives of the mentally retarded*. Berkeley: University of California, 1967.

Edgerton, R. B. Issues related to the quality of life among mentally retarded persons. In M. J. Begab & S. A. Richardson (Eds.), *The mentally retarded and society: A social science perspective*. Baltimore: University Park Press, 1975.

Edgerton, R. B., & Bercovici, S. M. The cloak of competence: Years later. *American Journal of Mental Deficiency*, 1976, *80*, 485-490.

Eyman, R. K., Demaine, G. C., & Lei, T. Relationship between community environments and resident changes in adaptive behavior: A path model. *American Journal of Mental Deficiency*, 1979, *83*, 330-338.

General Accounting Office. Returning the mentally disabled to the community: Government needs to do more. Washington, DC: United States Government Printing Office, 1977.

Gerbner, G., & Gross, L. The scary world of TV's heavy viewer. *Psychology Today*, 1976, *9*, 41-45, 89.

Glass, G. Policy for the unpredictable (uncertainty research and policy). *Educational Researcher*, 1979, *8*, 12-14.

Goffman, E. *Asylums*. New York: Doubleday, 1961.

Goffman, E. *Stigma: Notes on the management of spoiled identity*. Englewood Cliffs, NJ: Prentice-Hall, 1963.

Gollay, E., Freedman, R., Wyngaarden, M., & Kurtz, N. R. *Coming back: The community experiences of deinstitutionalized mentally retarded people*. Cambridge, MA: Abt Books, 1978.

Harlow, H. F. Experimental analysis of behavior. *American Psychologist*, 1957, *12*, 485-490.

Henshel, A. *The forgotten ones: A sociological study of Anglo and Chicano retardates*. Austin: University of Texas Press, 1972.

Herson, P. F. Biasing effects of diagnostic labels and sex of pupil on teachers' views of pupils' mental health. *Journal of Educational Psychology*, 1974, *66*, 117-122.

Hill, B. K., & Bruininks, R. H. Leisure time and social activities of mentally retarded people in residential facilities. Paper presented at the annual meeting of the American Association on Mental Deficiency, San Francisco, May 1980.

Kasanovich, J. An ethnography of bureaucratized service for the mentally retarded. Unpublished masters thesis, Department of Anthropology, University of Minnesota, 1980. (a)

Kasanovich, J. The conduct of empirical fieldwork research within a residential M. R. independence training program (Report #1 of Independent Living Skills Training Project). St. Paul: Minnesota Department of Public Welfare, 1980. (b)

Kasonovich, J. *Performance of M. R. client types in achieving independence* (Report #2 of Independent Living Skills Training Project). St. Paul: Minnesota Department of Public Welfare, 1980. (c)

King, R. D., Raynes, N. V., & Tizard, J. *Patterns of residential care: Sociological studies in institutions for handicapped children*. London: Routledge & Kegan Paul, 1971.

Kirk, S. A. *Educating exceptional children* (2nd ed.). Boston: Houghton Mifflin, 1972.

Landesman-Dwyer, S., Stein, J. G., & Sackett, G. P. *Group homes for the mentally retarded: A behavioral and ecological study* (Report #2). Olympia, WA: Department of Social and Health Services, 1976.

Landesman-Dwyer, S., Stein, J. G., & Sackett, G. P. A behavioral and ecological study of group homes. In G. P. Sackett (Ed.), *Observing behavior* (Vol. 1): *Theory and application in mental retardation*. Baltimore: University Park Press, 1978.

Light, R. J. Capitalizing on variation: How conflicting research findings can be helpful for policy. *Educational Researcher*, 1979, *8*, 7-11.

Matthews, M. A. One hundred institutionally trained mental defectives in community under supervision. *Mental Hygiene*, 1922, *6*, 332-342.

McCarver, R. B., & Craig, E. M. Placement of the retarded in the community. In N. R. Ellis (Ed.), *International review of research in mental retardation* (Vol. 7). New York: Academic Press, 1974.

Mead, G. H. *Mind, self and society*. Chicago: University of Chicago Press, 1934.

Mills, C. W. *The sociological imagination*. New York: Grove Press, 1961.

Moores, B., & Grant, G. W. B. On the nature and incidence of staff-patient interactions in hospitals for the mentally handicapped. *International Journal of Nursing Studies*, 1976, *13*, 69-81.

Murphy, H., Penner, B., & Luchins, D. *Foster homes: The new backwards*. Canada's Mental Health, 1972, *72*. (Monograph Supplement)

Nirje, B. The normalization principle. In R. B. Kugel & A. Shearer (Eds.), *Changing patterns in residential services for the mentally retarded* (rev. ed.). Washington, DC: President's Committee on Mental Retardation, 1976.

O'Connor, G. *Home is a good place: A national perspective of community residential facilities for the mentally retarded*. Washington, DC: American Association on Mental Deficiency, 1976.

Piaget, J. *The child's conception of the world*. New York: Harcourt, Brace, 1928.

Rosen, M., Diggory, J. C., & Werlinsky, B. E. Goal-setting and expectancy of success in institutionalized mental subnormals. *American Journal of Mental Deficiency*, 1966, *71*, 249-255.

Schalock, R. L., & Harper, R. S. Placement from community-based mental retardation programs: How well do clients do? *American Journal of Mental Deficiency*, 1978, *83*, 240-247.

Scheerenberger, R. C. *Public residential services for the mentally retarded* (1977). Minneapolis: Department of Psychoeducational Studies, University of Minnesota, 1978.

Scheerenberger, R. C. *Public residential services for the mentally retarded* (1979). Minneapolis: Department of Psychoeducational Studies, University of Minnesota, 1979.

Schroeder, S. R. & Henes, C. *An evaluation of the effectiveness of group homes in the North-Central Region of North Carolina*. Raleigh: North Carolina Division of Mental Health Research, 1976.

Seevers, C. T. An evaluation of the effects of group home living. *REAP*, 1975, *1*, 51-65.

Sigford, B. B., & Bruininks, R. H. Characteristics of residents released from public residential facilities, in preparation.

Stebbins, I. F. An evaluation of homes for parole placement of mental defectives. *Journal of Psycho-asthenics*, 1931, *36*, 50-67.

Wolfensberger, W., & Glenn, L. PASS: A method for the quantitative evaluation of human services (Handbook). Toronto: National Institute on Mental Retardation, 1973.

Wyatt vs. Stickney. 344 F. Supp. 387 (1972)

Zigler, E., Butterfield, E. C., & Capobianco, F. Institutionalization and the effectiveness of social reinforcement: A five- and eight-year follow-up study. *Developmental Psychology*, 1970, *3*, 255-263.

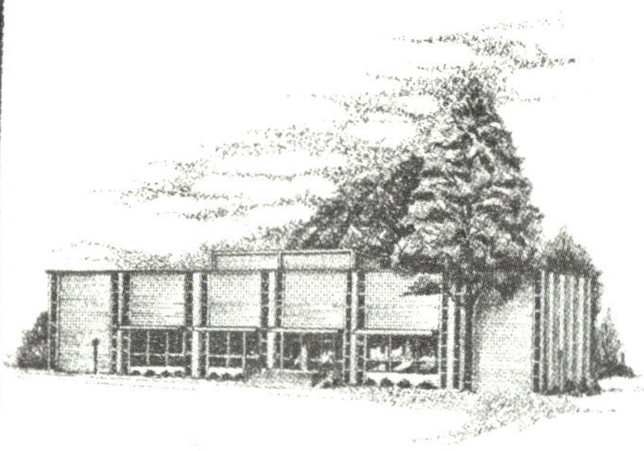